CRISIS INTERVENTION

Theory and Methodology

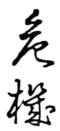

ABOUT THE COVER

The Chinese pictograms shown on the cover symbolize crisis, through the juxtaposition of figures that traditionally represent danger and opportunity. They were graciously supplied by Peter Berton, Professor Emeritus, University of Southern California School of International Relations, and member of the Far Eastern Society of Southern California.

CRISIS INTERVENTION

Theory and Methodology

DONNA C. AGUILERA, PHD, FAAN, FIAEP

Disaster Mental Health Services, American Red Cross
Consultant and Private Practice
Beverly Hills and Sherman Oaks, California

Eighth Edition
with 57 illustrations

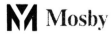 Mosby

An Affiliate of Elsevier

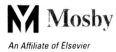

An Affiliate of Elsevier

Vice President and Publisher: Nancy L. Coon
Managing Editor: Jeff Burnham
Developmental Editor: Linda Caldwell
Associate Developmental Editor: Jeff Downing
Project Manager: John Rogers
Production Editor: Cheryl Abbott Bozzay
Designer: Yael Kats
Manufacturing Supervisor: Don Carlisle
Cover Art: Jacob Shapiro

EIGHTH EDITION
Copyright © 1998 by Mosby, Inc.

Previous editions copyrighted 1970, 1974, 1978, 1982, 1986, 1990, and 1994

Permissions may be sought directly from Elsevier's Health Sciences Rights Department in Philadelphia, PA, USA: phone: (+1) 215 239 3804, fax: (+1) 215 239 3805, e-mail: healthpermissions@elsevier.com. You may also complete your request on-line via the Elsevier homepage (http://www.elsevier.com), by selecting 'Customer Support' and then 'Obtaining Permissions'.

Transferred to Digital Printing 2008

Mosby, Inc.
11830 Westline Industrial Drive
St. Louis, Missouri 63146

ISBN-13: 978-0-8151-2604-1
ISBN-10: 0-8151-2604-2

07 08 / 10 9

*To all from whom I have learned
and all who will yet forever teach me.*

CONTENTS

FOREWORD

Biological evolution has prepared humans to survive even in the most challenging of life's threats and traumas, both physical and psychological. We have learned, however, that the *alarm reaction,* first described in full detail by Hans Selye during the 1940s, is associated with trauma and threats of trauma by the flow of stress hormones and neurotransmitters and also with other rapidly changing bodily physiology that, if unmodulated, can produce illness (physical or emotional) from *overreaction* to trauma. We also now know that trauma and threat of trauma can lead to changes in the immune system, which may operate against survival if such changes are unmodulated. Oftentimes, the threat of trauma can be more devastating than the actual trauma itself, especially in the cases of children (for example, in the witnessing of home violence) and anyone else who is helpless and is without well-timed social and psychological support when the trauma threat occurs.

Humankind's physical and psychic survival require both physical and emotional supports from others in the environment. This modulating influence from the environment is a part of our biological and social heritage. Humans are social mammals and are predisposed toward social responses to others and integrated joint activity, ensuring survival of the species. This social predisposition toward shared experience in humans makes it possible for an individual suffering pain, trauma or distress, or threats of these traumas to be understood and acknowledged directly or intuitively by another person. Thus one person's pain and trauma or threat becomes a shared threat or a shared trauma for others in the community.

Even before the days of technically equipped emergency services, "911," the paramedics, mountain rescue teams, as well as the crisis intervention hot lines and professional societies mobilized to respond to massive trauma in the community (referred to in this volume), the lives of many men, women, and children were saved because someone noticed and responded to them and provided a safe haven and a protective environment for the person in trouble or threat. What was provided before our more sophisticated methods of life-saving technology was primarily psychological, together with warmth and protection. Such support provided by our unsophisticated ancestors worked then and still works now. We now know *why* it works, which is because a supportive psychological and physical environment actually does modulate the overreactive responses of the body and the mind to a trauma or threat; thus the feeling of helplessness is diminished and does not escalate into an exaggerated, nonadaptive illness-producing response. For example, during a recent backpacking trip to the high Sierras, one of our party was stung on the finger by a wasp. Her whole hand began to swell, and she was frightened of dying and not easily reassured, even after she received some Benadryl and cold packs were applied to the hand. Luckily, we met a pleasant, uniformed forest ranger who had also been attacked by a swarm of wasps when he inadvertently disturbed their nest on the forest floor. He told us of his experience and of his recovery and reaffirmed the correctness of the treatment given and indicated further that the danger period for more complicated events had now passed.

Appropriate response to a crisis in the present helps individuals clearly distinguish between a minor stress and an impending catastrophe in the future. Learning to make this distinction is extremely important for each individual and can be helped by an understanding person who is knowledgeable and helpful to a person who has been traumatized. Making this distinction then prepares the person to truly emerge from the present situation with knowledge and understanding, such that the anxiety signal that alerts the person to a danger then also brings to mind the appropriate response to the danger, taking into account its magnitude. Not all dangers are of equal magnitude. A modulated response is required.

The helping professions must have and must be able to convey to others their presence and emotional availability in a timely fashion to the person in crisis. The professional must be able to understand the peculiar nature of each individual in crisis and out of such understanding must be able to help the patient gain hope and increased confidence in being able to survive the crisis. Another important asset of the professional is the capacity to understand that the person himself contains the forces that can lead to recovery. The implication is that the helping person helps the traumatized individual see and understand how to make use of his most strongly developed coping capacities. Well-timed warmth, caring, love, information leading to understanding, good communication, and the capacity of the injured party to distinguish between a minor transient incident and a more serious long-term incapacity provide a powerful holding environment that allows the individual to recover, even though temporarily overwhelmed with feelings of helplessness.

Many people have gone through traumatic experiences during their formative years without remembering such experiences. Overreactions later on to a faintly similar experience can be understood as a maladaptive response to the actual present reality, including the tendency to provoke and repeat the traumatic experience. Unrecognized posttraumatic effects coming late on the heels of earlier trauma are sources of considerable pain, suffering, and maladaptation in adolescent and adult life. They are the result of poorly resolved early traumatic experience, inadequately responded to by the environment, and with an inadequate convalescence of the person from the traumatic experience. Convalescence after any illness or trauma is the most important variable that determines whether the illness becomes chronic or whether it becomes fully resolved. It is worth pointing out here that life is full of eu traumas (health-producing traumas), which were fully incorporated in Selye's theory of adaptation in the fifties. A recent well-controlled study by Andrews and others (1993) shows that students going to foreign countries under AFS International Exchange programs show a long-term decline in vulnerability to neurotic symptoms as compared with a well-matched control group. Parmalee (1993) has written on the importance of helping families of young acute and chronically ill children adapt to situations such as being in the hospital, experiencing crisis, and preparing for potentially traumatic surgeries, emphasizing that successfully traversing these rather common potentially traumatic situations in childhood actually leaves the child and family in a stronger, more resilient psychological state.

Human beings inherently strive to attain new understanding and new meaning in every life experience. New meaning is critical for recovery from trauma and helps prevent the long-term consequences of repressed traumatic experience. Many cases of posttraumatic stress disorder have been hidden by this repression for many years.

This book will be a valuable resource for those who help or who want to help. It will soon be learned and acknowledged by anyone in the field, however, that helping is not as simple as it might seem on the surface. Sometimes "help" can add to distress and trauma rather than lead to a resolution of it. The complexity of both conscious and unconscious motivations of the persons providing help should be required as part of the training of anyone espousing skills in helping others. This book will help individuals achieve that kind of understanding. Insight, however, is a long, hard, and difficult road. The working through of insight in the helping professions requires constant vigilance and continuing psychological work.

Justin D. Call, MD
Newport Beach, California
University of California, Irvine

REFERENCES

Andrews G, Page AC, Neilson M: Sending your teenagers away: controlled stress decreases neurotic vulnerability, *Arch Gen Psychiatr* 50:585, 1993.

Parmalee AH: Children's illnesses and normal behavioral development: the role of care giver, *Zero to Three* 13(4):1, 1993.

PREFACE

The eighth edition of this text acknowledges the fact that crisis intervention is being widely used by those in the helping professions. Individuals from all walks of life and age groups and with diverse problems and varying cultural backgrounds have responded to the skilled use of crisis intervention. It is being used by professionals and nonprofessionals with a wide range of skills.

It was felt that there was still a need for an overview and a guide to crisis intervention, from its historical development to its present utilization. The techniques and skills of a therapist must be learned and practiced under professional supervision. However, it is believed that an awareness of the basic theory and principles of crisis intervention will be valuable to all who are involved in the helping professions. This book should be a particularly meaningful mode of intervention for those who have constant and intimate contact with individuals and families in stressful situations (those who seek help because they are unable to cope alone and situations that may be biological, sociological, or psychological in origin).

Chapter 1 presents the historical development of crisis intervention methodology. Its intent is to create an awareness of the broad base of knowledge incorporated in its present practice. Looking to the future, a discussion of potential crises that may result from society's technological advances is new to this edition.

Chapter 2 deals with the differences between psychotherapeutic techniques of psychoanalysis and psychoanalytic psychotherapy and between brief psychotherapy and crisis intervention methodology. It presents the major goals of these methods of treatment, foci, activities of the therapist, indications for treatment, average length of treatment, and the approximate cost to the individual. New to this chapter is the introduction of cognitive therapy and its utilization in crisis intervention with depressed patients.

Chapter 3 introduces the paradigms and illustrates their utilization in case studies. It focuses on the problem-solving process and introduces the reader to basic terminology used in this method of treatment. The paradigm clarifies the sequential steps of crisis development. Two case studies, with paradigms, illustrate its application as a guide to the case studies that are presented in subsequent chapters. New to this chapter is a discussion of the biophysiological components of stress, since individuals in crisis are under stress.

Also new to this edition are blank paradigms for the reader to complete for each case study in the text. The reader can then compare that paradigm with completed paradigms that are presented in Appendix D to evaluate his knowledge of crisis intervention. It is hoped that this interactive method will prove useful in learning and applying knowledge about the crisis intervention process.

Chapter 4 discusses the legal and ethical issues inherent in psychotherapy. Discussed are the legal aspects of malpractice. Sexual harassment is presented as it is related to psychotherapy and the relationship between the therapist and patient. A case study is presented that demonstrates the use of crisis intervention techniques in a case of sexual harassment. The first paradigm for the reader to complete accompanies this case study.

Chapter 5 presents posttraumatic stress disorder and, new to this edition, acute stress disorder. The American Psychiatric Association's *Diagnostic and Statistical Manual of Mental Disorders* (DSM-IV) criteria places these two disorders in separate categories. They are presented here to clarify and distinguish between them. A case study is included with a paradigm for the reader to complete.

Chapter 6, Violence in Our Society, is a new chapter that discusses concerns that individuals and therapists are confronted with daily: child abuse and neglect, violence in the home, violence in schools, and elder abuse and neglect. Case studies and paradigms are presented for each issue discussed.

Chapter 7, the Psychological Trauma of Infertility, is also a new chapter. Individuals are reluctant to discuss this topic with those who have had one or several spontaneous abortions ("miscarriages"). Infertility is presented as a life crisis. A case study and paradigm are included.

Chapter 8 deals with stressful events that could precipitate a crisis in individuals regardless of socioeconomic or sociocultural status. These events include role and status changes, rape, physical illness, Alzheimer's disease, and suicide. Case studies based on factual experience are presented to illustrate the techniques used by therapists in crisis intervention. Theoretical material preceding each case study is presented as an overview to the crisis situation.

Chapter 9, Life Cycle Stressors, presents stressors that occur during concomitant physiological and social transitions: prepuberty, adolescence, adulthood, and old age. Case studies are included with appropriate theoretical material.

Chapter 10 is a new chapter that is devoted to substance abuse. It includes the older and better known substances such as marijuana, heroin, and cocaine, as well as the newer "designer" drugs that are cheap and easy to obtain or manufacture but that can be deadly. A case study is presented. There is also a section that addresses the abuse and misuse of prescription drugs by the elderly and its consequences.

Chapter 11 delineates the concerns of the public toward individuals who are HIV-positive or who have AIDS and emphasizes the increase of this disease in youth, women, and those who do not use drugs. Two case studies are presented.

Chapter 12 is devoted to the burnout syndrome that occurs frequently in high-stress work situations. Theoretical material is presented, as well as a case study about a nurse who works in a hospice.

Postscriptum.   According to Webster's dictionary: "A postscript is a note . . . appended to a completed letter, book or the like." The postscript in this text is for me, as the author, to share with you, the reader, my thoughts, feelings, and beliefs regarding the future of patients and mental health professionals as we approach the twenty-first century.

Five appendixes have been added to this edition to provide key information that supplements text content. Appendix A is a key of terms used in legal disciplinary hearings. Appendix B contains terms associated with the mental status examination. Appendix C is a detailed list of organizations and other resources for couples dealing with infertility. Appendix D provides completed paradigms for each case study that the reader may consult after filling out the blank paradigm in each chapter. Appendix E is a register of authors quoted in this book.

Acknowledgments

I am greatly indebted to many individuals who have been of direct and indirect assistance in writing this edition. I wish to specifically thank the following individuals for their roles in bringing this manuscript to fruition:

My editors, Jeff Burnham, for his enthusiasm and encouragement, and
  Linda Caldwell, for her patience and understanding.

Cheryl Abbott Bozzay, Production Editor, and Jeff Downing, Associate Developmental Editor, for their expertise, wisdom, and knowledge.

Yael Kats, Designer, for creating such original artwork and a wonderful cover.

Dorothy and Norman Karasick (well-known writers), two very special friends who were always there when I needed them. They gave me advice about content, grammar, and my Macintosh.

Leslie Moffett, who typed the rough and completed drafts and edited as needed. If not for her, this manuscript would not have been completed.

Laurel Stine, my research assistant, for all her efforts and the help she provided.

Peter Berton, for providing me with the Chinese pictographs to use on the cover of the book.

Janice Messick, former co-author, especially for her moral support and continued friendship.

Justin D. Call, MD, well-known and famous child psychiatrist. (It is a particular honor to have him write the foreword. Our collegial friendship goes back many happy years.)

To my family, who are still my kindest critics and strongest supporters, for letting me take time away from them to write, I owe a very special debt—my eternal love.

Donna Conant Aguilera

CONTENTS

5. Posttraumatic Stress Disorder and Acute Stress Disorder, 62

6. Violence in Our Society, 76

7. The Psychological Trauma of Infertility, 122

8. Situational Crises, 138

9. Life Cycle Stressors, 186

10. Substance Abuse, 221

CRISIS
INTERVENTION
Theory and Methodology

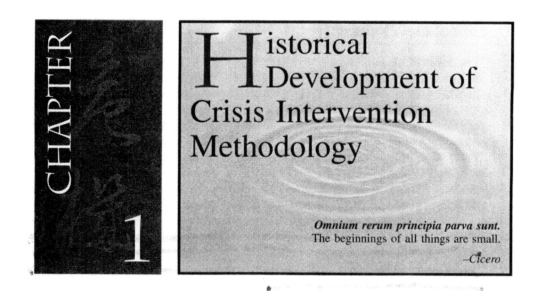

CHAPTER

1

Historical Development of Crisis Intervention Methodology

Omnium rerum principia parva sunt.
The beginnings of all things are small.

—Cicero

A *psychological crisis* refers to an individual's inability to solve a problem. We all exist in a state of emotional equilibrium, a state of balance, or homeostasis. When something that is different (either positive or negative), a change, or a loss that creates a state of disequilibrium occurs, we strive to regain and maintain our previous level of equilibrium. A person in crisis is at a turning point. He* faces a problem that he cannot readily solve by using the coping mechanisms that have worked before. As a result, his tension and anxiety increase, and he becomes less able to find a solution. A person in this situation feels helpless—he is caught in a state of great emotional upset and feels unable to take action *on his own* to solve the problem.

In a 1959 address John F. Kennedy stated, "When written in Chinese the word *crisis* is composed of two characters—one represents danger and the other represents opportunity."

Crisis is a *danger* because it threatens to overwhelm the individual or his family, and it may result in suicide or a psychotic break. It is also an *opportunity* because during times of crisis individuals are more receptive to therapeutic influence. Prompt and skillful intervention may not only prevent the development of a serious long-term disability but may also allow new coping patterns to emerge that can help the individual function at a higher level of equilibrium than before the crisis.

Crisis intervention can offer the immediate help that a person in crisis needs to reestablish equilibrium. It is an inexpensive, short-term therapy that focuses on solving the immediate problem. Increasing awareness of sociocultural factors that could precipitate crisis situations has led to the rapid evolution of crisis intervention methodology.

---

*For the sake of clarity, male pronouns have been used throughout this book except where the name of the patient or therapist denotes female gender.

Historical Development

The origin of modern crisis intervention dates back to the work of Eric Lindemann and his colleagues after the Coconut Grove fire in Boston on November 28, 1942. In what was at that time the worst single-building fire in the country's history, 493 people perished when flames swept through the crowded nightclub. Lindemann and others from the Massachusetts General Hospital played an active role in helping survivors who had lost loved ones in the disaster. His clinical report (Lindemann, 1944) on the psychological symptoms of the survivors became the cornerstone for subsequent theorizing on the grief process, a series of stages through which a mourner progresses on the way toward accepting and resolving loss. Lindemann came to believe that clergy and other community caretakers could play a critical role in helping bereaved people through the mourning process and thereby head off later psychological difficulties. This concept was further operationalized with the establishment of the Wellesley Human Relations Service (Boston) in 1948, one of the first community mental health services noted for its focus on short-term therapy in the context of preventive psychiatry.

Lindemann's (1956) initial concern was to develop approaches that might contribute to the maintenance of good mental health and the prevention of emotional disorganization on a community-wide level. He chose to study bereavement reactions in his search for social events or situations that would predictably be followed by emotional disturbances in a considerable portion of the population. In his study of bereavement reactions among the survivors of those killed in the Coconut Grove nightclub fire, he described both brief and abnormally prolonged reactions occurring in different individuals as a result of the loss of a significant person in their lives.

In his experiences working with grief reactions, Lindemann concluded that a frame of reference constructed around the concept of an emotional crisis, as exemplified by bereavement reactions, might be worthy of investigation and useful for the development of preventive efforts. Certain inevitable events in the course of the life cycle of every individual can be described as hazardous situations, for example, bereavement, the birth of a child, and marriage. He postulated that in each of these situations emotional strain would be generated, stress would be experienced, and a series of adaptive mechanisms would occur that could lead either to mastery of the new situation or to failure with more or less lasting impairment to function. Although such situations create stress for all people who are exposed to them, they become crises for those individuals who because of personality, previous experience, or other factors are especially vulnerable to this stress and whose emotional resources are taxed beyond their usual adaptive resources.

Lindemann's theoretical frame of reference led to the development of crisis intervention techniques, and in 1946 he and Caplan established a community-wide mental health program in the Harvard area, known as the Wellesley Project.

According to Caplan (1961), the most important aspects of mental health are the state of the ego, the stage of its maturity, and the quality of its structure. Assessment of the ego's state is based on three main areas:

1. The capacity of the person to withstand stress and anxiety and to maintain ego equilibrium

2. The degree of reality recognized and faced in solving problems
3. The repertoire of effective coping mechanisms the person can employ in maintaining a balance in his biopsychosocial field

Sigmund Freud was the first to demonstrate and apply the principle of causality as it relates to psychic determinism (Bellak and Small, 1965). Simply put, this principle states that every act of human behavior has its cause, or source, in the history and experience of the individual. It follows that causality is operative, whether the individual is aware of the reason for the behavior. Psychic determinism is the theoretical foundation of psychotherapy and psychoanalysis. The free association technique, dream interpretation, and assignment of meaning to symbols are based on the assumption that causal connections operate unconsciously.

A particularly important outcome of Freud's deterministic position was his construction of a developmental or "genetic" psychology (Ford and Urban, 1963). Present behavior is understandable in terms of the life history or experience of the individual; the crucial foundations for all future behavior are laid down in infancy and early childhood. The most significant determinants of present behavior are the "residues" of past experiences (learned responses, particularly those developed during the earliest years to reduce biological tensions).

Freud assumed that a reservoir of energy that exists in the individual initiates all behavior. Events function as guiding influences, but they do not initiate behavior; they serve to help mold behavior only in certain directions.

Since the end of the nineteenth century, the concept of determinism and the scientific bases from which Freud formulated his ideas have undergone many changes. Although the ego-analytic theorists have tended to subscribe to much of the Freudian position, they differ in several respects that seem to be extensions of Freudian theory rather than from direct contradictions. As a group they concluded that Freud neglected the direct study of normal or healthy behavior.

Heinz Hartmann was an early ego analyst who was profoundly versed in Freud's theoretical contributions (Loewenstein, 1966). He postulated that the psychoanalytic theories of Freud could prove valid for normal and pathological behavior. Hartmann began with the study of ego functions and distinguished between two groups: those that develop from conflict and those that are "conflict free," such as memory, thinking, and language, which he labeled "primary autonomous functions of the ego." He considered these important in the adaptation of the individual to the environment. Hartmann's conception of the ego as an organ of adaptation required further study of the concept of reality. Hartmann emphasized that a person's adaptation in early childhood and his ability to adapt to the environment in later life had to be considered. He also described the search for an environment as another form of adaptation—the fitting together of the individual and society. He believed that, although the behavior of the individual is strongly influenced by culture, a part of the personality remains relatively free of this influence.

Sandor Rado developed the concept of adaptational psychodynamics, providing a new approach to the unconscious, as well as new goals and techniques of therapy (Salzman, 1962). Rado saw human behavior as being based on the dynamic principles of motivation and adaptation. An organism achieves adaptation through interaction with culture. Behavior is viewed in terms of its effect on the welfare of the individual, not just in terms of cause and effect. The organism's patterns of interaction improve through adaptation, with the goal being the increase of possibilities for survival. Freud's classical psychoanalytic technique emphasized the developmental past and the uncovering of unconscious memories, yet he attached little if any importance to the reality of the present. Rado's adaptational psychotherapy, however, emphasizes the immediate present without neglecting the influence of the developmental past. Primary concern is with failures in adaptation "today," what caused them, and what the patient must do to learn to overcome them. Interpretations always begin and end with the present; preoccupation with the past is discouraged. As quickly as insight is achieved, it is used as a beginning to encourage the patient to enter into the present real-life situation repeatedly. Through practice, the patient automatizes new patterns of healthy behavior. According to Rado, this automatization factor—not insight—is ultimately the curative process. He believes that it takes place not passively, in the therapist's office, but actively, in the reality of daily living (Ovesy and Jameson, 1956).

Erik H. Erikson further developed the theories of ego psychology, which complement those of Freud, Hartmann, and Rado, by focusing on the epigenesis of the ego and on the theory of reality relationships (Rappaport, 1959). Epigenetic development is characterized by an orderly sequence of development at particular stages, each depending on the previous stage for successful completion. Erikson perceived eight stages of psychosocial development spanning the entire life cycle of the individual and involving specific developmental tasks that must be solved in each phase. The solution achieved in each phase is applied in subsequent phases. Erikson's theory is important because it offers an explanation of the individual's social development as a result of encounters with the social environment. Another significant feature is his elaboration on the normal rather than on the pathological development of social interactions. He dealt in particular with the problems of adolescence and saw this period in life as a "normative crisis," that is, a normal maturational phase of increased conflicts and one with apparent fluctuations in ego strength (Pumpian-Mindlin, 1966). Erikson integrated the biological, cultural, and self-deterministic points of view in his eight stages of human development and broadened the scope of traditional psychotherapy with his theoretical formulations concerning identity and identity crises. His theories have provided a basis for the work of others who further developed the concept of maturational crises and began serious consideration of situational crises and individual adaptation to the current environmental dilemma.

Caplan believes that all of the elements that comprise the total emotional milieu of the person must be assessed in an approach to preventive mental health. The material, physical, and social demands of reality, as well as the needs, instincts, and impulses of the individual, must all be considered important behavioral determinants. As a result of his work in Israel (1948) and his later experiences in Massachusetts with Lindemann and with the Community Mental Health Program at Harvard University, he evolved the concept of the importance of *crisis* periods in individual and group development (Caplan, 1951).

Caplan defined crisis as occurring "when a person faces an obstacle to important life goals that is, for a time, insurmountable through the utilization of customary methods of problem solving. A period of disorganization ensues, a period of upset, during which many abortive attempts at solution are made" (Caplan, 1961). In essence the individual is viewed as living in a state of emotional equilibrium, with the goal always to return to or to maintain that state. When customary problem-solving techniques cannot be used to meet the daily problems of living, the balance or equilibrium is upset. The individual must either solve the problem or adapt to nonsolution. In either case a new state of equilibrium develops, sometimes better and sometimes worse insofar as positive mental health is concerned. There is a rise in inner tension, there are signs of anxiety, and there is disorganization of function resulting in a protracted period of emotional upset. This he refers to as "crisis." The outcome is governed by the kind of interaction that takes place during that period between the individual and the key figures in his emotional milieu.

Evolution of Community Psychiatry

In today's healthcare environment, community psychiatry has emerged and has been changed due to economics, need, and demographics. More women, the traditional caretakers of the family, are employed outside the home. This is due in part to the necessity of the family to have two incomes to survive. It is also due to the reality that many spouses have lost their jobs. Because of economic conditions, many plants and businesses have closed, putting many men out of work (Janoff, 1992). This shift has significantly influenced the nature of the demands on the family and the availability of internal resources to meet these demands.

The increasing number of the elderly in our society has created a generation gap within families. Communities face the dilemma of how to cope with the tremendous number of people over the age of 65. Families do not always have the resources available and neither does the community. The burden thus becomes another problem for community psychiatry (Ravenscroft, 1994).

According to Bellak (1964), community psychiatry evolved from multiple disciplines and is intrinsically bound to the development of psychoanalytic theory. The social and behavioral sciences that advanced during the first half of the century were predicated on psychodynamic hypotheses. At the same time, concepts of public health and epidemiology were advancing in community health programs.

After World War II the general public's increasing awareness and acceptance of the high incidence of psychiatric problems created changes in attitudes and demands for community action. The discovery and use of psychotropic drugs were important steps forward; they resulted in opportunities for open wards and rehabilitation of the hospitalized patient in his home milieu.

It would be incorrect to assume that all of these factors merged spontaneously, creating a successful, structured cure for mental illness. Rather, it was a slow process of trial and error. Widely different programs—each striving to solve problems involving different cultures, interests, knowledge, and skills—were developed and related to other programs similarly initiated. Disciplines once separated in their goals became aware of their interdependence in attaining mutually recognized goals. New allied disciplines developed; roles changed and expanded. Tasks were diffused, and lines between disciplines became more flexible.

The origin of day hospitals for the care of psychiatric patients grew out of a shortage of hospital beds (Ross, 1964), which forced premature discharges of patients to their homes, rather than treatment innovation. The first reported day hospital was associated with the First Psychiatric Hospital in Moscow in 1933. As Dzhagarov (1937) states: "The need to continue treatment and for special observation in a setting similar to that of a hospital suggested a practical solution in the form of admission to the preventive section of the hospital. In time a transformation took place; the day hospital was created, proving to be adequately prepared to meet the new needs." In referring to this day hospital in Moscow, Kramer, as quoted by Ross (1964), says: "While this day center is little known and probably had little effect on later developments in the Western world, it is accurate to say that this was the first organized Day Hospital for individuals with severe mental illness."

In the late 1930s Bierer (1964) began the Marlborough Experiment in England. Patients, as members of a "therapeutic social club," lived outside the hospital and were treated at day hospitals or part-time facilities. According to Bierer, the primary goal of the program was to change the patient's role concept from that of a passive object of treatment to one of an active participant-collaborator. At the same time, the psychiatrist and staff had to reconceptualize the patient as a human being accessible to reason and emphasize his assets rather than concentrating on his psychopathology and conflicts. The reality of the "here and now" was the focus of attention.

These innovations in attitude gave rise to the concept of "therapeutic community." The patient became a partner and collaborator with the staff and was granted equal rights, opportunities, and facilities. The medical staff and their assistants functioned as advisors. The patient group assumed responsibility for the behavior of its members, as well as for planning activities, planning their futures, and offering support to each other. Group and social methods were used that encouraged the constant interaction of the members. Other complementary projects developed in the Marlborough Program were the Day Hospital, the Night Hospital, the Aftercare Rehabilitation Center, the Self-Governed Community Hotel, Neurotics Nomine, and the Weekend Hospital.

Linn (1964) describes Cameron's first day hospital in Montreal, Canada, in 1946, in which he and others were responsible for defining and giving formal structure to the program as a treatment innovation.

With this frame of reference, it was only natural that the general hospital added to the various roles in which it serves the community that of becoming a focal point of preventive medicine and public health functions in psychiatry.

In 1958 a "Trouble-Shooting Clinic" was initiated by Bellak (1960) as part of City Hospital of Elmhurst, New York, a general hospital with 1000 beds. The clinic was designed to offer first aid for emotional problems and was not limited to urgent crises. It combined two aspects of service on a walk-in basis around the clock: major emergencies, as well as minor problems involving guidance, legal problems, and marital relations.

After the passage of the California Community Mental Health Act in 1958, the California Department of Mental Hygiene established the first state agency in the country (1961) to undertake the training of specialists in community psychiatry. It was recognized that clinics were needed to accommodate those individuals in the community who were unfamiliar with established forms of psychiatric treatment. The cause for these individuals' exclusion from treatment conceivably could have been divergence in social or cultural background, lack of communication, or lack of recognition of the need for services by both the population and the existing agencies.

In January 1962 the Benjamin Rush Center for Problems of Living, a division of the Los Angeles Psychiatric Service, was opened as a no-wait, unrestricted intake, walk-in crisis intervention center. The center is currently under the direction of the Didi Hirsch Community Mental Health Center. After more than 30 years of operation, the Benjamin Rush Center has accumulated considerable evidence that persons who come to the center are often those who would not typically seek treatment in a traditional clinic. The approach has been to attract persons who, although judged to be genuinely in need of psychiatric treatment, would not have sought traditional treatment because of reluctance to consider themselves "sick," to assume the patient role, or to accept the stigma of psychiatric treatment.

In 1967 crisis intervention replaced emergency detention at the San Francisco General Hospital. On each of the psychiatric units, interdisciplinary teams were established whose primary goal was to reestablish independent functioning of the patients as soon as possible. In a follow-up study, Decker and Stubblebine (1972) concluded that the crisis intervention program achieved the anticipated reduction in psychiatric inpatient treatment.

In the early 1970s the Bronx Mental Health Center (Centro de Hygiene Mental del Bronx) (Morales, 1971) was created for crisis intervention for Spanish-speaking people of low socioeconomic status; it was staffed by Spanish-speaking psychiatrists.

At about the same time, suburban churches in Montreal, Canada, offered brief crisis intervention services on an experimental basis (Lecker and others, 1971). The goal of the program was to reach families undergoing a variety of stresses through a mobile walk-in clinic. The clinics served to facilitate delivery of these services to a latent population at risk, not reached by other means, and at a point early in the evolution of a life crisis.

The first hot line was started at Children's Hospital in Los Angeles in 1968. Hot lines and youth crisis centers have been created in recognition of the failure of traditional approaches to make contacts among adolescents. Twenty-four-hour crisis telephone services, free counseling with a minimum of red tape, walk-in contacts, crash pads, and young people serving as volunteer staff in such services continue to be increasingly attractive to youth who have emerged as the locus of a counterculture.

Trends such as these are being repeated around the country as community mental health programs recognize the value of providing primary and secondary prevention services unique to the needs of their particular clients. Increasing recognition is also being given to the need for more services for those clients who need continuing support in rehabilitation after resolution of the immediate crisis. The major concern of community mental health centers is no longer that of discerning just what services are appropriate for the needs of potential clients. It is not even that of recruiting clients for the services provided. The centers are faced with the problems of maintaining an adequate staff to meet the demands for their services and obtaining the finances to pay for these services. Professionals and nonprofessionals alike have been recruited and trained to fill the gap between supply and demand for these services. This has led to the deprofessionalization of many mental health functions previously considered to be solely within the scope of the professional's skills. Role boundaries have undergone increasing diffusion as the needs of the individual client and his community have become the determining factors in establishing appropriate services.

In most cities hot lines have increased for those seeking anonymous help. The hot lines are usually available 24 hours a day, 7 days a week. In most cities one seldom has strong and constant family support. One works with virtual strangers, lives among unknown neighbors, or shares an apartment with a "roommate," again a stranger. There is seldom anyone available to share their thoughts, concerns, and fears.

Hot lines may be used to provide assistance to rape victims or to give information about sexually transmitted diseases. There are hot lines established to provide information about acquired immunodeficiency syndrome (AIDS) and human immunodeficiency virus (HIV). Most metropolitan cities have Psychiatric Emergency Teams (PET) who respond to calls in the community when a visit to a home is necessary. Suicide hot lines are available in most cities as a result of the high incidence of suicide (Brent and others, 1993; Herman, 1992; Goh, 1993; Jones, 1990; Shneidman, 1993; Foa, 1992; and Janoff, 1992).

Crises Related to Technological Advances

Rapid increases in the use of technology have contributed to new challenges that could instigate the development of crises. Stress has increased in some families as a result of the use of personal computers. In some cases the computer, with its Internet and Cyberspace, has limited the communication between family members and possibly created new and different crises within the family unit.

The first and only study, to this author's knowledge, to examine the possible pathological uses of the Internet was presented at the American Psychological Association's annual meeting in Toronto, Ontario, Canada, in August of 1996. Kimberly S. Young, a clinical psychologist at the University of Pittsburgh at Bradford, presented a study on the dependency of individuals on the Internet (Roan, 1996).

Dr. Young in her study suggests that there is accumulating psychological evidence that people can become dependent on Internet use in ways very similar to drug, alcohol, and gambling addictions. This study is the first to propose pathological uses of Internet addiction as a legitimate clinical disorder that carries serious consequences.

These addicts "reported significant problems in their lives because they had simply lost control over their ability to limit the time they used the Internet." They typically tried to reduce their Internet use but couldn't, and when they tried to stop using the Internet, they showed signs of physical withdrawal, such as anxiety and shakiness.

Consequences of overuse ranged from not being able to pay their on-line service provider (one monthly bill was $1400) to a formerly happily married mother who was given an ultimatum by her husband—"me or the computer"—and chose her computer.

Dr. Young placed an advertisement on-line seeking "avid Internet users" and placed flyers around local college campuses. The respondents completed surveys and participated in telephone or personal interviews. She recruited 396 individuals whom she later classified as 296 dependent users and 100 nondependent users.

Her findings suggested that Internet dependence can happen to both men and women. The ages ranged from 14 to 71, but most were middle age. Many of the dependent users did not match the stereotypical "computer nerd." "Forty-two percent said they were currently not employed because they were homemakers, retired, or disabled."

The people who became dependent seemed to have more time on their hands. Many were new to the Internet—they had been accessing for an average of 8 months—and were discovering this new world, which then became enticing. So enticing, in fact, that although nondependent users in the survey said they spent 1 to 2 hours a day on-line, dependent users spent about eight times longer. Young's study pointed to another telltale characteristic of dependence. Users spent most of their time in "chat rooms" or playing Multiuser Dungeons, which allows users to take on a different persona. In contrast, the nondependent users logged on mostly for e-mail or to access the World Wide Web to gather information.

For the people who are addicted, the Internet is not an information database. It is an emotional attachment, a fantasy created on-line. Chat rooms can give people a feeling of power or status or camaraderie. For the most part, dependent users did not identify themselves as having current or past mental problems. A weakness of the study is that "it relies on the respondents' own reports, which may be biased." Dr. Young states that "Internet addiction could be a manifestation of some other underlying clinical disorder."

She also states that " . . . there were few warning signs that a dependence was developing." This, Young says, is another area in need of more research. The respondents said it was very insidious; that the problem grew quickly over time. The 2 hours in which they intended to stay on turned into 6 or 7 hours. They were staying up late, then they were getting up in the middle of the night. Most people who overuse on-line services change their behavior after they receive their first shocking bill; however, dependent users found that they could not cut back. Many dismantled their computers but felt compelled to reassemble them.

SIGNS OF AN ON-LINE ADDICT

A "dependent" Internet user may meet as few as four of the following criteria (similar to those used to identify alcohol and drug addiction) over a 1-year period (Young, 1996):
- Thinks about the Internet while off-line
- Has an increasing need to use the Internet to achieve satisfaction
- Unable to control Internet use
- Feels restless or irritable when attempting to cut down or stop Internet use

- Uses the Internet as a way of escaping from problems or relieving a poor mood
- Lies to family members or friends to conceal the extent of Internet involvement
- Jeopardizes or risks loss of a significant relationship, job, educational, or career opportunity because of the Internet
- Keeps coming back for more, even after spending an excessive amount of money for on-line fees
- Goes through withdrawal when off-line
- Stays on-line longer than intended

Although Young's study suggests some interesting possibilities, the population of her study (i.e., unemployed, homemakers, retired, or disabled) does not represent the majority of those who currently use the Internet. Those who seek information on the World Wide Web to communicate with others in their profession or field of interest do so because of the instant access otherwise unavailable through conventional mail delivery service. They can receive information from all over the world instantaneously. It may be a recent medical breakthrough, research in genetics, medications, or theories or treatments being used in fields such as psychiatry, psychology, nursing, social work, ophthalmology, and dentistry.

The Internet is the communication domain of the future. This writing is already obsolete—passé. The Internet is mushrooming to the point that anything written today is already "old." As with anything new and novel, there will always be those who cannot cope and will seek out methods by which to abuse this otherwise highly productive mode of communication and learning. The Internet is here to stay, to bring knowledge to mankind from all over the world.

REFERENCES

Bellak I, Small L: *Emergency psychotherapy and brief psychotherapy,* New York, 1965, Grune & Stratton.

Bellak L: A general hospital as a focus of community psychiatry, *JAMA* 174:2214, 1960.

Bellak L, editor: *Handbook of community psychiatry and community mental health,* New York, 1964, Grune & Stratton.

Bierer J: *The Marlborough experiment.* In Bellak L, editor: *Handbook of community psychiatry and community mental health,* New York, 1964, Grune & Stratton.

Brent DA and others: Adolescent witnesses to a peer suicide, *J Am Acad Child Adolesc Psychiatry* 32:1184, 1993.

Caplan G: *An approach to community mental health,* New York, 1961, Grune & Stratton.

Caplan G: A public health approach to child psychiatry, *Ment Health* 35:235, 1951.

Decker JB, Stubblebine JM: Crisis intervention and prevention of psychiatric disability: a follow-up study, *Am J Psychiatry* 129:101, 1972.

Dzhagarov MA: Experience in organizing a day hospital for mental patients, *Neurapathologia Psikhiatria* 6:147, 1937 (translated by G Wachbrit).

Foa E: National Victim Center and the Crime Victims Research and Treatment Center. *Rape in America: a report to the nation (Research Report #1992-1),* Washington, DC, 1992.

Ford D, Urban H: *Systems of psychotherapy,* New York, 1963, John Wiley & Sons.

Goh DS: The development and reliability of the attitudes toward AIDS scale, *Coll Student J* 27(2):208, 1993.

Herman JL: *Trauma and recovery,* New York, 1992, Basic Books.

Janoff BR: *Shattered assumptions,* New York, 1992, Free Press.

Jones J: Psychology's role in AIDS crisis grows, *APA Monitor* 20:6, June 1990.

Kennedy JF: Address, United Negro College Fund Convocation, Indianapolis, April 12, 1959.

Lecker S and others: Brief interventions: a pilot walk-in clinic in suburban churches, *Can Psychiatr Assoc J* 16:141, 1971.

Lindemann E: The meaning of crisis in individual and family, *Teachers Coll Rec* 57:310, 1956.

Lindemann E: Symptomatology and management of acute grief, *Am J Psychiatry* 101:101, 1944.

Linn L: Psychiatric program in a general hospital. In Bellak L, editor: *Handbook of community psychiatry and community mental health,* New York, 1964, Grune & Stratton.

Loewenstein RM: Psychology of the ego. In Alexander F, Eisenstein S, Grotjahn M, editors: *Psychoanalytic pioneers,* New York, 1966, Basic Books.

Morales HM: Bronx Mental Health Center, NY State Division, *Bronx Bull* 13:6, 1971.

Ovesy L, Jameson J: Adaptational techniques of psychodynamic therapy. In Rado S, Daniels G, editors: *Changing concepts of psychoanalytic medicine,* New York, 1956, Grune & Stratton.

Pumpian-Mindlin E: Contributions to the theory and practice of psychoanalysis and psychotherapy. In Alexander F, Eisenstein S, Grotjahn M, editors: *Psychoanalytic pioneers,* New York, 1966, Basic Books.

Rappaport D: A historical survey of psychoanalytic ego psychology. In Klein GS, editor: *Psychological issues,* New York, 1959, International Universities Press.

Ravenscroft T: After the crisis, *Nurs Times* 90(12):26, 1994.

Roan S: *Los Angeles Times;* Los Angeles, August 13, 1996.

Ross M: Extramural treatment techniques. In Bellak L, editor: *Handbook of community psychiatry and community mental health,* New York, 1964, Grune & Stratton.

Salzman L: *Developments in psychoanalysis,* New York, 1962, Grune & Stratton.

Shneidman ES: Some controversies in suicidology: toward a mentalistic discipline, *Suicide Life Threat Behav* 23(4):292, 1993.

Young KS: Personal communication, 1996, University of Pittsburgh.

ADDITIONAL READING

American Journal of Nursing: *Health care reform* (video), 32nd Biennial Convention of Sigma Theta Tau, 1993, Alan Trench/Helene Fuld Trust.

Bachrach LL: Community psychiatry's changing role, *Hosp Community Psychiatry* 42:573, 1991.

Beeber LS: The one-to-one relationship in nursing practice: the next generation. In Anderson CA, editor: *Psychiatric nursing 1974 to 1994: a report on the state of the art,* St. Louis, 1995, Mosby.

Betemps E, Ragiel C: Psychiatric epidemiology: facts and myths on mental health and illness, *J Nurs* 32:23, 1994.

Bishop JB: The university counseling center: an agenda for the 1990s, *J Counsel Dev* 68:408, 1990.

Clark MJ: *Nursing in the community,* Norwalk, Conn, 1992, Appleton & Lange.

Dazord A and others: Pretreatment and process measures in crisis intervention as predictors of outcome, *Psychother Res* 1(2):135, 1991.

Fontes LA: Constructing crises and crisis intervention theory, *J Strat Syst Ther* 10:59, 1991.

Grob GN: Mental health policy in America: *Health Aff* Fall, p 7, 1992.

Huffman K, Vernoy M, Williams B: *Psychology in action,* ed 2, New York, 1995, John Wiley & Sons.

Kaplan H, Sadock B: *Synopsis of psychiatry,* ed 6, Baltimore, 1994, Williams & Wilkins.

Kocmur M, Zavasnik A: Patients' experience of the therapeutic process in a crisis intervention unit, *Crisis* 12(1):69, 1991.

Miller WR and others: The helpful responses questionnaire: a procedure for measuring therapeutic empathy, *J Clin Psychol* 47:444, 1991.

Olsen DP, Rickles H, Travlik K: A treatment team model of managed mental health care, *Psychiatr Serv* 46(3):252, 1995.

Pollin IS: Linda Pollin Foundation NIMH workshop attendees: model curriculum in medical crises counseling super (SM). A model for counseling the medically ill: the Linda Pollin Foundation approach, Chevy Chase, MD, *Gen Hosp Psychiatry* 14(suppl 6):11, 1992.

Redick R and others: Expansion and evolution of mental health care in the United States, *Ctr Ment Health Serv Publ* No. #210, 1994.

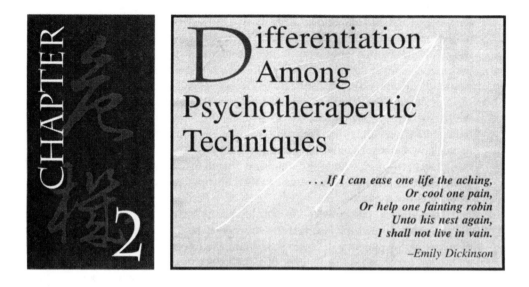

CHAPTER 2

Differentiation Among Psychotherapeutic Techniques

...If I can ease one life the aching,
Or cool one pain,
Or help one fainting robin
Unto his nest again,
I shall not live in vain.

—Emily Dickinson

Psychotherapy as a form of treatment has had many definitions, some conflicting and others concurring. Areas of divergence are generally those of methodology, therapeutic goals, length of therapy, and indications for treatment. There is general agreement, however, that psychotherapy is a set of procedures for changing behaviors based primarily on the establishment of a relationship between two (or more) people.

Psychoanalysis and Psychoanalytic Psychotherapy

The original theories of Sigmund Freud, the founder of psychoanalysis, passed through several phases as he subjected changing hypotheses to the tests of experience and observation, all directed toward the goal of making the unconscious available to the conscious.

In collaboration with Breuer, Freud first developed the psychotherapeutic technique of "cathartic hypnosis." Recognizing that ego control of the unconscious was released under the influence of hypnosis, Freud used hypnotism to induce the patient to answer direct questions in an effort to uncover the unconscious causes of the symptomatology and to allow free expression of pent-up feelings.

Freud observed, however, that to obtain therapeutic results, the procedure had to be repeated. He recognized that material brought to consciousness during hypnosis returned to the unconscious as the awakening patient regained control over his emotions. The therapeutic task of making the conscious patient recall and face repressed emotions to gain insight and increased ego strength was only transiently achieved by this technique.

Freud then experimented with what he referred to as "waking suggestion." Laying his hand on the patient's forehead, he would strongly suggest that the patient could recall the past if he tried. Freud soon learned that a person could not be forced to recall repressed, conflictual emotional events through this approach. He next devised an indirect method of freeing unconsciously repressed material for confrontation by the conscious. Using the process of "free association," the patient was expected to verbalize whatever thoughts came into his mind, freely associating events from his whole life span of experiences, feelings, fantasies, and dreams without concern for logic or continuity. Freud concentrated on gaining an intellectual understanding of the patient's psychogenic past. He insisted on the "basic rule" that the patient tell the therapist everything that came into his mind during each interview. Nothing, no matter how inconsequential the patient might think it was, could be withheld from the analyst. In this search for repressed memories, Freud found that repressed emotions were gradually discharged as they emerged, although not as dramatically as in cathartic hypnosis.

"Transference phenomena" is considered to be one of the most important discoveries by Freud. He deemed transference to be a valuable therapeutic tool in overcoming the patient's defenses in resisting the release of unconscious, repressed emotional experiences. He thought of transference as an emotional reaction of the patient to the therapist in which the patient would relive his conflicts and emotions as they emerged from the past, from his unconscious. He would transfer to the therapist emotions he had felt toward authority figures in his childhood.

Freud referred to this reliving of the neurotic past in a present relationship with the therapist as *transference neurosis*. The principal factor in this process was that the patient expressed his aggressions against the therapist without any fears of the reprisal or censure that he may have been subjected to by the authority figure in his childhood. Through the therapist's nonjudgmental acceptance, the patient was encouraged to face new material released from his own unconscious with reduced fear and anxiety. As these new experiences were assimilated into the conscious ego, coping skills increased, which in turn facilitated further release of repressed material. Alexander (1956) refers to this process as a "corrective emotional experience."

Psychoanalysis is concerned with theory as well as techniques. Alexander and French (1946) also state that the traditional approach in psychoanalytic therapy has been nondirective. The therapist is a passive observer who follows the lead of the patient's verbal expressions as they unfold. Tarachow (1963) indicates that psychoanalytic therapy is for those whose personalities and ego strengths are relatively intact, despite neurotic symptoms or mild to moderately severe characterological disturbances due to unconscious conflicts.

Stone (1951) lists eight factors in the situation and technique of psychoanalysis from which technical variations have derived.

1. Practically exclusive reliance during the hour of the patient's free associations for communications
2. Regularity of the time, frequency, and duration of appointments and clearly defined financial agreement
3. Three to five appointments a week (originally six), with daily appointments the dominant tendency
4. Recumbent position of the patient, in most instances with some impediment against seeing the analyst directly

5. Confinement of the analyst's activity essentially to interpretation or other purely informative interventions such as reality testing or an occasional question
6. Emotional passivity and neutrality (benevolent objectivity) of the analyst, specifically abstention from gratifying the patient's transference wishes
7. Abstention by the analyst from advice or any other direct intervention or participation in the patient's daily life
8. No immediate emphasis by the analyst on curing symptoms, the procedure being guided by the patient's free associations from day to day; in a sense, regarding the whole scope of the patient's psychic life as the field of observation

In psychoanalytic psychotherapy the therapist is more active than in psychoanalysis. The therapist interacts more with the patient and does not interpret the transference attitudes as completely as in analysis. The most helpful attitude is one of calmness, continued interest, and sympathetic, understanding helpfulness; this differs from the neutral attitude of the analyst in psychoanalysis. The contention is that this calm, helpful, interested attitude of the therapist in psychotherapy provides support for the patient in dealing with tension, sustains contact with reality, and provides gratifications and rewards in the therapeutic relationship that provide incentives for the patient to continue to deal with emerging unconscious material.

Alexander (1956) has noted that in procedures that deviate from the classical psychoanalysis of Freud, one or another of the basic phenomena is emphasized from the standpoint of therapeutic significance and is often being dealt with in isolation. For example, Rank centered on the life situation, believing that insight into infantile history had no therapeutic significance. Feranczi placed emphasis on the emotional experience in transference (abreaction factor). Reich concentrated on the analysis of the resistances to allow, by their removal, the discharge of highly charged emotional experiences. He emphasized the importance of hidden forms of resistance and the understanding of the patient's behavior apart from his verbal communication. Psychoanalytic psychotherapy procedures have customarily been divided into two functional categories based on methodology; these are frequently referred to as *supportive* and *uncovering*.

According to Alexander (1956), the aim of the uncovering method is to intensify the ego's ability to handle repressed emotional conflict situations that are unconscious. Through the use of transference, the patient relives his early interpersonal conflicts in relation to the therapist. Supportive and uncovering methods overlap, but it is not difficult to differentiate between them. Primarily, supportive methods of treatment are indicated when functional impairment of the ego is temporary in nature and caused by acute emotional distress. Alexander designated therapeutic tasks in supportive methodology as follows:

1. Gratifying dependency needs of the patient during stress situations, thereby reducing anxiety
2. Reducing stress by giving the patient an opportunity for abreaction
3. Giving intellectual guidance by objectively reviewing with the patient his acute stress situation and assisting the patient in making judgments, thereby enabling him to gain proper perspective of the total situation

4. Supporting the patient's neurotic defenses until his ego can handle the emotional discharges
5. Actively participating in manipulation of the life situation when this might be the only hopeful approach in the given circumstances

Psychoanalysis and psychoanalytic psychotherapy require many years of intensive training on the part of the therapist; this in itself has limited the number of therapists available. Both methods may require that the individual remain in therapy over an extended period, often for years. The obligations of time and expense for such extensive treatment also limits its availability for many.

Brief Psychotherapy

Brief psychotherapy as a treatment form developed as the result of the increased demand for mental health services and the lack of personnel trained to meet this demand. Initially, much of it was conducted by psychiatric residents as part of their training. Later, psychiatric social workers and psychologists became involved in this form of treatment.

Brief psychotherapy has its roots in psychoanalytic theory but differs from psychoanalysis in terms of goals and other factors. It is limited to removing or alleviating specific symptoms when possible. Intervention may lead to some reconstruction of personality, although it is not considered the primary goal. As in more traditional forms of psychotherapy, the therapy must be guided by an orderly series of concepts directed toward beneficial change in the patient. It is concerned with the degree of abatement of the symptoms presented and the return to or maintenance of the individual's ability to function adequately. To attain this goal the individual may choose to get involved in a longer form of therapy. Another goal is assistance in preventing the development of deeper neurotic or psychotic symptoms after catastrophes or emergencies in life situations.

Free association, interpretation, and the analysis of transference are also used successfully in a modified manner. According to Bellak and Small (1965), free association is not a basic tool in short-term therapy. It may arise in response to a stimulus from the therapist. Interpretation is modified by the time limit and the immediacy of the problem. Although it may occur in brief psychotherapy, it is commonly used with medical or environmental types of intervention.

Bellak and Small also believe that positive transference should be encouraged. It is crucial in brief therapy that the patient see the therapist as being likeable, reliable, and understanding. The patient *must* believe that the therapist will be able to help. This type of relationship is necessary if treatment goals are to be accomplished in a short time. This does not mean that negative transference feelings are to be ignored; it does mean that these feelings are not analyzed in terms of defenses.

The therapist assumes a more active role than in the traditional methods. Trends not directly related to the presenting problem are avoided. The positive is accentuated, and the therapist acts as an interested, helpful person. The difficulties faced by the patient are circumscribed. The therapist uses the patient's environmental position to help him evaluate the reality of his situation in an attempt to modify and change it. Productive behavior is encouraged.

Diagnostic evaluation is extremely important in short-term therapy. Its aim is to understand the patient and his symptoms dynamically and to formulate hypotheses that can be validated by historical data. The results of the diagnosis enable the therapist to decide which factors are most susceptible to change and to select the appropriate method of intervention. Part of the evaluation should be the degree of discrepancy or accord between the patient's fantasies and reality. The patient's probable ability to tolerate past and future frustrations should also be considered; the adequacy of his past and present relationships is also pertinent. The question "Why do you come now?" must be asked and means not only "What is it that is going on in your life that distresses you?" but "What is it that you expect in the way of help?" It is reasonable to assume that a request for help is motivated by emotional necessities, both external and internal, that are meaningful to the patient. Short-term goals can be beneficial for *all* patients.

After determining the causes of the symptoms, the therapist elects the appropriate intervention. Interpretation to achieve insight is used with care. Direct confrontation is used sparingly. An attempt is made to strengthen the ego by increasing the patient's self-esteem. One facet of this approach is to help the patient believe that he is on the same level with the therapist and no less worthwhile. The patient's problems should not be seen as being more unusual than those of others. This technique not only relieves the patient's anxiety but also facilitates communication between the patient and the therapist. Other basic procedures used include catharsis, drive repression and restraint, reality testing, intellectualization, reassurance and support, counseling and guidance to move the patient along a line of behavior, and conjoint counseling (Bellak and Small, 1965).

The ending of treatment is an important phase in brief therapy. The patient must be left with a positive transference and the feeling that he may return if the need arises. The learning that has taken place during therapy must be reinforced to encourage the patient to realize that he has begun to understand and solve his own problems. This has a preventive effect that helps the patient recognize possible future problems.

As an adjunct, drug therapy may be used in selected cases, in contrast to pure psychoanalysis, where drugs are seldom used. Environmental manipulation is considered when it is necessary to remove or modify an element causing disruption in the patient's life pattern. Included might be close scrutiny of family and friends, job and job training, education, and plans for travel (Bellak and Small, 1965).

Brief psychotherapy is indicated in cases of acutely disruptive emotional pain, in cases of severely destructive circumstances, and in situations endangering the life of the patient or others. Another indication involves the life circumstances of the individual. If the person cannot participate in the long-term therapeutic situation, which implies a stable residence, job, and so forth, brief therapy is advocated to alleviate disruptive symptoms.

It is imperative that the patient feel relief as rapidly as possible, even during the first therapeutic session. The span of treatment can be any reasonable, limited number of sessions but usually is more than six. Most clinics expect the number of visits to be under 20. Treatment goals can be attained in this short time if the patient is seen quickly and intensively after requesting help. Circumstances associated with disrupted functioning are more easily accessible if they are recent. Only active conflicts are amenable to therapeutic intervention. Disequilibriated states are more easily resolved *before* they have crystalized, acquired secondary gain features, or developed into highly maladaptive behavior patterns.

Crisis Intervention

Crisis intervention extends logically from brief psychotherapy. The minimum therapeutic goal of crisis intervention is psychological resolution of the individual's immediate crisis and restoration to at least the level of functioning that existed before the crisis period. A maximum goal is improvement in functioning above the precrisis level.

Caplan (1964) emphasizes that crisis is characteristically self-limiting and lasts from 4 to 6 weeks. This time constitutes a transitional period, representing both the danger of increased psychological vulnerability and an opportunity for personality growth. In any particular situation the outcome may depend to a significant degree on the availability of appropriate help. On this basis the length of time for intervention is from 4 to 6 weeks, with the average being 4 weeks (Jacobson, 1965). Because time is at a premium, a therapeutic climate is generated that commands the concentrated attention of both therapist and patient. A goal-oriented sense of commitment develops, in sharp contrast to the more modest pace of traditional treatment modes.

METHODOLOGY

Jacobson and associates (1968, 1980) state that crisis intervention may be divided into two major categories, which may be designated as *generic* and *individual.* These two approaches are complementary.

Generic approach. A leading proposition of the generic approach is that there are certain recognizable patterns of behavior in most crises. Many studies have substantiated this thesis. For example, Lindemann's (1944) studies of bereavement found a well-defined process that a person goes through in adjusting to the death of a relative. He refers to these sequential phases as "grief work" and found that failure to grieve appropriately or to complete the process of bereavement could potentially lead a person to future emotional illness.

Subsequent studies of generic patterns of response to stressful situations have been reported. Kaplan and Mason (1960)* and Caplan (1964)* studied how the birth of a premature baby affects the mother and identified four phases or tasks that she must work through to ensure healthy adaptation to the experience. Janis (1958) suggests several hypotheses concerning the psychological stress of impending surgery and the patterns of emotional response that follow a diagnosis of chronic illness. Rapoport (1963)* defines three subphases of marriage during which unusual stress could precipitate crises. These are only a few of the broad research studies done in this field.

The generic approach focuses on the characteristic course of the *particular kind of crisis* rather than on the psychodynamics of each individual in crisis. A treatment

---

*These studies are also discussed in Chapters 8 and 9 of this text.

plan is directed toward an adaptive resolution of the crisis. Specific intervention measures are designed to be effective for all members of a given group rather than for the unique differences of one individual. Recognition of these behavioral patterns is an important aspect of preventive mental health.

Tyhurst (1957) has suggested that knowledge of patterned behaviors in transitional states occurring during intense or sudden change from one life situation to another might provide an empirical basis for the management of these states and the prevention of subsequent mental illness. He cites the studies of individual responses to community disaster, migration, and retirement of pensioners as examples.

Jacobson and associates (1968) state that generic approaches to crisis intervention include

. . . direct encouragement of adaptive behavior, general support, environmental manipulation and anticipatory guidance. . . . In brief, the generic approach emphasizes (1) specific situational and maturational events occurring in significant population groups, (2) intervention oriented to crisis related to these specific events, and (3) intervention carried out by non-mental health professionals.

This approach has been found to be a feasible mode of intervention that can be learned and implemented by nonpsychiatric physicians, nurses, social workers, and others. It does not require a mastery of knowledge of the intrapsychic and interpersonal processes of an individual in crisis.

Individual approach.   The individual approach differs from the generic in its emphasis on assessment, by a professional, of the interpersonal and intrapsychic processes of the person in crisis. It is used in selected cases, usually those not responding to the generic approach. Intervention is planned to meet the unique needs of the individual in crisis and to reach a solution for the particular situation and circumstances that precipitated the crisis. It differs from the generic approach, which focuses on the characteristic course of a particular kind of crisis.

Unlike extended psychotherapy, the individual approach deals relatively little with the developmental past of the individual. Information from this source is seen as relevant for the clues that may result in a better understanding of the present crisis situation only. Emphasis is placed on the immediate causes for disturbed equilibrium and on the processes necessary for regaining a precrisis or higher level of functioning.

Jacobson (1968, 1980) cites the inclusion of family members or other important persons in the process of the individual's crisis resolution as another area of differentiation from most individual psychotherapy methods. In comparison with the generic approach, the individual approach is viewed by Jacobson as emphasizing the need for greater depth of understanding of the biopsychosocial process, intervention oriented to the individual's unique situation, and intervention carried out only by mental health professionals.

Morley, Messick, and Aguilera (1967) recommend several attitudes that are important adjuncts to the specific techniques. In essence, these attitudes comprise the general philosophical orientation necessary for the full effectiveness of the therapist. These attitudes are vital for the therapist to have ingrained and inherent in his basic personality if they are to be effective in working with patients in crisis. If one cannot make changes in the way in which one interprets this philosophical orientation, it may be necessary to accept the fact that working with crisis patients is not for him. The recommended attitudes follow.

1. It is essential that the therapist view the work being done not as a "second-best" approach but as the treatment of choice with persons in crisis.
2. Accurate assessment of the presenting problem, *not* a thorough diagnostic evaluation, is essential to an effective intervention.
3. Both the therapist and the individual should keep in mind that the treatment is time limited and should persistently direct their energies toward resolution of the presenting problem.
4. Dealing with material that is not directly related to the crisis has no place as an intervention of this kind.
5. The therapist must be willing to take an active and sometimes directive role in the intervention. The relatively slow-paced approach of more traditional treatment is inappropriate in this type of therapy.
6. Maximum flexibility of approach is encouraged. Such diverse techniques as serving as a resource person or information giver and taking an active role as an established liaison with other helping resources are often appropriate in particular situations.
7. The goal toward which the therapist is striving is explicit. Energy is directed entirely toward returning the individual to at least his precrisis level of functioning.

STEPS IN CRISIS INTERVENTION

There are certain specific steps involved in the technique of crisis intervention (Morley, Messick, and Aguilera, 1967). Although each cannot be placed in a clearly defined category, typical intervention would pass through the following sequence of phases.

- **Assessment:** Assessment of the individual and his problem is the first phase. It requires the therapist to use active focusing techniques to obtain an accurate assessment of the precipitating event and the resulting crisis that brought the individual to seek professional help. The therapist may have to judge whether the person seeking help presents a high suicidal or homicidal lethality. If the patient is thought to show a high level of danger to himself or to others, referral is made to a psychiatrist for consideration of hospitalization. If hospitalization is not considered necessary, intervention proceeds.

- **Planning therapeutic intervention:** After accurate assessment is made of the precipitating event(s) and the crisis, intervention is planned. It is not designed to bring about major changes in the personality structure but to restore the person to at least the precrisis level of equilibrium. In this phase determination is made of the length of time since onset of the crisis. The precipitating event usually occurs from 1 to 2 weeks before the individual seeks help. Frequently, it may have occurred within the past 24 hours. It is important to know how much the crisis has disrupted the person's life and the effects of this disruption on others in his environment. Information is also sought to determine what strengths he has, what coping skills he may have used successfully in the past and is not using currently, and what other people he used as supports.

- **Intervention:** The nature of intervention techniques is highly dependent on the preexisting skills, creativity, and flexibility of the therapist. Morley, Messick, and Aguilera (1967) suggest some of the following, which have been useful.
1. *Helping the individual to gain an intellectual understanding of his crisis.* Often the individual sees no relationship between a hazardous situation occurring in life and the extreme discomfort of disequilibrium that he is experiencing. The therapist should use a direct approach, describing to the patient the relationship between crisis and the event in his life.
2. *Helping the individual become aware of his present feelings.* Frequently the person may have suppressed some very real feelings, such as anger or other inadmissible emotions toward someone he "should love or honor." It may also be denial of grief, feelings of guilt, or failure to complete the mourning process following bereavement. An immediate goal of intervention is the reduction of tension by providing means for the individual to recognize these feelings and bring them into the open. It is sometimes necessary to produce emotional catharsis and reduce immobilizing tension.
3. *Exploring coping mechanisms.* This approach requires assisting the individual to examine alternate ways of coping. If for some reason the behaviors used in the past for successfully reducing anxiety have not been tried, the possibility of their use in the present situation is explored. New coping methods are sought, and frequently the individual devises some highly original methods that he has never tried before.
4. *Reopening the social world.* If the crisis has been precipitated by the loss of someone significant to the individual's life, the possibility of introducing new people to fill the void can be highly effective. It is particularly effective if supports and gratifications provided in the past by the "lost" person can be achieved to a similar degree from a new relationship.
- **Resolution of the crisis and anticipatory planning:** In this last phase the therapist reinforces those adaptive coping mechanisms that the individual has used successfully to reduce tension and anxiety. As coping abilities increase and positive changes occur, they may be summarized to allow the person to reexperience and reconfirm the progress made. Assistance is given as needed in making realistic plans for the future, and there is discussion of ways in which the present experience may help in future crises.

USE OF COGNITIVE THERAPY IN CRISIS INTERVENTION

When patients seek help in a crisis, the two cardinal symptoms that the therapist usually observes are *anxiety* and/or *depression.* Cognitive therapy can appropriately be used in working with crisis patients with some modifications. The time line of 6 weeks must be given consideration, as well as the methodology.

Beck recognized the contributions of the behavioral therapies in the development of cognitive therapy (Beck, 1979). Beck places much more importance on the external, or mental, experiences of the patients than do behavioral therapists (Beck, 1979).

Beck believes, as do other theorists, that the way in which an individual structures the world through thoughts and evaluations largely influences both behavior and outcome. How one perceives a situation influences the emotions one has toward that situation. It then follows that behaviors and actions will match the emotions. Beck explored this concept and found a consistency in the way in which individuals who experience depression structure their experiences. He organized this into a cognitive model of depression with three components, which he named the "Cognitive Triad." The cognitive triad, the concept of schemas, and faulty patterns of processing information, is the basis of Beck's cognitive theory of depression.

Cognitive triad.   The cognitive triad is Beck's term to identify three common characteristics in the thinking of people with depression. First, depressed people hold a very negative view of themselves; they tend to see themselves as defective in some way, either psychologically, morally, or physically. Because of these presumed defects, they have a tendency to view themselves as worthless. Second, people with depression tend to evaluate ongoing life events in a negative way. The person with depression tends to misinterpret available data so as to always result in a negative outcome, for example, defeat, humiliation, rejection, or inadequacy. Third, the person with depression assumes that the future holds no promise and that the current difficulties will continue. He expects despair, frustration, and failure to persist.

The cognitive triad is basic to Beck's understanding of depression. He views all other symptoms of depression as connecting back to the cognitive patterns of negative self-image, negative interpretation of ongoing experiences, and the negative view of the future.

Schemas.   *Schema* refers to an individual's organization of incoming data into meaningful patterns. Beck (1971) points out that, although people tend to conceptualize situations in a variety of ways, an individual will be fairly consistent in interpreting similar sets of data. These schemas have been learned over time and represent attitudes or assumptions that have been formed on the basis of one's experiences. Schemas affect how an individual will cognitively respond to them. He proposes that in a state of depression, dysfunctional schemas become prevalent and the data from a situation are distorted to fit the dysfunctional schema. The individual is no longer able to match an appropriate schema to a situation because the dysfunctional schema predominates over so much of the thinking. In effect, any stimulus will trigger the negative, dysfunctional schema. This would then explain why people with depression cannot "see" or respond to the many positive aspects of their lives.

Faulty patterns of processing information.   This aspect of the cognitive theory of depression refers to the characteristics of a depressed individual's thinking. Beck (1971) calls depressed thinking "primitive," as opposed to more mature thinking.

Primitive thinking is more absolute than relative, more judgmental than flexible, and more invariable than variable. It is "black and white" thinking, with the emphasis on black. There are no shades of gray. Primitive thinking misses the context and variations of life and tends to be rigid and fixed. It locks the person with depression into a flat and unidimensional way of thinking—an "all-or-none" mentality whereby he views self and actions as "all-bad." Faulty patterns of processing information follow.

Arbitrary inference: Drawing a conclusion when evidence does not support it

Selective abstraction: Paying attention to only one detail of a situation, taking that detail out of context, and ascribing the meaning to the situation based on this single detail

Overgeneralization: The practice of drawing a conclusion based on one incident and then applying it in general

Magnification and minimization: The inability to evaluate the importance or significance of an event to the point of creating a distortion

Personalization: The tendency to assume that external events are related to one's self, when there is no reason to make such a connection

Absolute thinking: The habit of defining experiences in one or two opposite categories, for example, good or bad and perfect or imperfect

Summary

A differentiation among psychoanalysis, brief psychotherapy, and crisis intervention methodology has been explored. No attempt has been made to state that one type of therapy is superior to another. Table 2-1 shows some of the major differences.

In psychoanalysis the goal of therapy is restructuring the personality, and the focus of treatment is the genetic past and the freeing of the unconscious. Psychoanalytic psychotherapeutic procedures are usually divided into two functional categories:

Table **2-1**   Major Differences Among Psychoanalysis, Brief Psychotherapy, and Crisis Intervention Methodology

	Psychoanalysis	Brief psychotherapy	Crisis intervention
Goals of therapy	Restructuring the personality	Removal of specific symptoms	Resolution of immediate crisis
Focus of treatment	1. Genetic past 2. Freeing the unconscious	1. Genetic past as it relates to present situation 2. Repression of unconscious and restraining of drives	1. Genetic present 2. Restoration to level of functioning before crisis
Usual activity of therapist	1. Exploratory 2. Passive observer 3. Nondirective	1. Supportive 2. Participant observer 3. Indirect	1. Supportive 2. Active participant 3. Direct
Indications	Neurotic personality patterns	Acutely disruptive emotional pain and severely disruptive circumstances	Sudden loss of ability to cope with a life situation
Average length of treatment	Indefinite	1-20 sessions	1-6 sessions
Cost of treatment	$100-200	$75-100	$0-75

supportive and uncovering. The therapist's role is nondirective, exploratory, and that of a passive observer. This type of therapy is indicated for those individuals with neurotic personality patterns. The length of therapy is indefinite and depends on the individual and the therapist.

The goals in brief psychotherapy are to remove specific symptoms and aid in the prevention of deeper neurotic or psychotic symptoms. Its focus is on the genetic past as it relates to the present situation, repression of the unconscious, and restraining of drives. The role of the therapist is indirect, supportive, and that of a participant observer. Basic tools used are psychodynamic intervention coupled with medical or environmental types of intervention. Indications for brief psychotherapy are acutely disruptive emotional pain, severely disruptive circumstances, and situations endangering the life of the individual or others. It is also indicated for those who have problems that do not require psychoanalytic intervention. The average length of treatment is from 1 to 20 sessions.

The goal of crisis intervention is the resolution of an immediate crisis. Its focus is on the supportive, with the restoration of the individual to his precrisis level of functioning or possibly to a higher level of functioning. The therapist's role is direct, supportive, and that of an active participant. Techniques are varied and limited only by the flexibility and creativity of the therapist. Some of these techniques include helping the individual gain an intellectual understanding of the crisis, assisting the individual in bringing his feelings into the open, exploring past and present coping mechanisms, finding and using situational supports, and anticipatory planning with the individual to reduce the possibility of future crises. This type of therapy is indicated when a person (or family) suddenly loses the ability to cope with a life situation. The average length of treatment is from one to six sessions. The cost of each therapy is dependent on the geographic region.

When patients are in a crisis, they are usually depressed and/or anxious. Beck's (1971, 1979) theory of cognitive therapy with depressed patients can be used with these patients if certain guidelines are followed. His theory has been added to give the therapists more flexibility in working with crisis patients.

These recommended guidelines are inherent in the philosophy of crisis theory.
- The crucial time line of six sessions
- Focus on the immediate problem
- Use of the direct approach by the therapist
- Maximum flexibility and creativity of the therapist
- The belief that crisis theory is their treatment of choice—not a temporary bandage

REFERENCES

Alexander F: *Psychoanalysis and psychotherapy,* New York, 1956, WW Norton.
Alexander F, French TM: *Psychoanalytic therapy,* New York, 1946, Ronald Press.
Beck AT: *Depression: causes and treatment,* Philadelphia, 1971, University of Pennsylvania Press.
Beck AT and others: *Cognitive therapy of depression,* New York, 1979, Guilford Press.
Bellak L, Small L: *Emergency psychotherapy and brief psychotherapy,* New York, 1965, Grune & Stratton.

Caplan G: *Principles of preventive psychiatry,* New York, 1964, Basic Books. Strachey A, and Strachey J).

Jacobson G: Crisis theory, *New Dir Ment Health Serv* 6:1, 1980.

Jacobson G: Crisis theory and treatment strategy: some sociocultural and psychodynamic considerations, *J Nerv Ment Dis* 141:209, 1965.

Jacobson G, Strickler M, Morley WE: Generic and individual approaches to crisis intervention, *Am J Public Health* 58:339, 1968.

Janis IL: *Psychological stress, psychoanalytical and behavioral studies of surgical patients,* New York, 1958, John Wiley & Sons.

Kaplan DM, Mason EA: Maternal reactions to premature birth viewed as an acute emotional disorder, *Am J Orthopsychiatry* 30:539, 1960.

Lindemann E: Symptomatology and management of acute grief, *Am J Psychiatry* 101:101, 1944.

Morley WE, Messick JM, Aguilera DC: Crisis: paradigms of intervention, *J Psychiatr Nurs* 5:537, 1967.

Rapoport R: Normal crises, family structure, and mental health, *Fam Process* 2:68, 1963.

Stone L: Psychoanalysis and brief psychotherapy, *Psychoanal Q* 20:217, 1951.

Tarachow S: *An introduction to psychotherapy,* New York, 1963, International Universities Press.

Tyhurst JA: *Role of transition states—including disasters—in mental illness.* Paper presented at Symposium on Preventive and Social Psychiatry, sponsored by Walter Reed Institute of Research, Walter Reed Medical Center, and National Research Council, Washington, DC, April 15-17, 1957, U.S. Government Printing Office.

ADDITIONAL READING

Corrigan PW, Holmes EP, Huchins D: Identifying staff advocates of behavioral treatment innovations in state psychiatric hospitals, *J Behav Ther Exp Psychiatry* 24(3):219, 1993.

Ellis A: Reflections on rational-emotive therapy, *J Consult Clin Psychol* 61:199, 1993.

Mahoney JM: Introduction to special section: theoretical developments in the cognitive psychotherapies, *J Consult Clin Psychol* 61(2):187, 1993.

Mason EA: Method of predicting crisis outcome for mothers of premature babies, *Public Health Rep* 78:1031, 1963.

Maynard CK: Comparison of effectiveness of group interventions for depression in women, *Arch Psychiatr Nurs* 7(5):272, 1993.

Miller CR, Eisner W, Allport C: Creative coping: a cognitive-behavioral group for borderline personality disorder, *Arch Psychiatr Nurs* 8(4):280, 1994.

Newell R, Shrubb S: Attitude change and behaviour therapy in body dysmorphic disorder: two case reports, *Behav Cog Psychother* 22(2):163, 1994.

Nobily P, Herr KA, Kelley LS: Cognitive-behavioral techniques to reduce pain: a validation study, *Int J Nurs Stud* 30(6):537, 1993.

Ofman PS, Mastria MA, Steinberg J: Mental health response to terrorism: the World Trade Center bombing. Special Issue: disasters and crises: a mental health counseling perspective, *J Ment Health Counsel* 17(3):312, 1995.

Rickelman BL, Houfek JF: Toward an interactional model of suicidal behaviors: cognitive rigidity, attributional style, stress, hopelessness, and depression, *Arch Psychiatr Nurs* 9(3):158, 1995.

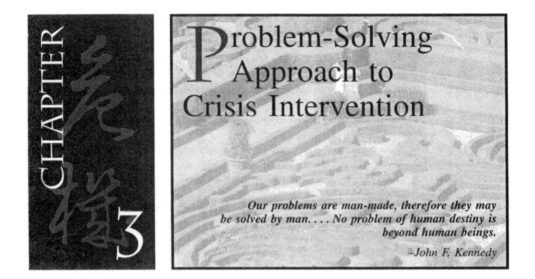

CHAPTER 3

Problem-Solving Approach to Crisis Intervention

Our problems are man-made, therefore they may be solved by man. . . . No problem of human destiny is beyond human beings.

—John F. Kennedy

According to Caplan (1964), a person is constantly faced with a need to solve problems to maintain equilibrium. When he is confronted with an imbalance between the difficulty (as he perceives it) of a problem and his available repertoire of coping skills, a crisis may be precipitated. If alternatives cannot be found or if solving the problem requires unusual amounts of time and energy, disequilibrium occurs. Tension rises and discomfort is felt, with associated feelings of anxiety, fear, guilt, shame, and helplessness.

One purpose of the crisis approach is to provide the consultation services of a therapist who is skilled in problem-solving techniques. The therapist will not have an answer to every problem; however, he will be expected to be competent in problem solving, guiding and supporting his client toward crisis resolution. The therapeutic goal for the individual seeking help is to establish a level of emotional equilibrium equal to or better than the precrisis level.

Problem solving requires that a logical sequence of reasoning be applied to a situation in which an answer is required for a question and in which there is no immediate source of reliable information (Black, 1946). This process may take place either consciously or unconsciously. Usually the need to find an answer or solution is felt more strongly when such a resolution is most difficult.

The problem-solving process follows a structured, logical order of steps, each depending on the one preceding. In the routine decision making required in daily living, this process is rarely necessary. Most people are unaware that they may follow a defined, logical sequence of reasoning in making decisions; often they remark that only some solutions seem to have been reached more easily than others. Finding out the time or deciding which shoe to put on first rarely calls for long, involved reasoning, and more often than not the question arises and the answer is found without any conscious effort.

Factors Affecting the Problem-Solving Process

Depending on past experience related to the immediate problem, some people are more adept at finding solutions than others. Both internal and external factors affect the process at any given time, although initially there may be a temporary lack of concrete information. For example, when a driver finds himself lost because of a missing road sign, how much finding the right directions means to him in terms of his physical, psychological, and social well-being could affect the ease with which he finds an answer to the problem. His anxiety will increase in proportion to the value he places on finding a solution. If he is out driving for pleasure, for example, he may feel casually concerned, but if he is under stress to be somewhere on time, his anxiety may increase according to the importance of his arrival at his immediate goals.

When anxiety is kept within tolerable limits, it can be an effective stimulant to action. It is a normal response to an unknown danger, experienced as discomfort, and helps the individual use his resources to solve the problem. As anxiety increases, however, perceptual awareness narrows and all perceptions are focused on the difficulty. When problem-solving skills are available, the individual is able to use this narrowing of perceptions to concentrate on the problem at hand.

If a solution is not found, anxiety may become more severe. Feelings of discomfort intensify, and perceptions are narrowed to a crippling degree. The ability to understand what is happening and to make use of past experiences gives way to concentration on the discomfort itself. The individual becomes unable to recognize his own feelings, the problem, the facts, the evidence, and the situation in which he finds himself.

Although problem solving involves a logical sequence of reasoning, it is not *always* a series of well-defined steps. It usually begins with a feeling that something has to be done. The problem area is general rather than specific and well defined. Next, the memory is searched in an attempt to come up with ideas or solutions from similar problems in the past. March and Simon (1963) refer to this as "reproductive problem solving," and its value greatly depends on past successes in finding solutions. When no similar past experiences are available, the individual may then turn to "productive problem solving." Here he is faced with the need to construct new ideas from more or less raw data. He will have to go to sources other than himself to get his facts. For example, the driver looking for the road sign may find someone nearby who can give him the needed new data—directions to the right road. If no one is nearby, he will have to find some other source of information. He may resort to trial and error and with luck and patience find the way himself. Finding a solution in this way may meet a present need, but the information gained may not always be applicable to solving a similar problem in the future.

Anxiety is created by some type of stress. Robinson (1990) has divided stress into three phases: *immediate, intermediate,* and *long term.* Since patients in crisis usually experience anxiety or depression, it would be of value to look at the biophysiological components.

- **Immediate physiological processes:** The autonomic nervous system is activated when an individual perceives a threat or demand from the environment. In the stress response the hypothalamus stimulates the sympathetic fibers. The body prepares for "fight or flight," increasing its likelihood of survival. The effects of sympathetic stimulation occur within 2 to 3 seconds and last between 5 and 10 minutes. Sympathetic nerve fibers release the catecholamines epinephrine and norepinephrine. Anxiety is experienced and can be observed both through a person's verbal report and through clinical signs, including perspiration, tremulousness, and rapid pulse and breathing.

- **Intermediate response:** Within 2 to 3 minutes after perception of the stressor, epinephrine and norepinephrine are secreted; these neurotransmitters travel to the end organs, where they maintain the processes already initiated. These sympathetic effects are maintained for 1 to 2 hours. The adrenal medulla does not continue its response but is reactive only after the central nervous system triggers the sympathetic nervous system again. The catecholamines also stimulate gluconeogenesis, which provides the body with additional energy.

- **Long-term response:** Three pathways of the endocrine system perpetuate the long-term effects of stress: the adrenocorticotropic, the thyroxine, and the vasopressin pathways. The adrenal cortex secretes two types of corticoids: mineralocorticoids and glucocorticoids. Aldosterone, a mineralocorticoid, raises the systemic blood pressure. Cortisol, representative of the three glucocorticoids, is pivotal to the breakdown of fats and proteins for energy. Their prolonged secretion, however, has negative effects. The effects of thyroxine are not observed until it peaks at about the tenth day after the stressful event, and the effect may last 6 to 8 weeks. Thyroxine increases the body's metabolism as much as 60% to 100%. Vasopressin is released from the posterior gland and elevates blood pressure.

The therapist should assess the crisis patient for stress and anxiety not only psychologically but also physiologically. With a high level of stress the patient will be unable to understand everything that the therapist is trying to elicit from him. This is just one more reason for the therapist to have solid problem-solving skills and use them wisely.

To summarize, problem solving is a process for settling a difficult situation or satisfying an unmet need, resolving the discrepancy between what is and what should be. Decision making is the process of arriving at a judgment about a need or problem, reaching a conclusion about what to do, and then choosing the action that should be taken. Both problem solving and decision making involve the following:

- Logical consideration of the relevant facts and feelings
- Reasoning characterized by analysis and evaluation of available information
- Use of memories
- Recognition of knowledge deficits

Effective decision making is the outcome of effective problem solving. Ineffective decision making is arrived at impulsively, without thoughtful consideration, or by relying on inaccurate information. Effective problem solving and decision making occur thoughtfully and involve acquisition, analysis, and the use of accurate information (Haber and others, 1992).

Problem Solving In Crisis Intervention

John Dewey (1910) proposed the classical steps or stages represented in different episodes of problem solving: (1) a difficulty is felt; (2) the difficulty is located and defined; (3) possible solutions are suggested; (4) consequences are considered; and (5) a solution is accepted. With minor modifications this approach to the steps in problem solving has persisted over the years. Johnson (1955) simplified problem solving by reducing the number of steps to three: preparation, production, and judgment.

In 1962, Merrifield and associates extensively researched the role of intellectual factors in problem solving. They advocated returning to a five-stage model: preparation, analysis, production, verification, and reapplication. The fifth stage was included in recognition of the fact that the problem solver often returns to earlier stages in a kind of revolving fashion.

According to Guilford (1967), the general problem-solving process involves the following:

- **Input:** From environment and soma
- **Filtering:** Attention aroused and directed
- **Cognition:** Problem sensed and structured
- **Production:** Answers generated
- **Cognition:** New information obtained
- **Production:** New answers generated
- **Evaluation:** Input and cognition tested, answers tested; new tests of problem structure, new answers tested

Fortinash and Holoday-Worret (1996) believe that *critical thinking* is more important in the therapeutic process and contains many of the components of keen judgment, intuition, and expertise. Critical thinking skills enhance and become a part of the therapist's continually expanding knowledge base and help the therapist decide which data are meaningful and which take priority.

When using this process, the therapist incorporates experience and knowledge from other fields to apply theories and principles in practice. Knowledge of basic human needs; anatomy and physiology; disease processes; growth and development; sociological patterns and trends; and various cultures, religions, and philosophies are all crucial components of the critical thinking framework. The following critical thinking skills are used in all phases of crisis intervention:

- *Observing*, which should be planned and continual versus casual and singular
- *Distinguishing* between relevant and irrelevant data
- *Validating* data through observations and communication
- *Organizing* data into meaningful parts
- *Categorizing* data for efficient retrieval and communication

ASSESSMENT OF THE INDIVIDUAL AND THE PROBLEM

When professional help is sought because a person is in crisis, the therapist must use logic and background knowledge to define the problem and plan the intervention. Mental health professionals should be familiar with the model for problem solving in the crisis approach.

The crisis approach to problem solving involves assessing the individual and the problem, planning of therapeutic intervention, intervention, and resolution of the crisis and anticipatory planning (Morley, Messick, and Aguilera, 1967).

The first therapy session is directed toward finding out what the crisis-precipitating event was and what factors are affecting the individual's ability to solve problems. It is important that both therapist and patient be able to define a situation clearly before taking any action to change it. Questions such as "What do I need to know?" and "What must be done?" are asked. The more specifically the problem can be defined, the more likely it is that the "correct" answer will be sought.

Clues are investigated to point out and explore the problem or what is happening. The therapist asks questions and uses observational skills to obtain factual knowledge about the problem area. It is important to know what has happened within the immediate situation. How the individual has coped in past situations may affect his present behavior. Observations are made to determine his level of anxiety, expressive movements, emotional tone, verbal responses, and attitudinal changes. It is important to remember that the therapist's task is to focus on the immediate problem. There is not enough time and no need to go into the patient's history in depth.

One of the therapist's first questions usually is "Why did you come for help today?" The word *today* should be emphasized. Sometimes the individual will try to avoid stating why he came by saying, "I've been planning to come for some time." The usual reply is "Yes, but what happened that made you come in *today?*" Other questions to ask are "What happened in your life that is *different?*" and "*When* did it happen?"

In crisis the precipitating event usually occurs 10 to 14 days before the individual seeks help. Frequently it is something that happened the day before or the night before. It could be almost anything, for example, threat of divorce, discovery of extramarital relations, finding out that a son or daughter is taking drugs, loss of a boyfriend or girlfriend, loss of job or status, or an unwanted pregnancy.

The next area on which to focus is the individual's *perception of the event:* What does it mean to him? How does he see its effect on his future? Does he see the event realistically, or does he distort its meaning? The patient is then questioned about *available situational supports:* Who in the environment can the therapist find to support the person? With whom does he live? Who is his best friend? Whom does he trust? Is there a member of the family to whom he feels particularly close? Crisis intervention is sharply time limited, and the more people involved in helping the person, the better. Also, if others are involved and familiar with the problem, they can continue to give support when therapy is terminated.

Next determined is *what the person usually does when he has a problem he cannot solve:* What are his coping skills? Has anything like this ever happened to him before? How does he usually reduce tension, anxiety, or depression? Has he tried the same method this time? If not, why not, if it usually works for him? If his usual method was tried and it did not work, why did it not work? What does he feel would reduce his symptoms of stress? The patient usually thinks of something; coping skills are individual. Methods of coping with anxiety that have not been used in years may be remembered. One patient recalled that he used to "work off tensions" by playing the piano for a few hours, and it was suggested that he try this method again. Because he did not have a piano, he rented one; by the next session his anxiety had reduced enough to enable him to begin problem solving.

One of the most important parts of the assessment is to find out whether the person is suicidal or homicidal. The questions must be very *direct* and *specific:* Is he planning to kill himself or someone else? How? When? The therapist must find out and assess the lethality of the threat. Is the person merely thinking about it or does he have a method selected? Is it a lethal method, for example, a loaded gun? Has he picked out a tall building or bridge? Can he tell the therapist when he plans to do it, for example, after the children are asleep? If the threat does not seem too imminent, the person is accepted for crisis therapy. If the intent is carefully planned and details are specific, hospitalization and psychiatric evaluation are arranged to protect the person or others.

PLANNING THERAPEUTIC INTERVENTION

After identifying the precipitating event and the factors that are influencing the individual's state of disequilibrium, the therapist plans the method of intervention. Determination must be made as to how much the crisis has disrupted the individual's life. Is he able to work? Go to school? Keep house? Care for his family? Are these activities being affected? This is the first area to examine for the degree of disruption. How is his state of disequilibrium affecting others in his life? How does his wife (or husband, boyfriend, girlfriend, roommate, or family) feel about this problem? What do they think he should do? Are they upset?

This is basically a search process in which data are collected. It requires the use of cognitive abilities and recollection of past events for information relative to the present situation. The last phase of this step is essentially a thinking process in which alternatives are considered and evaluated against past experience and knowledge, as well as in the context of the present situation.

Tentative solutions are advanced about *why* the problem exists. This step requires familiarity with theoretical knowledge and anticipation of more than one answer. In the study of behavior it is important to seek causal relationships. Clues observed in the environmental conditions are examined and related to theories of psychosocial behavior to suggest reasons for the individual's disturbed equilibrium.

INTERVENTION

In the third step, intervention is initiated. Action is taken with the expectation that, if the *planned action* is taken, the *expected result* will occur.

After the necessary information is collected, the problem-solving process is continued to initiate intervention. The therapist defines the problem from the information that has been given and reflects it back to the individual. This process clarifies the problem and encourages focusing on the immediate situation. The therapist then explores possible alternative solutions to the problem to reduce the symptoms produced by the crisis. At this time, specific directions may be given as to what should be tried as tentative solutions. Then the individual can leave the first session with some positive guidelines for going out and testing alternative solutions. At the next session the individual and therapist evaluate the results. If none of these solutions has been effective, they work toward finding others.

The therapist may validate observations and tentative conclusions by reviewing the case with another therapist, when he thinks it may be helpful or necessary. Briefly, the therapist identifies the crisis-precipitating event, symptoms that the crisis has produced in the individual, degree of disruption evident in the individual's life, and plan for intervention. Planned intervention may include one technique or a combination of several techniques. It may be helping the individual to gain an intellectual understanding of the crisis or helping him to explore and ventilate his feelings. Other techniques may be helping the individual to find new and more effective coping mechanisms or utilizing other people as situational supports. Finally, a plan is presented for helping the person establish realistic goals for the future.

ANTICIPATORY PLANNING

An evaluation determines whether the planned action has produced the expected results. Appraisal must be objective and impartial to be valid. Has the individual returned to his usual level or a higher level of equilibrium in his functioning? The problem-solving process is continued as the therapist and the individual work toward resolution of the crisis.

Paradigm of Intervention

According to Caplan (1964), a crisis has four developmental phases.
1. There is an initial rise in tension as the stimulus continues and more discomfort is felt.
2. There is a lack of success in coping as the stimulus continues and more discomfort is felt.
3. A further increase in tension acts as a powerful internal stimulus that mobilizes internal and external resources. In this stage, emergency problem-solving mechanisms are tried. The problem may be redefined, or there may be resignation, and certain unattainable aspects of the goal may be given up.
4. If the problem continues and can be neither solved nor avoided, tension increases and a major disorganization occurs.

Whenever a stressful event occurs, certain recognized *balancing factors* can effect a return to equilibrium; these factors are *perception of the event, available situational supports,* and *coping mechanisms* (Figure 3-1). The upper portion of the paradigm illustrates the "normal" initial reaction of an individual to a stressful event.

A stressful event is seldom so clearly defined that its source can be determined immediately. Internalized changes occur at the same time as the externally provoked stress. As a result, some events may cause a strong emotional response in one person, yet leave another apparently unaffected. Much is determined by the presence or absence of factors that can effect a return to equilibrium.

In column A of Figure 3-1, the balancing factors are operating and crisis is avoided. However, in column B the absence of one or more of these balancing factors may block resolution of the problem and thus increase disequilibrium and precipitate crisis.

Figure 3-2 demonstrates the use of the paradigm for presentation of subsequent case studies. Its purpose is to serve as a guideline to help the reader focus on the

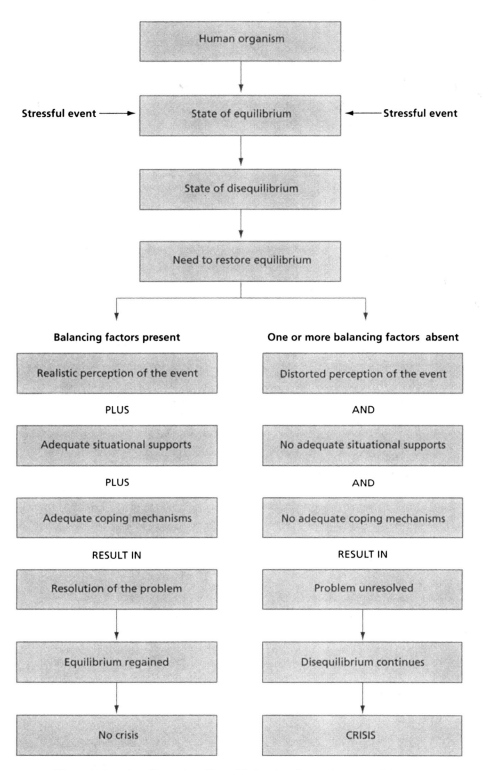

Figure 3-1   Paradigm: the effect of balancing factors in a stressful event.

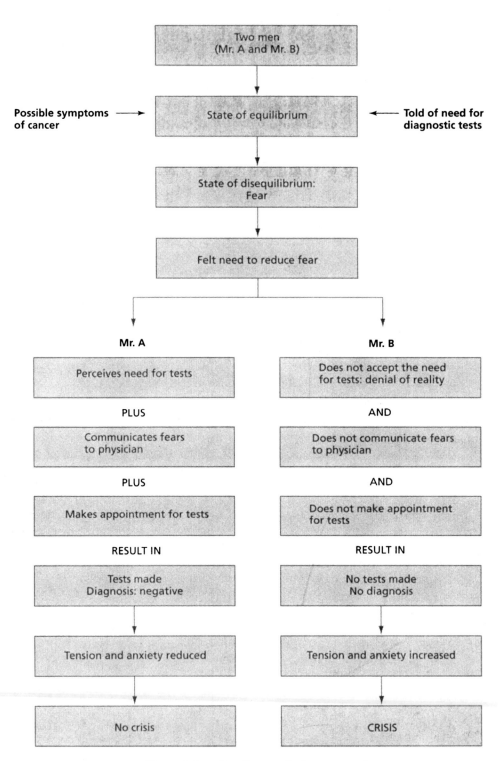

Figure 3-2 Paradigm applied to case study.

problem areas. An example of its applicability is presented in the cases of two people affected by the same stressful event. One resolved the problem and avoided crisis; the other did not.

Balancing Factors Affecting Equilibrium

Between the perceived effects of a stressful situation and the resolution of the problem are three recognized balancing factors that may determine the state of equilibrium. Strengths or weaknesses in any one of the factors can be directly related to the onset of crisis or to its resolution. These factors are perception of the event, available situational supports, and coping mechanisms.

Why do some people go into crisis when others do not? Figure 3-2 illustrates the case of two men, Mr. A and Mr. B. Both men have possible symptoms of cancer and are told of the need for diagnostic tests. Mr. A is upset but does not go into crisis, whereas Mr. B *does* go into crisis. Why does Mr. A react one way and Mr. B another? What "things" in their lives make the difference?

PERCEPTION OF THE EVENT

Cognition, or the subjective meaning, of a stressful event plays a major role in determining both the nature and degree of coping behaviors. Differences in cognition, in terms of the event's threat to an important life goal or value, account for large differences in coping behaviors. The concept of *cognitive style* (Cropley and Field, 1969) suggests uniqueness in the way people take in, process, and use information from the environment.

Cognitive styles, or the characteristic modes for organizing perceptual and intellectual activities, play an important role in determining an individual's coping responses to daily life stresses. According to Inkeles (1966), cognitive style helps to set limits on information seeking in stress situations. It also strongly influences perceptions of others, interpersonal relationships, and responses to various types of psychiatric treatment.

For example, in stressful situations a person whose cognitive style is identified as "field dependent" is very dependent on external objects in the environment for orientation to reality. This type of individual tends to use such coping mechanisms as repression and denial. In contrast, the "field-independent" person tends to prefer intellectualization as a defense mode.

If the event is perceived realistically, the relationship between the event and feelings of stress is recognized. Problem solving can be appropriately oriented toward reduction of tension, and successful resolution of the stressful situation is more probable.

Lazarus (1966) and colleagues (1974) focused on the importance of the mediating cognitive process, *appraisal,* to determine the various coping methods used by individuals. This approach recognizes that coping behaviors always represent an interaction between the individual and the environment and that environmental demands of each unique situation initiate, form, and limit coping activities that may be required in the interaction. As a result, people engage in widely diverse behavioral and intrapsychic activities to meet actual or anticipated threats. Appraisal, in this context, is an ongoing perceptual process by which a potentially harmful event is distinguished from a potentially beneficial or irrelevant event in one's life.

When a threatening situation exists, first a *primary* appraisal is made to judge the perceived outcome of the event in relation to one's future goals and values. This is followed by a *secondary* appraisal, whereby one perceives the range of coping alternatives available either to master the threat or to achieve a beneficial outcome. As coping activities are selected and initiated, feedback cues from changing internal and external environments lead to ongoing *reappraisals* or to changes in the original perception.

As a result of the appraisal process, coping behaviors are never static. They change constantly in both quality and degree as new information and cues are received during reappraisal activities. New coping responses may occur whenever new significance is attached to a situation.

If, in the appraisal process, the outcome is judged to be too overwhelming or too difficult to be dealt with by using available coping skills, an individual is more likely to resort to use of intrapsychic defensive mechanisms to repress or distort the reality of the situation. An appraisal of a potentially successful outcome, however, more likely leads to the use of direct action modes of coping such as attack, flight, or compromise.

If the perception of the event is distorted, a relationship between the event and feelings of stress may not be recognized. Thus attempts to solve the problem are ineffective, and tension is not reduced. In other words, what does the event mean to the individual? How is it going to affect his future? Can he look at it realistically or does he distort its meaning? In the example, Mr. A perceived the need for diagnostic tests; his perception of the event was realistic. Mr. B was unable to accept the need for tests to confirm or refute the possibility of having cancer; his perception was distorted, and he used denial.

SITUATIONAL SUPPORTS

By nature, human beings are social and dependent on others in their environment to supply them with reflected appraisals of their own intrinsic and extrinsic values. In establishing life patterns, certain appraisals are more significant to the individual than others because they tend to reinforce the perception the individual has of himself. Dependency relationships may be more readily established with those whose appraisals tend to support the individual against feelings of insecurity and with those who reinforce feelings of ego integrity.

These meaningful relationships with others provide a person with nurturance and support, which are vital resources for coping with a wide variety of stressors. Social isolation, whatever the cause, denies a person the availability of social interactions and opportunities to develop meaningful relationships. Sudden or unexpected social isolation results in the loss of usual resource supports. With these lacking, a person is much more vulnerable to daily living stressors.

Loss, threatened loss, or feelings of inadequacy in a supportive relationship may also leave a person in a vulnerable position. Confrontation with a stressful situation, combined with a lack of situational support, may lead to a state of disequilibrium and possible crisis.

Appraisal of self varies across ages, sexes, and roles. The belief system that forms the basis of the self-concept and self-esteem develops out of experiences with significant others in a person's life. Although self-esteem is fairly static within a certain range, it does fluctuate according to internal and external environmental variables that impinge on it at a specific time and in a specific situation. To achieve and maintain a sense of value and self-worth, a person must feel loved by others and capable of achieving an ideal self, one that is strong, capable, good, and loving of others.

When self-esteem is low or when a situation is perceived as particularly threatening, the person is strongly in need of and seeks out others from whom positive reflective appraisals of self-worth and ability to achieve can be obtained. The lower the self-esteem or the greater the threat, the greater the need to seek situational supports. Conversely, a person avoids or withdraws from contacts with those he perceives as threatening to his self-esteem, whether the threat is real or imagined. Any potentially stressful situation can set off questions of self-doubt about how one is perceived by others, the kind of impression being made, and the real or imagined inadequacies that might be disclosed (Mechanic, 1974).

Success or failure of a coping behavior is always strongly influenced by the social context in which it occurs. The environmental variable most centrally identified is the person's significant others. From them, a person learns to seek responses such as advice and support in solving daily problems in living. Confidence in being liked and respected by these peers is based on past testing and reaffirmation of their expected supportive responses. Any perceived failure to obtain adequate support to meet psychosocial needs may provoke, or compound, a stressful situation. Negative support could be equally detrimental to a person's self-esteem.

Situational supports are those persons who are available in the environment and who can be depended on to help solve the problem. In the example, Mr. A talked to his physician and told him of his fear of having cancer. He asked about the tests that would be conducted and what would be done if the tests did reveal that he had cancer. He talked with his wife and children about the possibility of having cancer. He received reassurance from his family and his physician. In effect, he had strong support during this stressful event. Mr. B did not feel close enough to his physician to discuss his fears about the possibility of having cancer, and he did not talk to his family or friends about his symptoms. His denial made him isolate himself. He did not have anyone to turn to for help; therefore he felt overwhelmed and alone.

COPING MECHANISMS

Through the process of daily living, people learn to use many methods to cope with anxiety and reduce tension. Lifestyles are developed around patterns of response, which in turn are established to cope with stressful situations. These lifestyles are highly individual and quite necessary to protect and maintain equilibrium.

The early work of Cannon (1929, 1939) provided a basis for later systematic research on the effects of stress on the human organism. According to Cannon's "fight or flight" theory, reactions of acute anxiety, similar to those of fear, are vital to prepare the individual physiologically to meet any real or imagined threat to self. From his studies of homeostasis, Cannon described the mechanisms whereby human and other animal life systems maintain steady life states, with the goal always to return to such states whenever conditions force a temporary departure.

Over the years it has been unusual to find the term *coping* used interchangeably with such similar concepts as adaptation, defense, mastery, and adjustive reactions. Coping activities take a wide variety of forms, including all the diverse behaviors that people engage in to meet actual or anticipated challenges. In psychological stress theory, *coping* emphasizes various strategies used, consciously or unconsciously, to deal with stress and tensions arising from perceived threats to psychological integrity. It is not synonymous with mastery over problematical life situations; rather, it is the *process* of attempting to solve them (Lazarus, 1966).

Coleman (1950) defined *coping* as an adjustive reaction made in response to actual or imagined stress in order to maintain psychological integrity. Within this concept human beings are perceived as responding to stress by either attack, flight, or compromise reactions. These reactions become complicated by various ego-defense mechanisms whenever the stress becomes ego involved.

Attack reactions usually attempt to remove or overcome the obstacles seen as causing stress in life situations. They may be primarily constructive or destructive in nature. Flight, withdrawal, or fear reactions may be as simple as physically removing the threat from the environment (such as putting out a fire) or removing oneself from the threatening situation (running away from the fire area). They might also involve much more complex psychological maneuvering, depending on the perceived extent of the threat and the possibilities for escape.

Compromise or substitution reactions occur when either attack or flight from the threatening situation is thought to be impossible. This method is most commonly used to deal with problem solving and includes accepting substitute goals or changing internalized values and standards.

Masserman (1946) demonstrated that, in situations of extended frustration, individuals find it increasingly possible to compromise for substitute goals. This often involves use of *rationalization,* a defense mechanism whereby "half a loaf" does indeed soon appear to be "better than none."

Tension-reducing mechanisms can be overt or covert and can be consciously or unconsciously activated. They have been generally classified into such behavioral responses as aggression, regression, withdrawal, and repression. The selection of a response is based on tension-reducing actions that successfully relieved anxiety and reduced tension in similar situations in the past. Through repetition the response may pass from conscious awareness during its learning phase to a habitual level of reaction as a learned behavior. In many instances the individual may not be aware of *how,* let alone *why,* he reacts to stress in given situations. Except for having vague feelings of discomfort, the individual may not notice the rise and consequent reduction in tension. When a novel stress-producing event arises and learned coping mechanisms are ineffectual, discomfort is felt on a conscious level. The need to "do something" becomes the focus of activity, narrowing perception of all other life activities.

Normally, defense mechanisms are used constructively in the process of coping. This is particularly evident whenever there is danger of becoming psychologically overwhelmed. Almost all defense mechanisms are seen as important for survival.

· None is equated with a pathological condition unless it interferes with the process of coping, such as being used to deny, to falsify, or to distort perceptions of reality.

According to Bandura and others (1977), the strength of the individual's conviction in his own effectiveness in overcoming or mastering a problematical situation determines whether coping behavior is even attempted. People fear and avoid stressful, threatening situations that they believe exceed their ability to cope. They behave with assurance in those situations where they judge themselves able to manage, and they expect eventual success. It is the perceived ability to master that can influence the choice of coping behaviors, as well as the persistence used once one is chosen.

Available coping mechanisms are what people *usually* use when they have a problem. They may sit down and try to think it out or talk it out with a friend. Some cry it out or try to get rid of their feelings of anger and hostility by swearing, kicking a chair, or slamming doors. Others may get into verbal battles with friends. Some may react by temporarily withdrawing from the situation to reassess the problem. These are just a few of the many coping methods people use to relieve their tension and anxiety when faced with a problem. Each has been used at some time in the developmental past of the individual, has been found effective in maintaining emotional stability, and has become part of his life style in meeting and dealing with the stresses of daily living.

Continuing with the example, Mr. A made an appointment for the tests recommended by his physician. The tests were conducted; the diagnosis was negative for cancer. His tension and anxiety were reduced, equilibrium was restored, and he did not have a crisis. Mr. B withdrew; he had no coping skills. He did not make an appointment for the needed tests, no tests were made, and, as a result, he had no definitive diagnosis, and his tension and anxiety increased. Unable to solve the problem and to function, Mr. B went into crisis.

The balancing factors that affect equilibrium were demonstrated in Figure 3-2. Mr. A had a *realistic* perception of the event and returned to his original state of equilibrium. He did not have a crisis. Mr. B had a *distorted* perception of the event, used denial, remained in a state of disequilibrium, and went into crisis.

What if Mr. A's tests had been *positive* instead of negative? Figure 3-3 presents a new paradigm of comparative cases and introduces Mr. C, whose balancing factors are identical to Mr. A's with one exception: Mr. C had the diagnostic tests for cancer and his results were *positive*. His tension and anxiety increased, and he had surgery that successfully removed the cancer. He did not have a crisis. The balancing factor that made the difference was his realistic perception of the event. The relationship between the event and his feelings of stress was recognized. His problem solving was appropriately oriented toward reduced tension, and his stressful situation was resolved successfully.

It can be seen how the paradigm helps the therapist focus on the essential areas that have created the problem for Mr. B in Figure 3-2. The utilization of the paradigm can also be seen in the comparative cases in Figure 3-3. In subsequent chapters there will be actual case studies followed by a paradigm with a blank right column for the reader to complete using the format of those in this chapter.

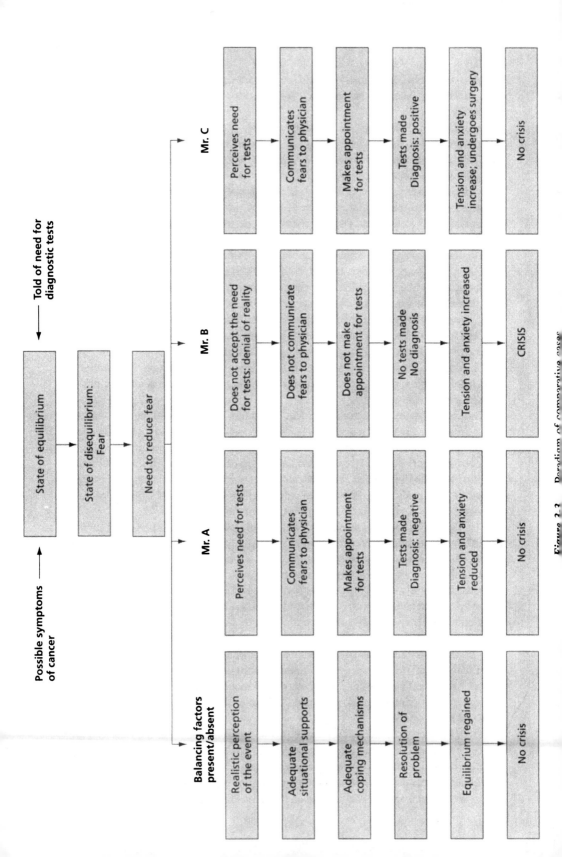

Figure 3.2 Paradigm of comparative cases.

The reader will be able to compare his paradigm with the completed one in Appendix D. This chapter should be used as a resource when the reader completes the blank paradigm. This exercise should enhance skills in resolving crises.

REFERENCES

Bandura A and others: Cognitive processes mediating behavioral change, *J Pers Soc Psychol* 35:125, 1977.

Black M: *Critical thinking: an introduction to logic and scientific method,* Englewood Cliffs, NJ, 1946, Prentice-Hall.

Cannon WB: *Bodily changes in pain, hunger, fear, and rage,* New York, 1929, D Appleton.

Cannon WB: *The wisdom of the body,* ed 2, New York, 1939, WW Norton.

Caplan G: *Principles of preventive psychiatry,* New York, 1964, Basic Books.

Coleman JC: *Abnormal psychology and modern life,* Chicago, 1950, Scott, Foresman.

Cropley A, Field T: Achievement in science and intellectual style, *J Appl Psychol* 53:132, 1969.

Dewey J: *How we think,* Boston, 1910, DC Heath.

Fortinash KM, Holoday-Worret PA: *Psychiatric-mental nursing,* St. Louis, 1996, Mosby.

Guilford JP: *The nature of human intelligence,* New York, 1967, McGraw-Hill.

Haber J and others: *Comprehensive psychiatric nursing,* ed 4, St. Louis, 1992, Mosby.

Inkeles A: Social structure and the socialization of competence, *Harv Ed Rev* 36:265, 1966.

Johnson DM: *The psychology of thought and judgment,* New York, 1955, Harper & Row.

Lazarus RS: *Psychological stress and the coping process,* New York, 1966, McGraw-Hill.

Lazarus RS and others: The psychology of coping: issues in research and assessment. In Coehlo GV and others, editors: *Coping and adaptation,* New York, 1974, Basic Books.

March JG, Simon HA: *Organizations,* New York, 1963, John Wiley & Sons.

Masserman JH: *Principles of dynamic psychology,* Philadelphia, 1946, WB Saunders.

Mechanic D: Social structure and personal adaptation: some neglected dimensions. In Coehlo GV and others, editors: *Coping and adaptation,* New York, 1974, Basic Books.

Merrifield PR and others: The role of intellectual factors in problem-solving, *Psychol Monogr* 76:1, 1962.

Morley WE, Messick JM, Aguilera DC: Crisis: paradigms of intervention, *J Psychiatr Nurs* 5:538, 1967.

Robinson L: Stress and anxiety, *Nurs Clin North Am* 25:(4)935, 1990.

ADDITIONAL READING

Altmaier EM: Linking stress experiences with coping resources and responses: comment on Catanzaro, Horaney, and Creasey (1995), Long and Schutz (1995), Heppner and others (1995), and Bowman and Stern (1995), *J Counseling Psychol* 42(3):304, 1995.

Antonietti A, Gioletta MA: Individual differences in analogical problem solving, *Pers Individual Differences* 18(5):611, 1995.

Bergan JR: Evolution of a problem-solving model of consultation, *J Educational Psychol Consultation,* 6(2):111, 1995.

D'Zurilla T, Chang EC: The relations between social problem solving and coping, *Cognitive Ther Res* 19(5):547, 1995.

D'Zurilla TJ, Maydeu-Olivares A: Conceptual and methodological issues in social problem-solving assessment, *Behav Ther* 26(3):409, 1995.

Davila J and others: Poor interpersonal problem-solving as a mechanism of stress generation in depression among adolescent women, *J Abnorm Psychol* 104(4):592, 1995.

Diehl M, Willis SL, Schaie K Warner: Everyday problem-solving in older adults: observational assessment and cognitive correlates, *Psychol Aging* 10(3):478, 1995.

Goodman SH, Gravitt GW, Kaslow NJ: Social problem solving: a moderator of the relation between negative life stress and depression symptoms in children, *J Abnorm Child Psychol* 23(4):473, 1995.

Littlepage GE and others: An input-process-output analysis of influence and performance in problem-solving groups, *J Pers Soc Psychol* 69(5):877, 1995.

Nickols FW: Reengineering the problem-solving process (finding better solutions), *Performance Improvement Q* 7(4):3, 1994.

Nystul MS: A problem-solving approach to counseling: integrating Adler's and Glasser's theories, *Elementary School Guidance Counseling* 29(4):297, 1995.

Powell CA: Cognitive hurdles in the use of decision support systems to enhance problem understanding. Special issue: decision making under conditions of conflict, *Group Decision Negotiation* 3(4):413, 1994.

Rooney EF and others: I can problem solve: an interpersonal cognitive problem-solving program, *J Sch Psychol* 31(2):335, 1993.

Sautter FJ, Heaney C, O'Neill P: A problem-solving approach to group psychotherapy in the inpatient milieu, *Hosp Community Psychiatry* 42:814, 1991.

Sternberg JA, Bry BH: Solution generation and family conflict over time in problem-solving therapy with families of adolescents: the impact of therapist behavior, *Child Fam Behav Ther* 16(4):1, 1994.

Stewart SL, Rubin KH: The social problem-solving skills of anxious-withdrawn children, *Dev Psychopathol* 7(2):323, 1995.

Tomic W: Training in inductive reasoning and problem solving, *Contemporary Educational Psychol* 20(4):483, 1995.

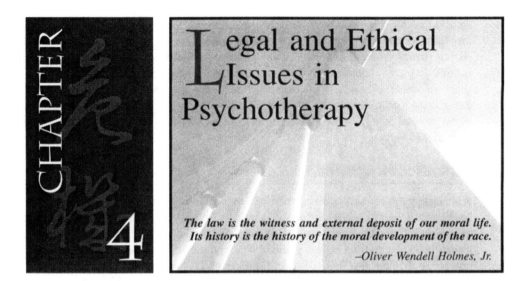

CHAPTER 4

Legal and Ethical Issues in Psychotherapy

The law is the witness and external deposit of our moral life.
Its history is the history of the moral development of the race.

—Oliver Wendell Holmes, Jr.

If mental health professionals are to be expected to know the relevant law, it is important to provide a definition of mental health law that sets boundaries for the field. Mental health law is defined as the field of inquiry that is concerned with the intersection of the law with the mental health status of individuals: the operation of the mental health system and of other public or private systems in their provision of services to individuals with mental illness (e.g., education and child welfare systems and private psychiatric hospitals) and the roles, functions, and responsibilities of mental health professionals, who need to be familiar with the law as it operates in each of these contexts (Sales and Shuman, 1994).

Law and mental health care are now so interconnected that it is difficult to remember a time when they did not interact. For better or for worse, mental health professionals are both directly and indirectly affected by the law. Their practice is directly controlled by laws that regulate such matters as licensure and certification, third-party reimbursement, and professional incorporation. The quality of their services is subject to review by courts in malpractice actions. Indirectly, the law affects mental health professionals through the increasingly frequent involvement of their patients in legal entanglements in which mental status issues are pivotal (e.g., divorce proceedings, child custody disputes, litigation over mental and emotional injury, and involuntary civil commitment) (Sales and Shuman, 1994).

Laws relating to the competence of a patient to consent to mental health services focus on the patient's mental status, as well as on the patient's legal right to consent or refuse to consent to these services. Laws focusing on the authority of the state to operate a public mental health system that includes both voluntary and involuntary services are an important component of mental health law and continue to raise significant legal controversy. Mental health professionals' roles, functions, and responsibilities are also an important component of mental health law because patients' rights (e.g., a right to confidentiality of information revealed during therapy) concomitantly involve mental health professionals' responsibilities (e.g., to maintain confidences) and because laws specify the involvement of mental health professionals in their administration (e.g., evaluating defendants who claim that they were insane when they committed the crime) and affect mental health professionals' practices (e.g., malpractice law) (Sales and Miller, 1993).

Therapeutic Jurisprudence

Although some of the key components of the stated definition of mental health law have been exemplified, there is still a need to clarify the goals of that law. The generation of mental health law scholarship and legal decision making that began in the early 1960s and has recently ended was dominated by a moral perspective that conceives of the law as advancing important values, often ensconced within normative constitutional principles (e.g., the right to an attorney, right to a hearing, and privilege against self-incrimination). The deontological (moral obligation) perspective contrasts with the utilitarian, consequentialist perspective that espouses legal rules as important to achieve some end. For example, from the moral perspective, recognition of the patient's right to a judicial hearing preceding involuntary civil commitment should turn on whether commitment is a deprivation of liberty under the Fourteenth Amendment to the U.S. Constitution; from the utilitarian perspective, the right to a hearing should turn on its consequences, such as the accuracy of the hearing's results or patient compliance with the hearing's decision (Tyler, 1993).

Although much of the previous generation of mental health law scholarship and decision making was deontologically oriented, there developed concurrently a significant body of literature that arose from a utilitarian perspective, with roots in the early twentieth-century Legal Realist movement (Monahan and Walker, 1990). It was concerned with empirically testing whether laws were achieving their explicit and implicit goals. This approach to law and behavioral and social science interactions asserts that almost all laws are based on behavioral, social, and economic assumptions, the validity of which can be empirically determined (Sales, 1993; Sales and Hafemeister, 1985; Shuman, 1993). When a federal court ordered that mentally ill persons who reside in state hospitals be accorded their right to privacy, utilitarian-driven research was able to demonstrate that the institutional changes aimed at fulfilling the court order did not achieve their goal (O'Reilly and Sales, 1986, 1987). The findings of this type of research can be used to argue for changes in the law or in its implementation.

Building on this empirical heritage, a new school of thought in mental health law has evolved called *therapeutic jurisprudence* (Wexler and McGrath, 1993). Rather than exclusively relying on moral-driven legal rules, this new movement looks to analyze the consequences of legal rules and incorporate this information in legal decision making. The overarching goal of therapeutic jurisprudence is that mental health law realize its potential to advance therapeutic outcomes, at least when it is possible to do so without offending other important considerations (e.g., constitutional principles). The notion is not that therapeutic considerations should trump all others but rather that legal decisions involving both mentally ill and non-mentally ill individuals take into account their therapeutic or antitherapeutic consequences (Sales and Shuman, 1994).

LIMITS OF THERAPEUTIC JURISPRUDENCE

Therapeutic jurisprudence seeks to advance therapeutic outcomes by encouraging legal decision makers to consider therapeutic consequences; it does not dictate the selection of legal rules that advance a therapeutic outcome. Therapeutic jurisprudence clarifies the decisional stakes but does not purport to resolve them; balancing of values is not given to a simplistic formulaic analysis. If empirical research reveals that recognition of a right to refuse treatment is antitherapeutic, a court or legislature may, because of this finding, refuse to recognize that right or, notwithstanding this finding, recognize that right based on a moral valuation of the importance of autonomy (Schopp, 1993).

When legal decision makers choose to recognize a rule that is therapeutic or refuse to recognize a rule that is antitherapeutic, the judgments of the legal system and the mental health system are congruent. The congruence in the judgments of the two disciplines can occur either because legal decision makers use a utilitarian approach that accepts the empirical outcomes as dispositive or because legal decision makers use a deontological approach that coincidentally concurs with the empirical research. The absence of congruence occurs when, for moral reasons, legal decision makers choose laws that are antitherapeutic or reject laws that are therapeutic. It is this absence of congruence that has understandably troubled mental health professionals, whose language and professional values do not share the legal system's deontological concerns. Mental health professionals should not expect from therapeutic jurisprudence a change in legal values or orientation that subordinates normative constitutional values to therapeutic values (Sales and Shuman, 1994).

Even when attempts are made to achieve appropriate communication, tensions can result when, in an attempt to avoid addressing various normative and policy questions head on, legal decision makers erroneously recast them as technical or scientific issues to be answered by "experts." Even when issues require scientific rather than normative judgments, legal reliance on mental health expertise is problematic because mental health professionals often lack available, relevant, empirically grounded knowledge or are willing to render opinions beyond their areas of expertise (Grisso, 1986).

There can be tensions and conflicts based on the different values, interests, and needs among key participants in law and mental health interactions (e.g., policymakers, institutions and organizations providing services, program administrators and providers, patients, family members, and researchers). What if a state institution wishes to deinstitutionalize a minor, but the parents do not wish to have the minor returned to the home (Frohboese and Sales, 1980)? And what if the mental health professional providing services objects to being used for social control purposes by prison administrators, for example, when they ask the mental health professional to conduct evaluations to determine for security purposes whether the patient is dangerous.

ALLIANCE OF MENTAL HEALTH LAW AND CARE

In what ways can a therapeutic jurisprudence perspective serve to form a working relationship between law and practice in mental health? Both mental health professionals and lawyers may find some benefit in a therapeutic jurisprudence perspective, since it explicates the tensions between law and mental health, even if it does not always resolve them. Therapeutic jurisprudence serves to remind lawyers and mental health professionals that therapeutic consequences of legal decision making need examination and helps to make the rationale for these decisions more explicit. As mental health professionals well know, talking openly about conflict has therapeutic value.

In those areas of the law in which false conflicts now exist between the goals of mental health law and mental health care, therapeutic jurisprudence may advance shared therapeutic goals previously frustrated by ill-conceived legal rules (Wexler and McGrath, 1993). Consider the matter of plea bargaining by sex offenders, in which the defendant is often allowed to plead no contest without acknowledging the specific acts of abuse, thereby avoiding the danger of losing at trial. If research reveals that not acknowledging one's guilt promotes the abuser's cognitive distortions and makes treatment less likely to succeed, changing the legal rule to require acknowledgment of the abusive acts in the plea may advance the shared therapeutic goal of reducing abuse.

Therapeutic jurisprudence reveals that legal rules often have explicit or implicit therapeutic agendas that sometimes get lost in the tumult of day-to-day application. By focusing its therapeutic lens, therapeutic jurisprudence assists the law to achieve its own therapeutic agenda. Malpractice laws, though often caught up in a political diatribe, are intended to improve the quality of care delivered by mental health professionals and to aid in making whole those injured by substandard care. By understanding the impact of these laws on providers and consumers of mental health services, legal decision makers can better develop rules that accomplish these goals (Shuman, 1993).

Perhaps most important, a therapeutic jurisprudence view of mental health law is needed, since the traditionally deontologically driven mental health law perspective has advanced about as far as it can go (Shuman, 1992). For example, the deontological approach has substantially succeeded in establishing for mentally ill persons who face involuntary hospitalization many of the constitutional rights applicable to persons facing criminal prosecution; the recognition of more rights is unlikely at this time given our national temperament (Perlin, 1994). Now, the accomplishments of this morally driven analysis need examination to determine how the imposition of the law affects the interests of its intended beneficiaries and whether therapeutic outcomes have been advanced. Such work should (1) use feedback from mental health professionals and patients, mental health scholars, and empirical research and (2) focus on the availability and delivery of effective systems of mental health services.

The next generation of mental health law and scholarship would ideally have the law participate with mental health professionals in making their services available to consumers who seek them. Without abandoning normative constitutional values, such efforts should include a plan for mental health services that incorporates the following*:

- Identification of those in need of services and those not being served and the reasons for discrepancy
- Development of a comprehensive plan of integrated services
- Provision of services with clear outcome goals
- Systematic collection of accurate information on delivery of services and operation of systems providing those services, and the reporting of those data in a meaningful fashion
- Use of these data to aid in decision making on mental health care
- Provision of appropriate services to ethnic minorities
- Provision of sufficient funding to support legally mandated entitlements

This shift in focus should help to reorient mental health law to the core concerns of those consumers who need and want mental health services and of mental health professionals who are devoted to providing those services. The plan would support a rational planning and implementation process by legal and public policymakers and administrators who are responsible for interpreting and implementing legal guidelines. In addition, it would facilitate effectiveness and efficiency in the delivery of mental health services (Sales and Shuman, 1994).

Legal and Ethical Defined

According to Black's (1990) Law Dictionary there are several definitions of the term *legal*. The following are included.

1. Conforming to the law; according to law; required or permitted by law; not forbidden or discountenanced by law; good and effectual in law; of or pertaining to the law; lawful
2. Proper or sufficient to be recognized by the law; cognizable in courts; competent or adequate to fulfill the requirements of the law
3. Cognizable in courts, as distinguished from courts of equity; construed or governed by the rules and principles of law, in contradistinction to rules of equity (with the merger in most states of law and equity courts, this distinction generally no longer exists)
4. Created by law

Now that *legal* is more than sufficiently defined, it is only equitable to examine the definition of *ethics* by Karasu (1984) as it pertains to psychotherapy. Karasu states that ethics is a code of morality of a person or group of people, such as a professional group. Morality is the distinction between right and wrong conduct. The mental health sciences, on the other hand, are concerned with the establishment of facts and knowledge. From one point of view, ethics and psychotherapy are two separate areas

---

* National Institute of Mental Health, 1991.

of study and are almost opposite in focus. Psychotherapy is concerned with describing human nature and validating its ideas about what "is true" about human nature. Ethics is concerned with prescribing actions, and forming judgments, based on "what ought to be."

Related to ethical concerns, Karasu states that society is now experiencing an "Age of Ethical Crisis" compared with our previous "Age of Anxiety." This age of ethical crisis has many components, including the following:

- Progressive loss of faith in traditional institutions
- Mistrust of authority
- Renewed concern for human rights
- Disappointment with mental health care sciences and their inability to solve the problems of society
- Anti-elitism, the professionals' misuse of power to maintain the unequal distribution of resources in society

Questions related to psychotherapeutic intervention may include the following:

- Whether traditional mental health care institutions meet the needs of the population
- Whether professionals, entrusted with responsibility for providing care, have the interests of patients in mind
- Whether the rights of patients are protected in mental health care

These questions should be expected. Traditionally, the treatment of the mentally ill has evoked an image of "controller" and "vulnerable victim" who cannot provide consent for treatment because of illness. Also, both psychiatry and philosophy, traditionally the fields in which ethical matters are extensively studied, have discussed ethical concerns in their fields in highly abstract terms and principles. The pressing everyday concerns of patients seem removed from these abstract discussions.

Therapists in psychotherapeutic practice were once removed and left undisturbed in the confines of their offices. Now therapists are questioned by other therapists about their methods, ideas of mental illness, and other topics. This is not surprising, since there are more than 250 models of psychotherapeutic methods, with the proponents of each claiming that theirs is the correct method of treatment. Therapists are also questioned by patients themselves, who are confused about methods of therapy, as well as about the power of the therapist. Increasingly, patients expect, and have the right to, treatment that is understandable. They demand that therapists be held accountable. Patients expect to have a part in planning and evaluating their treatment with the therapist. Therapists can no longer expect blind reverence.

Professionals in mental health care cannot ignore ethical questions. Historically, professionals have been relatively blind to ethical concerns. Ethical issues are often overlooked because they are not apparent. Therapists may ignore ethical topics because they, like all human beings, have internal forces that motivate people toward both right and wrong.

Legal Issues

The landmark case establishing that therapists have a legal duty to warn potential victims of their patient's behavior is *Tarasoff v. Regents of University of the*

California (1976). The details of the case are well known. In the course of therapy, Prosenjit Poddar threatened to kill Tatiana Tarasoff, a fellow student in his square dancing class. Poddar was held for observation and released. No one notified Tarasoff of the threat Poddar had made against her. Two months later, Poddar murdered Tarasoff, and the Tarasoff family filed suit. The court held that "when a therapist determines, or pursuant to the standards of his profession should determine, that his patient presents a serious danger of violence to another, he incurs an obligation to use reasonable care to protect the intended victim against such danger" (*Tarasoff v. Regents of the University of California,* 1976).

DUTY TO WARN

The *Tarasoff* case identifies three elements central to therapists' legal duty to warn. One element is the likelihood that patients will cause physical harm to themselves or others. The second is the special relationship between the therapist and client (patient) (Schopp and Quattrocchi, 1985); therapists have special duties to control the actions of their patients and to protect patients from harm. The third element is the existence of an identifiable victim (Lamb and others, 1989). That a special relationship exists between patients and therapists is rarely disputed. This relationship is referred to as *fiduciary,* that is, related to a confidence or trust. The other elements may be less clear.

Privilege, confidentiality, and disclosure statements. To understand the impact of the *Tarasoff* ruling, therapists must understand the relationships among privilege, confidentiality, and disclosure statements.

Confidentiality is the therapist's ethical obligation to safeguard patient communications (Ciccone, 1985; Stein, 1990). Confidentiality is a general ethical duty, a feature of many professional organizations' code of ethics, and a component of many licensing and certifying agencies' regulations.

Privilege constitutes the particular legal rights that state law gives to patients (Kamenar, 1984). According to Black's Law Dictionary (1990), privileged communications are "those statements made . . . within a protected relationship . . . which the law protects from forced disclosure." Privilege, notes Ciccone (1985), "is a legal right belonging to the patient" not the therapist. Gumper and Sprenkle (1981) define privilege as "a limited, legal right, usually vested in the patient rather than the professional, to refuse or prevent disclosure of therapy communications." In most states the therapist's general duty of confidentiality must give way when disclosure is necessary to warn or prevent harm to an identifiable third party.

A *disclosure statement* is a written document detailing the policy, negotiated between the therapist and patient, concerning therapist disclosure of patient information. Frequently, the document expresses the standard policy of the therapist and is signed by the patient. It should inform the patient of the therapist's legal responsibilities and indicate how the therapist will use discretion within the limits of the law.

The relationships among confidentiality, privilege, and a therapist's disclosure policy may be summarized as follows:
1. The duty to safeguard confidential information is a general duty of the therapist's. As a general duty, it may give way to other duties or rights.

Box 4-1

EXAMPLE OF A DISCLOSURE STATEMENT

Although the information you give me is generally confidential, there are important exceptions of which you should be aware.

1. If, in my opinion, therapy cannot profitably proceed unless something you tell me is shared with other family members, I may need to give you the choice of telling the other family members yourself, having me tell them, or terminating therapy.

2. I have an ethical obligation to balance the interests of all family members. If you inform me of a situation that, in my opinion, is blatantly harmful, unfair, or unethical, I may, at my discretion, give you the choice of correcting the situation when that is feasible, informing other family members of the situation, having me tell them, or terminating therapy.

3. If, in my opinion, you pose a danger to yourself or others, I have a legal duty to intervene. For example, if you threaten someone's life, I am legally obligated to warn that person, even if you terminate therapy. If you threaten to commit suicide, I may have to notify members of your family and/or the police or other agencies.

4. In general, I will follow, to the best of my ability, all state laws and regulations, as well as the policies and codes of ethics of (the relevant licensing agency and/or professional society). (Here, set forth a clear summary of the relevant laws, codes of ethics, and any other appropriate information.)

5. Please feel free to ask for clarification about any of these matters at any time, either now, during therapy, or before you tell me something I might have to share with others.

---

2. A privilege is a specific right owned by the patient; privilege exists when the law protects the patient's communication from disclosure.
3. A written disclosure statement indicates to the patient the policy the therapist will follow concerning disclosure of patient information and communications.

An example of the relevant section of a disclosure statement is provided in Box 4-1. Any sample statement, including this one, may be inconsistent with state law or licensing agency policy in some areas. Statement 3, in the example, may be invalid in Maryland. Therapists must review (or preferably, seek legal advice in reviewing) local requirements before adopting a disclosure statement.

In the oral discussion of the policy, the therapist should provide several examples of each sort of patient information that the therapist might need to disclose.

Legal and Ethical Consequences of Therapist Malfeasance

Therapist-patient sexual involvement is increasingly being acknowledged as the most common and prolific problem for all mental health professions. More disciplinary actions are taken for therapist-patient sexual involvement than for all other unethical discrepancies combined (Pope and Vetter, 1991). It should be noted here that the term *psychotherapist* refers to any licensed therapist, including psychologists; psychiatrists; psychiatric social workers; psychiatric nurses; and marriage, family, and child counselors. The harm that may occur for a patient has become the focus for clinical inquiry.

Psychotherapists can obtain information relevant to ethical practice and standards from a large number of sources. These sources include the American Psychiatric Association; the American Psychological Association; the Board of Behavioral Science Examiners; the formal ethics committees of all major health disciplines; and published research, clinical, and theoretical works (Conte and others, 1989). Most people are usually unfamiliar with the terms used in disciplinary actions, unless it is a highly publicized incident or involves high-profile and well-known or popular individuals. Therefore the Disciplinary Key in Appendix A defines important legal terms used in disciplinary actions.

Case law (*Roy v. Hartogs,* 1976; Kardener and others, 1976) has reflected agreement with the ethical codes of all mental professional societies that sexual relations between therapists and their patients are at least unethical and under rare circumstances criminal. Such relations represent a deviation from the standard of care and a basis for the finding of malpractice if the other requisite elements (e.g., damages) are present (Gutheil, 1982). Case law dramatically fails, however, to reflect the actual scope of the problem (Gartrell and others, 1986) because of the large number of episodes never reported at all and the substantial number of filed legal cases—probably the majority—that are settled out of court. False accusations represent a small fraction of total allegations: accusations are usually true. Therapists can benefit from being aware of certain repeating patterns of errors in therapy and countertransference responses. With this awareness, they can avert the serious outcomes that result from these errors, such as trauma to the patient and/or highly destructive litigation (Aguilera, 1996).

One caveat is necessary to prevent misunderstanding. To study the patient-therapist dyad in clinical terms is not the same as indicting the patient (blaming the victim) for some depravity, nor is it the same as explaining away (exoneration) or excusing the therapist's behavior. Sex with a patient is never acceptable.

Codes of ethics covering the practice of professional psychotherapists have been adopted by at least 18 of the 45 national members of the International Union of Psychological Science and by all but 1 of the 16 members of the European Federation of Professional Psychologists' Associations. These codes cover basic values such as the protection and promotion of human dignity and welfare, assumption of responsibility for professional action, restriction of practice to areas of competence, confidentiality, and honesty in all matters. In most countries the codes are implemented by ethics committees and usually enforced by appropriate sanctions (Pope and Vetter, 1991).

Differences among nations in the definition of those qualified to provide psychological services make the estimation of human resources in psychotherapy a very uncertain endeavor. However, certain broad differences in the employment patterns of psychological health service providers can be noted among the industrialized countries of the West, the socialist countries, the dynamically developing countries, and the less developed countries.

In the United States, for which data are most readily available, 31% of doctoral-level psychotherapists work full time in independent practice, followed by

20% in hospitals, and 14% in clinics. Another 19% work in academic or educational settings, with the remainder distributed among business, government, and other human service settings (Stapp and Fulcher, 1983). Counseling therapists are found in the same general fields but in greater concentration in academic settings (40%), where they counsel students in addition to teaching and performing research.

Throughout Europe the great majority of professional psychotherapists are salaried employees of public agencies. Private practice is practically nonexistent in the socialist countries and fairly rare in many countries of the industrialized West (e.g., the United Kingdom), where high-quality public health and welfare services may be available. There are wide variations in the specialties in which psychotherapists may be employed.

When examining urban areas and rural towns throughout the world, it is important to keep in mind the heterogeneity of communities. Many cities require people of different backgrounds to live close together and independently. This heterogeneity may involve language, race, religion, social class, nationality, or a preferred lifestyle. Stress is sometimes associated with this diversity and with pressures and conflicts that may accompany acculturation. Factors such as national policies that force assimilation or historical and economic factors that generate intergroup conflict are predictive of high stress, and their absence is predictive of low stress (Berry and others, 1984). The weakening of traditional support systems makes such stress especially difficult to handle.

Increases in the rates of divorce, child abuse, crime, and mental illness within urban centers of the world are requiring more services from psychotherapists than has been typical in the past. To be effective such services must take the cultural background of the patient into account. Psychotherapists who are competent to deal with cross-cultural issues in health and human development have developed techniques for measuring and reducing personal alienation, for adapting psychotherapy to local conditions, and for improving the mental health of diverse populations (Triandis and Draguns, 1980).

Crisis intervention is a relatively recent "frontline" mental health specialty with obvious implications for physical health. Experience acquired in providing assistance to ordinary well-functioning individuals on occasions of intense stress (e.g., rape, assault, combat shock or panic, and transitory episodes of depression related to changes in personal relationships or circumstances of employment) has enabled psychotherapists to become involved in large-scale efforts to lessen the harmful effects of human-created and natural disasters.

Therapist-patient sexual involvement confronts us with a pressing problem that has far-reaching implications for the professions. It may also involve increased understanding of the sexualization of teaching relationships and the ways in which training programs provide education and modeling regarding sexual issues (Pope and Vetter, 1991).

SEXUAL HARASSMENT

The effect of role modeling on the development of professional ethics and behavior cannot be dismissed (Pope, Levenson, and Schover, 1980). According to Sandler (1990),

One of the most striking aspects of sexual harassment is that the victim feels quite powerless in the situation. Students rely on the professors not only for grades but for future recommendations, as well as academic and career opportunities. In a very real sense, a student's life chances are at stake.

It is rare, then, that a victim exhibits the courage and willingness to take the risk to confront the harasser and, once the complaint process is complete, to share the experience with others.

The *Thomas-Hill* case (October 1991) attracted the attention not only of the nation but also of the world. The media had a proverbial field day. The results are still being debated today. In Las Vegas, September 1991, the "Tailhook" reunion for Navy pilots was another graphic example of blatant sexual harassment.

Institutional administrators, managers, and supervisors attempting to formulate strategies for the prevention and remediation of sexual harassment may feel caught in a similar muddle: How are we to prevent what we cannot clearly define? How can we be responsible for that which we did not know was occurring? The confusion is due to the range of possible behaviors and judicial findings of sexual harassment. Determinations as to whether sexual harassment has taken place necessarily proceed on a case-by-case basis as courts and enforcement agencies consider circumstances ranging from the outright demand for sexual favors at one extreme to complaints about sexual innuendos at the other. Interpretation of such behavior is closely related to context (Padgitt and Padgitt, 1986); the finding in one case is unlikely to predict the finding in another. In addition, the fact that institutions and supervisors can be liable for sexual harassment that "they anticipated or reasonably should have anticipated" (Wetherfield, 1990) is not reassuring.

Although an honest case can be made for the difficulty of developing an absolute definition of sexual harassment (Walker and Woolsey, 1985), neglecting to formulate institutional policy is hazardous, and disciplinary employment decisions made without pertinent written policy may not be defensible. Apart from concern about legal liability, schools and human service providers should be as eager as they are obligated to provide working and learning environments that are not hostile to students and employees. Resorting to definitional difficulties to explain the absence of policies and procedures concerning sexual harassment neither protects nor empowers its potential victims, and the institutional climate may be expected to remain unchanged.

Blanshan (1982) defined *sexual harassment* as "the unwanted imposition of sexual requirements in the context of a relationship of unequal power." A wide range of behaviors constitutes sexual harassment, including verbal (jokes, innuendos, and catcalls), nonverbal (winks, leers, and the presence of visual sexual materials), and physical (patting, stroking, and blocking one's path). In *Sexual Harassment* (1978), the Project on the Status and Education of Women described and elaborated on the varieties of such behavior, and the 1980 guidelines of the U.S. Equal Employment Opportunity Commission (EEOC) include representative examples. What all working definitions have in common is the emphasis in such behavior on the sex of the recipient and the unwelcomeness of the attention (Cammaert, 1985).

Specifically, the guideline definition of the EEOC (1980) is as follows.

Unwelcome sexual advances, requests for sexual favors, and other verbal or physical conduct of a sexual nature constitute sexual harassment when one or more of the following occur.

1. Submission to such conduct is made either explicitly a term or condition of employment.
2. Submission to or rejection of such conduct by an individual is used as a basis for employment decisions affecting such individuals.
3. Such conduct has the purpose or effect of unreasonably interfering with an individual's work performance or of creating an intimidating, hostile, or offensive working environment.

Definitions 1 and 2 are quid pro quo harassment; definition 3 is hostile environment harassment.

In 1986 the U.S. Supreme Court adopted the EEOC's definition and found sexual harassment to be a violation of the victim's civil rights as protected by Title VII of the 1964 Civil Rights Act (*Meritor Savings Bank v. Vinson;* Aguilera, 1996). The Court also alerted employers (and, by extension, educational institutions) to their potential liability not only for quid pro quo harassment in the workplace but also for acts of hostile environment harassment under certain circumstances. This finding and related decisions applying it in lower courts have stimulated growing numbers of employers and educational institutions to formulate sexual harassment policies and to establish pertinent grievance procedures.

Thoughtfully written sexual harassment policies and procedures, widely disseminated, arguably constitute the best legal protection that may be available and may reasonably be expected to provide a preventive influence as well. Organizations lacking such policies should be guided by their affirmative action personnel and legal counsels in formulating appropriate statements.

An adequate sexual harassment policy includes all relevant conduct of a sexual or gender-based nature that may be visited on an unwilling person. The examples that come most readily to mind, especially with respect to quid pro quo harassment, tend to involve persons of unequal status (e.g., the harassment of students by faculty or workers by their supervisors). It is also important, however, to anticipate those relationships in which the inequality of power is less apparent. Although less obvious, the power of graduate teaching assistants over their students, for example, should be considered in the formulation of an adequate policy.

It is also important to be aware of the growing attention being paid to peer harassment. As with sexual harassment in general, such conduct may range from innuendo and jokes to sexual assault (Project on the Status of Women, 1988). Peer harassment appears to be widespread and can have devastating effects. An adequate policy statement identifies it as a form of prohibited activity along with those previously cited (Aguilera, 1996).

Students or others wishing to file a complaint of sexual harassment need easy access to nonthreatening grievance procedures that should be described as part of the policy statement. The procedures may be modeled on other grievance procedures within the organization but should include the proviso that grievants may avoid presenting the complaint to their immediate supervisors, who may be the source of the problem (Van Tol, 1986).

Wagner (1990) suggested that a comprehensive policy and effective procedures feature "informal channels that include mediation, and formal avenues which are impartial and confidential, and protect the complainant and witnesses against retaliation." Most organizations have a designated person (or persons), such as an equal opportunity or affirmative action officer, who acts in an official capacity to receive and investigate formal complaints. This individual (or individuals) should be specified in the policy.

With respect to informal channels, victims may be encouraged to report the incident to another appropriate individual, such as a personnel officer, division supervisor, department chair or dean, faculty member, health service personnel, or counselor. For such informal means of resolution to work, persons likely to receive these complaints must be provided with guidelines for resolving them and with easy access to consultation with the organization's equal opportunity or affirmative action officer.

Persons complaining of sexual harassment are entitled to a prompt and impartial investigation, which should both protect the complainant from retaliation and observe the due process rights of the alleged harasser.

Case Study   *Therapist-Patient Involvement*

Jennine stated on her form at the Crisis Clinic that she would like to see a woman therapist. One was available, so the therapist went out, met Jennine, and took her to her office. Jennine stated that she was 32 years old, lived alone, was originally from another state, and was considering getting engaged to Neil. She further stated that she was a school teacher at a local middle school and that she truly enjoyed her work.

The therapist asked her why she had come to the clinic. Jennine hesitated briefly and then explained why she needed help. She had been in psychotherapy for 18 months with a licensed social worker named Jim. Jim was in his early 40s, married, with two children. Jennine said that she was very lonely at the time when she entered therapy with Jim. She explained that she had been in the state approximately 6 weeks and was having difficulty meeting and making new friends. All of the other teachers knew each other well and most were considerably older than she. She felt that something must be "wrong" with her, because she was encountering so much trouble getting to know people—a problem, she said, that she never had before.

One night, while looking through the telephone directory, she found herself looking at the advertising section for psychotherapists. Jim's ad caught her attention because he not only had a large ad, but he also had his picture in it. Jennine said that he had a "kind face and was smiling slightly." On impulse she called his telephone number, expecting to get a "machine" or even an exchange. Jim answered the telephone himself. Jennine said that he had a "nice, soothing voice." She explained that she had not expected to have him answer the telephone. He laughed and said, "I always answer. If someone has a problem, they don't want to talk to an anonymous machine. Why did you call? You must have a problem. What is your first name?"

Jennine said he sounded so nice that she began talking to him. She told Jim "my entire life history. We must have talked for at least 20 minutes. He told me that it was more difficult to meet new people in a large city and that it would take a little while to adjust." He asked her if she felt she needed psychotherapy and she had answered, "I certainly don't think it could hurt—and I would have someone to talk to." She asked if he could see her in therapy, and he said that he had an opening at 4:00 PM on Thursday (in 2 days). Jennine asked him to book her for the appointment and said she would bring her insurance forms.

Jennine began seeing Jim in therapy every Thursday at 4:00 PM. She thought he was a competent therapist because she always felt "so good" after she left their sessions. After their first five sessions, Jim walked her to the door and handed her a card for her next appointment. Jennine said she laughed and said that she really didn't need an appointment card because she always looked forward to seeing him on Thursdays. Jim smiled, took her in his arms and kissed her lightly on the lips. She felt herself responding to his kiss. He kissed her again and said that he, too, "looked forward to seeing her."

Jennine left his office in a daze. She couldn't believe that he had kissed her and that she had responded so strongly. She said that she knew he was married and had children—there was a picture of them on his desk. He told her that it was a picture of his wife and children—he certainly did not try to hide them.

On her next appointment, the minute she walked into his office he took her in his arms and kissed her. He told her that since the last time he had seen her she was all he could think about. He said that he wanted to make love to her and began to unbutton her blouse. She admitted that she responded by taking off his tie and unbuttoning his shirt. In a few minutes they were on his couch making love. It was "wonderful," he was gentle, very considerate of her needs, and, in essence, a wonderful lover. They had remained lovers for approximately the entire time she was in therapy. She said, bitterly, "If you can call what we were doing therapy!"

Jennine went on to explain that 3 months ago he started canceling their appointments, saying, for example, that he had to attend a meeting or a lecture. Then she went to an appointment, and he told her that he wouldn't be able to make any more appointments with her because his wife had just had a baby, and he wanted to spend as much time as possible with her and his new daughter.

"I sat there and felt like a fool! I had some fantasy in my mind that one day he would divorce his wife, and we would get married!" She said she stood up and told him, "I guess I won't be needing any more therapy," and walked out. Jim didn't say a word.

Jennine went to her apartment and cried for hours, then began to get angry. She wanted to hurt him, too, but she didn't want to call his wife. "I am not *that* vindictive," she stated. "Besides, it was as much my fault as his."

Three weeks later one of the teachers at school introduced Jennine to her younger brother, Neil, who was in the process of moving to their city. Neil had accepted a great job as corporate attorney for a well-known company—something that he had wanted ever since he left law school. He asked Jennine to have dinner with him to help him celebrate. She declined, saying that she had already made plans for the evening. She admitted that she thought Neil was very nice looking and seemed friendly. She said she felt "something" about Neil she couldn't describe, but if she could, she would have to say that she felt that she had fallen in love "at first sight." Jennine told Neil to call her when he got settled and gave him her telephone number. She said she did not want to get hurt again and was afraid that she was responding "on the rebound" from Jim.

The therapist asked if Jennine felt that she had been in love with Jim. She was quiet for a few moments and then answered, "No, I think I was lonely and needed someone, and he happened to be the one I met at that time."

The therapist asked Jennine why she had come to the Crisis Clinic that day. Jennine responded saying that Neil had called her once he was settled in his new job and town house, and they had gone to dinner. She said they seemed to have much in common. They were both from small Midwestern towns, both came from large close-knit families. She related that after dinner they went back to her apartment and sat up drinking coffee and talking until 4:00 AM. She said that she felt as if she had known him forever. He had a marvelous sense of humor, and he didn't try to make a "pass" at her. As Neil was leaving, he asked her out the next day to a picnic. She agreed. "Jennine, do you believe in love at first sight?" he asked. "Maybe, I don't know," she responded. "I do. . . I knew that I loved you the day we met," confessed Neil. "Don't worry, I'll give you all the time you need to get to know me . . . but I think you feel the same."

They continued seeing each other almost every day, at the very least talking to each other every evening. Jennine said she knew she had fallen in love with him, but she felt she had to tell him about Jim, and she was very concerned about how he would react. Finally, she got up her courage and told Neil about Jim. Neil was furious; however, not at her, as she had expected. He was furious at Jim for having taken advantage of her. Speaking as an attorney, he told Jennine that what Jim had done was not only unethical but illegal. He took money from her insurance company under false pretenses. Neil told Jennine that she must report him to his licensing board and to the ethics committee. She said she wanted only to forget about Jim and didn't want to cause any trouble. Neil told her that she must think of others who would be seeing Jim "in therapy"—that he should be disciplined for what had occurred between them.

Her reason for coming to the Crisis Clinic was to verify that what Neil had told her was the correct thing to do. She was reassured by the therapist that what Neil had told her was indeed accurate and that Jim should be reported to the appropriate board and ethics committee.

Jennine was apparently relieved to hear that Neil had been correct in his advice. She told the therapist that she understood she could have six therapy sessions. "Is that correct?" she asked. "Yes, Jennine, you have five more sessions. Do you want to keep them?" Jennine smiled and said very firmly, "Yes, very much. It helps to have another woman to talk to . . . and I will need your support after Neil reports Jim! I will never go to a male therapist again."

"And what else won't you do?" asked the therapist.

"I won't see any professionals without first checking them out with their professional boards!"

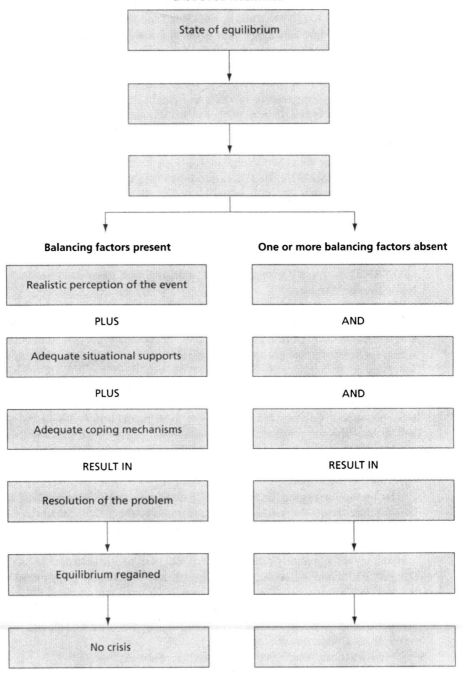

CASE STUDY: JENNINE

State of equilibrium

Balancing factors present

Realistic perception of the event

PLUS

Adequate situational supports

PLUS

Adequate coping mechanisms

RESULT IN

Resolution of the problem

Equilibrium regained

No crisis

One or more balancing factors absent

AND

AND

RESULT IN

Figure 4-1

Jennine was seen for the full five sessions. The ethics committee found that there had been two prior complaints against Jim. Jim's disposition was *license revoked, effective* _____, and he was placed on probation for 2 years.

Jennine and Neil became engaged to be married. She brought Neil to meet the therapist, and Neil expressed his gratitude for the help and support that the therapist gave to Jennine through the hearing. The therapist wished them well and a long and happy life together.

The conscience does make cowards of us all.

–William Shakespeare

Complete the paradigm in Figure 4-1 for this case study, then compare it with the completed one in Appendix D. Refer to the paradigms in Chapter 3 as needed.

REFERENCES

Aguilera BA, Esq., Vice President and General Counsel, The Mirage, Las Vegas, Personal communication, September 1996.

Berry JW and others: Acculturation and mental health. In Dasen PR, Berry JW, Sartorius NS, editors: *Health and cross cultural psychology,* London, 1984, Sage.

Black's Law Dictionary, St. Paul, Minn, 1990, West.

Blanshan S: Activism, research and policy: sexual harassment, *J NAWDAC* 46:16, 1982.

Cammaert L: How widespread is sexual harassment on campus? *Int J Women's Stud* 8:388, 1985.

Ciccone JR: Privilege and confidentiality: psychiatric and legal considerations, *Psychiatr Med* 2(3):272, 1985.

Conte HR and others: Ethics in the practice of psychotherapy: a survey, *Am J Psychother* 43:32, 1989.

Equal Employment Opportunity Commission: *Sexual harassment guidelines 29CFR,* chap XIV, part 1604.11(a), Washington, DC, 1980, U.S. Government Printing Office.

Frohboese RF, Sales BD: Parental opposition to deinstitutionalization: a challenge in need of attention and resolution, *Law Hum Behav* 4:1, 1980.

Gartrell N and others: Psychiatrist-patient contact: results of a national survey, *Am J Psychiatry* 143:1126, 1986.

Grisso T: *Evaluating competencies: forensic assessments and instruments,* New York, 1986, Plenum Press.

Gumper LL, Sprenkle DH: Privileged communication in therapy: special problems for the family and couples therapist, *Fam Process* 20:1123, 1981.

Gutheil TG, Appelbaum PS: *Clinical handbook of psychiatry and law,* New York, 1982, McGraw-Hill.

Holmes, OW Jr: Speech, Boston, January 8, 1897.

Karasu T: Ethical Aspects of Psychotherapy. In Bloch S, Chodoff P, editors: *Professional ethics,* Oxford, 1984, Oxford University Press.

Kamenar PD: Psychiatrists' duty to warn of a dangerous patient: a survey of the law, *Behav Sci Law* 2(3):259, 1984.

Kardener SH, Fuller M, Mensh IN: Characteristics of "erotic" practitioners, *Am J Psychiatry* 133:1324, 1976.

Lamb DH and others: Applying Tarasoff to AIDS-related psychotherapy issues, *Prof Psychol Res Pract* 20(1):37, 1989.

Monahan J, Walker L: *Social science in law: cases and materials,* Westbury, NY, 1990, Foundation Press.

National Institute of Mental Health: *Caring for people with severe mental disorders: a national plan of research to improve services* (DHHS Pub No. [ADM]91-1762), Washington, DC, 1991, U.S. Government Printing Office.

O'Reilly J, Sales B: Setting physical standards for mental hospitals: to whom should the courts listen? *Int J Law Psychiatry* 8:301, 1986.

O'Reilly J, Sales B: Privacy for the institutionalized mentally ill: are court-ordered standards effective? *Law Hum Behav* II, p 41, 1987.

Padgitt S, Padgitt J: Cognitive structure of sexual harassment: implications for university policy, *J College Students Personnel* 27:34, 1986.

Perlin ML: Law and the delivery of mental health services in the community, *Am J Orthopsychiatry* 64:194, 1994.

Pope K, Levenson H, Schover L: Sexual intimacy training: results and implications of a national survey, *Am Psychologist* 34:682, 1980.

Pope KS, Vetter VA: Prior therapist-patient sexual involvement among patients seen by psychologists, *Psychother* 28:429, 1991.

Project on the Status and Education of Women: *Sexual harassment: a hidden issue,* Washington, DC, 1978, Association of American Colleges.

Project on the Status of Women: *Peer harassment: hassles for women on campus,* Washington, DC, 1988, Association of American Colleges.

Roy v. Hartogs, 366 NYS 2d297 (Civ Ct, NY, 1975): *affirmed on condition of remittitur,* 381 NYS 2d587 (Sup Ct, NY, 1976).

Sales BD, Hafemeister T: Law and psychology. In Altmaier E, Meyer M, editors: *Applied specialties in psychology,* Boston, 1985, Random House.

Sales BD, Miller MO: *Law and mental health professionals* [series], Washington, DC, 1993, American Psychological Association.

Sales BD, Shuman DW: Mental health law and mental health care: introduction, *Am J Orthopsychiatry* 64(2):172, 1994.

Sandler BR: Sexual harassment: a new issue for institutions, *Initiatives* 52:5, 1990.

Schopp RF: Therapeutic jurisprudence and conflicts among values in mental health law, *Behav Sciences Law* 11:31, 1993.

Schopp RF, Quattrocchi MR: Tarasoff, the doctrine of special relationships, and the psychotherapist's duty to warn, *J Psychiatry Law* 12(1):13, 1985.

Shuman DW: Making the world a better place through tort law: through the therapeutic looking glass, *NY Law Sch J Hum Rights* 10:739, 1993.

Shuman DW: Therapeutic jurisprudence and tort law: a limited subjective standard of care, *South Methodist University Law Rev* 46:409, 1992.

Stapp J, Fulcher R: The employment of APA members: 1982, *Am Psychol* 38:1298, 1983.

Stein RH: *Ethical issues in counseling,* Buffalo, NY, 1990, Prometheus.

Tarasoff v. Regents of the University of California, 529 P 2d553 (Cal 1974) and 551 P 2d553 (Cal 1976).

Triandis HC, Draguns J, editors: *Handbook of cross-cultural psychology,* Boston, 1980, Allyn & Bacon.

Tyler TR: The psychological consequences of judicial procedures: implications for civil commitment hearings, *South Methodist University Law Rev* 46:433, 1993.

Van Tol J, editor: *Sexual harassment on campus: a legal compendium,* 1986, American Council on Education, p 123, 1986, National Association of College and University Attorneys.

Wagner KC: Programs that work: prevention and intervention: developing campus policy procedures, *Initiatives* 52:37, 1990.

Walker GE, Woolsey L: Sexual harassment: ethical research and clinical implications in the academic setting, *Int J Women's Stud* 8:424, 1985.

Wetherfield A: Sexual harassment: the current state of the law governing educational institutions, *Initiatives* 52:23, 1990.

Wexler HK, McGrath E: Family member stress reactions to military involvement separation, *Psychother* 28:515, 1993.

ADDITIONAL READING

Bulletin of the World Health Organization, vol 65, Geneva, 1987, The Organization.

Ethics Committee of the American Psychological Association: Report of the ethics committee: 1986, *Am Psychol* 42:730, 1987.

LaFond JQ: Law and the delivery of involuntary mental health services, *Am J Orthopsychiatry* 64(2):409, 1994.

Schlossberger E, Stokes L: HIV and family therapists' duty to warn: a legal and ethical analysis: *J Marital Fam Ther,* vol 22, No. 1, p 27, 1996.

Weiner BA, Wettstein RM: *Legal issues in mental health care,* New York, 1993, Plenum Press.

Weiner MF: Privilege: a comparative study, *J Psychiatry Law* 12:373, 1989.

Williams MH: Therapist-patient sex as sex abuse: six scientific professional and practice dilemmas in addressing victimization and rehabilitation: comment, *Prof Psychol Res Pract* 21:420, 1990.

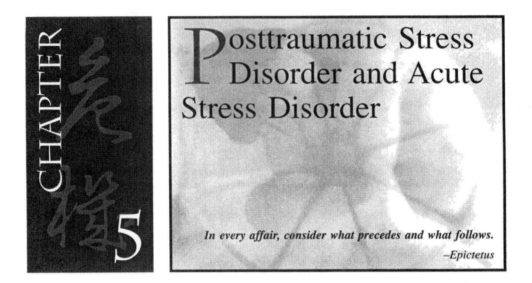

CHAPTER 5

Posttraumatic Stress Disorder and Acute Stress Disorder

In every affair, consider what precedes and what follows.

–Epictetus

The American Psychiatric Association criteria from the Diagnostic and Statistical Manual of Mental Disorders (DSM—IV) (1994) has placed *posttraumatic stress disorder* and *acute stress disorder* into two separate categories. Table 5-1 compares these two disorders. A brief review of the major differences is presented in this chapter. The terms applicable to the mental status examination are defined in Appendix B.

Posttraumatic Stress Disorder

Posttraumatic stress disorder (309.81) (PTSD) has been called *shell shock, battle fatigue, accident neurosis,* and *post rape syndrome.* It has often been misunderstood or misdiagnosed, even though the disorder has very specific symptoms that form a definite psychological syndrome.

PTSD affects hundreds of thousands of people who have been exposed to violent events such as rape, domestic violence, child abuse, war, accidents, natural disasters, and political torture. Psychiatrists estimate that from 1% to 3% of the population have clinically diagnosable PTSD. More still show some symptoms of the disorder. It was once thought to be a disorder of war veterans who had been involved in heavy combat, although research shows that PTSD can result from many types of trauma, particularly those that include a threat to life. PTSD can affect both females and males (Bile, 1993; Symes, 1995).

Not all individuals who experience PTSD require treatment. Some will recover with the help of strong situational supports such as their family, friends, or a pastor, priest, or rabbi. Many do require professional help to successfully recover from the psychological damage that can result from experiencing, witnessing, or participating in an overwhelming traumatic event.

Table 5-1   Comparison of Posttraumatic Stress Disorder and Acute Stress Disorder

	PTSD	ASD
NATURE OF THE TRAUMA		
Individual experienced, witnessed, or was confronted with an event that involved actual or threatened death or serious injury or a threat to the physical integrity of self or others	Yes	Yes
Individual's response involved intense feelings of fear, horror, or helplessness	Yes	Yes
SYMPTOM CRITERIA		
Persistent reexperiencing of the trauma	Yes	Yes
Avoidance of reminders of the trauma	Yes	Yes
Physical symptoms of hyperarousal	Yes	Yes
Symptoms of dissociation during or immediately after the trauma	No	Yes
Clinically significant distress	Yes	Yes
TIME REQUIREMENTS		
Duration of symptoms	1 Month	2 Days to 4 weeks
Onset of symptoms in relation to trauma	Any time after trauma	Within 2 days to 4 weeks

SYMPTOMS OF PTSD

The symptoms of PTSD may initially seem to be part of a normal response to an overwhelming experience. Only if those symptoms persist beyond 3 months are they considered part of the disorder. Sometimes the disorder surfaces months or even years later.

Although PTSD is based primarily on studies of trauma in adults, it also occurs in children. It is known that traumatic occurrences (e.g., sexual or physical abuse, loss of parents, or the disaster of war) often have a profound effect on the lives of children. In addition to PTSD symptoms, children may develop learning disabilities and problems with attention and memory. They may become anxious or cling and may also abuse themselves or others.

Individuals suffering from PTSD often have an episode when the traumatic event "intrudes" into their current life. This can happen in sudden, vivid memories that are accompanied by painful emotions. Sometimes the trauma is "reexperienced." This is called a *flashback*, a recollection that is so strong that the individual thinks he is actually experiencing the trauma again or seeing it unfold before his eyes. In traumatized children this reliving of the trauma often occurs in the form of repetitive play. At times the reexperiencing occurs in nightmares. In young children, distressing dreams of the traumatic event may evolve into generalized nightmares of monsters, of rescuing others, or of threats to self or others.

The reexperiencing may come as a sudden, painful onslaught of emotion, seemingly without cause. These emotions are often of grief that bring tears, fear, or anger. Individuals say these emotional experiences occur repeatedly, much like memories or dreams about the traumatic event.

Another set of symptoms involves what is called *avoidance phenomena*. This affects the individual's relationships with others because he often avoids close emotional ties with family, colleagues, and friends. The person feels numb, has diminished emotions, and can complete only routine, mechanical activities. When the symptoms of "reexperiencing" occur, people seem to spend their energies on suppressing that flood of emotion. Often, they are incapable of mustering the necessary energy to respond appropriately to their environment; individuals who suffer posttraumatic stress disorder say frequently that they can't feel emotions, especially toward those to whom they are the closest. As the avoidance continues, the individual seems bored, cold, or preoccupied. Family members often feel rebuffed by the person because he lacks affection and acts mechanically (Blake, Cook, and Keane, 1992).

Emotional numbness and diminished interest in significant activities may be difficult concepts to explain to a therapist. This is especially true for children. For this reason the reports of family members, friends, parents, teachers, and other observers are particularly important. The person with PTSD also avoids situations that are reminders of the traumatic event because the symptoms may worsen when a situation or activity occurs that reminds them of the original trauma. An individual who survived a prisoner-of-war camp might overreact to seeing people wearing uniforms. Over time, people can become so fearful of particular situations that their daily lives are ruled by their attempts to avoid them.

Many war veterans, for example, avoid accepting responsibility for others because they think they failed in ensuring the safety of people who did not survive the trauma. Some people also feel guilty because they survived a disaster while others— particularly friends or family—did not. In combat veterans or with survivors of civilian disasters, this guilt may be manifested if they witnessed or participated in behavior that was necessary to survival but unacceptable to society. Such guilt can deepen depression as the person begins to look on himself as unworthy, a failure, a person who violated his predisaster values. Children suffering from PTSD may show a marked change in orientation toward the future. A child, for example, may not expect to marry or to have a career. He may exhibit "omen formation," the belief in an ability to predict future untoward events.

The PTSD patient's inability to work out grief and anger over injury or loss during the traumatic event means the trauma will continue to control his behavior without his being aware of it. Depression is a common product of this inability to resolve painful feelings (Symes, 1995).

PTSD can cause those who suffer with it to act as if they are still threatened by the trauma that caused their illness. Individuals with PTSD may become irritable, have trouble concentrating or remembering current information, and may develop insomnia. Because of their chronic hyperarousal, many people with PTSD have poor work records, trouble with their bosses, and poor relationships with their family and friends (Henry, 1993).

The persistence of a biological alarm reaction is expressed in startle reactions. War veterans may revert to their war behavior, such as diving for cover when they hear a car backfire or a string of firecrackers exploding. At times those with PTSD suffer panic attacks, whose symptoms include extreme fear resembling that which they felt during the trauma. Many traumatized children and adults may have physical symptoms, such as stomachaches and headaches, in addition to symptoms of increased arousal (Herman, 1992).

PTSD can be defined as *acute* if symptoms have occurred from between 1 and 3 months and *chronic* if the symptoms have persisted for at least 3 months or more. When the onset of symptoms is more than 6 months after the traumatic event, the disorder can be further defined as *delayed onset* (APA, 1994).

SPECIAL NEEDS OF CHILDREN WITH PTSD

Children are less likely than adults to speak directly about their problems or even to know they are having them. Their stress-related difficulties may instead emerge in their schoolwork, their relations with peers, or in their interactions with family members. Children who have PTSD are very vulnerable because they have less experience in coping with stressful events. Lack of prior experience may lead them to exaggerate their problems and prevent them from seeing light at the end of the tunnel.

Specific coping patterns need to be adjusted for children at their age-appropriate level. The following apply specifically to children.

- Parents and teachers should be encouraged to listen in a nonjudgmental fashion to children's thoughts, concerns, and ideas about the stressful event, for example, the war and reunion of the family.
- Adults should provide warmth and reassurance to children without minimizing their concerns. Children need to feel that there is a safe haven provided by strong adults.
- Adults should not impose their fears or burdens on children. Children should not be entirely sheltered from family difficulties, but they should not be made to feel that it is up to them to shoulder responsibilities that are beyond their developmental capability.
- Most adults cope effectively, even if there are rough roads to travel in the process of adjustment. Children, too, need to be given this positive expectation. Because of their limited experience and the length of stressors like separation from parents, it is vital that children gain this perspective.
- Children's reactions often mirror the reactions of their parents. If their parents are combating stressors effectively, the children gain a sense that they, too, can overcome their difficulties. If, however, their parents are not adjusting successfully, children develop a sense that problems are insurmountable, and they lose their key support link. It is critical that parents see that seeking help for themselves when it is needed is the best therapy for their troubled children.
- Children need accurate information about what has happened and why, but this information should be appropriate to their developmental stage. This information should be provided before, during, and after stressful events. Children also need to know why certain behaviors are required of them and usually need behavioral examples and sometimes rehearsal of behaviors that are not in their repertoire. It should not be assumed that children do not know the "dark side"

of current events. Given that they have seen horrible events on television or have overheard serious discussions, it is incumbent on adults to help them work through the meaning and significance of these events through discussion, support, and—in cases in which a child is traumatized—professional treatment.
- As with adults, children should be involved in helpful behaviors. By being part of the solution in their own classrooms, families, and communities, children develop an enhanced sense of mastery and control over their lives and cope more effectively with war and other severe stressful events.

The overall message must be that adjustment is not a short-term process and that commitment to these individuals cannot be short term (Milgran, 1989).

Acute Stress Disorder

Acute stress disorder (308.3) (ASD) (APA, 1994) is differentiated from PTSD in three ways: the individual experiences at least three of the symptoms indicating dissociation; the development time frame and the duration of symptoms is shorter; and the dissociative symptoms may prevent the individual from adaptively coping with the trauma.

Dissociative symptoms
Subjective sense of numbing or detachment
Reduced awareness of surroundings (e.g., being in a daze)
Derealization
Depersonalization
Dissociative amnesia

In terms of time, the symptoms may last from 2 days to 1 month. The onset of the dissociative experience may occur during the trauma experience or develop immediately thereafter. The defining characteristic of significant distress causation or social and occupational functioning impairment is that the individual is prevented from pursuing some necessary task, such as obtaining needed medical or legal assistance (Fortinash and Holoday-Worret, 1996). The clinical profile of symptoms of both PTSD and ASD include varying degrees of symptoms in the cognitive, affective, physiological, behavioral, and relationship categories (Haber, 1997).

Cognitive symptoms
Difficulty concentrating
Recurrent and intensive recollections of traumatic experiences
Sudden reliving of traumatic experiences (illusions, hallucinations)
Dissociative experiences; psychogenic amnesia; inability to recall important
    aspects of trauma
Anniversary reaction associated with traumatic event
Avoidance of thoughts associated with the traumatic event
Impaired career-related future orientation, marriage, family
Recurring vivid dreams/nightmares
Unconventional and often distorted perception of reality
Self-blame
Lack of cognitive integration of traumatic event perceived vulnerability:
    perception of threat and danger in innocuous/neutral situations

Absolutist thinking

Problem solving overridden by anger and anxiety

Affective symptoms

Irritability, explosive angry outbursts

Intense distress when confronted with events symbolizing, or in some aspect resembling, the traumatic experience

Avoidance of feelings associated with traumatic event

Restricted range of affect

Inability to experience loving feelings

Diminished or constricted responsiveness (emotional anesthesia or psychic blunting)

Emotional lability

Feelings of guilt

Inability to enjoy activities

Feelings of depression

Symptoms of anxiety (nervousness, jumpiness, jitteriness, or panic attacks)

Feelings of alienation

Phobias

Physiological reactions

Difficulty falling or staying asleep

Exaggerated startle response

Physiological reactivity in the presence of stimuli that reactivate memories, feelings, or sensations associated with the trauma

Hypervigilance/hyperalertness

High resting heart beat, blood pressure; increased urinary catecholamines

Behavioral symptoms

Phobic avoidance of situations that elicit recall of the traumatic event

Diminished interest and participation in significant activities

Psychogenic fugue (unexpected travel away from home; assumption of a new identity)

Restlessness

Impulsiveness (sudden trips, unexplained absences, changes in lifestyle or residence)

Difficulty completing tasks

Episodes of unpredictable aggressiveness

Substance abuse (alcohol, street drugs)

Chemical dependency on prescribed antianxiety or pain relief medications used to treat emotional distress and/or physical pain after the traumatic event

Self-mutilation (attempt to end feelings of depersonalization)

Sexual dysfunction

Relationship symptoms

Detachment, estrangement and isolation from others

Impaired ability to experience intimacy, tenderness, and sexuality

Impaired marital relationships

Impaired parent relationships

Excessive interpersonal distance from others related to fear of a past experience of betrayal (e.g., an officer who put a partner in unnecessary danger,
a physically or sexually abusive parent or husband, or a mugger or rapist)

Avoidance of personal disclosure related to mistrust of others and fear of
rejection

Treatment of Stress Disorders

At present, psychiatrists and other mental health professionals have effective
psychological and pharmacological treatments available for these two psychological
disorders. These treatments can restore a sense of control and diminish the power of
past events over current experiences. The sooner individuals are treated, the more
likely they are to recover from a traumatizing experience. Appropriate therapy can
help with other chronic trauma-related disorders, as well (Shelby and Tredinnick,
1995).

Psychotherapists help individuals with stress disorders to accept the traumatic
experience without being overwhelmed by memories of the trauma and without
arranging their lives to avoid being reminded of it. It is important to reestablish
a sense of safety and control in the individual's life. This helps him to feel strong
and secure enough to confront the reality of what has happened. For individuals
who have been badly traumatized, the support and safety provided by loved ones
is critical. Friends and family should resist the urge to tell the traumatized person
to "snap out of it" and instead should allow the individual time and space for
intense grief and mourning. Being able to talk about what happened and to get
help with feelings of guilt, self-blame, and rage about the trauma usually is very
effective in helping individuals put the event behind them. Psychotherapists know
that loved ones can make a significant difference in the long-term outcome of
the traumatized individual by being active participants in creating a treatment
plan—helping him to communicate and anticipating what he needs to restore a sense
of equilibrium to his life. If treatment is to be effective, it is also important that the
traumatized individual feel that he is a part of the planning process (Glynn and others,
1995).

Sleeplessness and other symptoms of hyperarousal may interfere with recovery
and increase preoccupation with the traumatizing experience. Psychiatrists have
several medications, including benzodiazepines and the new class of serotonin
re-uptake blockers, that can help people sleep and to cope with their hyperarousal.
These medications, as part of an integrated treatment plan, can help prevent the
development of long-term psychological problems in a traumatized individual
(Herman, 1992).

With individuals whose trauma occurred years or even decades before, the
treating psychotherapist must pay close attention to the behaviors—often deeply
entrenched—that the individual has developed to cope with his symptoms. Many
people whose trauma happened long ago have suffered in silence with symptoms
without ever having been able to talk about their trauma, nightmares, numbing, or
irritability. During treatment, being able to talk about what has happened and making

the connection between past trauma and current symptoms provides these individuals with the increased sense of control needed to manage their current lives and develop meaningful relationships.

Relationships are often a trouble spot for individuals with stress disorders. They often resolve conflicts by withdrawing emotionally or by becoming physically violent. Therapy can help them to identify and avoid unhealthy relationships. This is vital to the healing process; only after the feeling of stability and safety is established can the process of uncovering the roots of the trauma begin.

To make progress in easing flashbacks and other painful thoughts and feelings, most individuals with PTSD need to confront what has happened to them and, by repeating this confrontation, learn to accept the trauma as part of their past. Psychiatrists and other psychotherapists use several techniques to facilitate this process.

One important form of therapy for those who struggle with a stress disorder is *cognitive/behavioral therapy,* which is a form of treatment that focuses on correcting painful and intrusive patterns and thoughts by teaching the individual relaxation techniques and by examining—and challenging—his mental processes. A therapist using behavioral therapy to treat an individual with PTSD might, for example, help a patient who is provoked into panic attacks by loud street noises by setting a schedule that gradually exposes the patient to such noises in a controlled setting until he becomes "desensitized" and is no longer prone to terror. Using other techniques, the patient and therapist explore the patient's environment to determine what might aggravate the PTSD symptoms, and they work to reduce sensitivity and learn new coping skills.

Psychiatrists and other mental health professionals also treat cases of stress disorder with psychodynamic psychotherapy. Stress disorders result, in part, from the difference between the individual's personal values or view of the world and the reality experienced during the traumatic event. Psychodynamic psychotherapy, then, focuses on helping the individual examine personal values and how behavior and experience during the traumatic event violated those personal values. The goal is resolution of the conscious and unconscious conflicts that were created. In addition, the individual works to build self-esteem and self-control, develops a good and reasonable sense of personal accountability, and renews a sense of integrity and personal pride.

Whether patients with stress disorder receive cognitive/behavioral treatment, psychodynamic treatment, or crisis intervention, they need to identify the triggers for their memories of trauma, as well as to identify those situations in their lives that promote feelings of being out of control and the conditions that need to exist for them to feel safe. Therapists can help patients construct ways of coping with the hyperarousal and painful flashbacks that come over them when they are around reminders of the trauma. The trusting relationship between patient and therapist is crucial in establishing this necessary feeling of safety (Davidson, 1992).

PTSD and ASD treatment is usually done on an outpatient basis. For some individuals whose symptoms make it impossible for them to function, or for those who have developed additional symptoms as a result of their stress disorder, inpatient treatment is sometimes necessary to create the vital atmosphere of safety in which they can examine their flashbacks, reenactments of the trauma, and self-destructive behavior. Inpatient treatment is also important for patients with PTSD or ASD who have developed alcohol or other drug problems as a result of their attempts to "self-medicate." Occasionally, also, inpatient treatment is very useful in helping a patient with stress disorder get past a particularly painful period in his therapy.

The recognition of PTSD and ASD as major health problems in the United States is fairly recent. Over the past 20 years, research has produced a major explosion of knowledge about the ways people deal with trauma—what places them at risk for the development of long-term problems, and what helps them to cope. Mental health professionals are working hard to disseminate this understanding, and an increasing number of mental health professionals are receiving specialized training to help them reach out to persons in their communities with posttraumatic stress disorder.

Many entire communities have experienced traumatic situations in the past few years. There have been massive floods, major earthquakes, and devastating hurricanes and tornados. There have also been an unusual number of human-created disasters, for example, the tragic bombing in Oklahoma City, the complete destruction of Trans World Airlines flight 800, and the bombing at the 1996 Olympic games in Atlanta—and these are just a few of the traumas that affected men, women, and children who are all vulnerable to a stress disorder.

PHYSIOLOGICAL REACTIONS

A mental health professional, either in a community mental health crisis center or in an emergency room trauma center, must become familiar with the physiological symptoms of possible stress disorders. Some of the reactions, emotions, and observations to be aware of are increased heart rate, raised blood pressure, rapid breathing, a sluggish digestive process, inhibited salivation, tightened muscular tone, dilated pupils, increased blood sugar, and cold skin and extremities.

Assessment data

OBSERVATIONS	SUBJECTIVE REPORTS
Sweating	Feeling of weakness
Increased pulse	Desire to escape situation
Increased respiratory rate	Feelings of generalized fatigue
Increased blood pressure	Trembling or shaking
Overeating or anorexia	Complaints of dry mouth or thirst
Difficulty sleeping	Feelings of restlessness
Flushed face	Feelings of unsteadiness
Cold hands and extremities	Empty stomach
Dilated pupils	Bad taste, dry mouth
Unsteady voice	Clammy hands, feet
Urinary urgency	
Tense or rigid muscles	
Less pain perception	

Relationship to other emotions

SOURCE	MANIFESTATION	RELATION TO PTSD/ASD
Guilt (violation of conscience)	Feeling of self-unworthiness	Fear of punishment
Shame (disapproved action or wish exposed to others)	Feeling of unworthiness to others	Fear of being discovered and disapproved
Grief (loss of love object)	Feelings of sadness or aloneness	Fear of separation
Anger (being hostile and demanding)	Feelings of frustration or resentment	Fear of control by authority

From a clinically descriptive standpoint, PTSD and ASD may be seen as a multifaceted set of psychological and biological symptoms assumed to be associated with extreme trauma and thought to be exacerbated by stress and experiences of various kinds. Kolb (1987) urged the classification of these disorders into mild, moderate, and severe forms, depending on the number of symptoms, their expression, and the potential for intensification on reexposure to emotional stress.

There appears to be no overriding agreement regarding the most appropriate theoretical framework for understanding these disorders, particularly in accounting for causation, expression, and course. Stress disorders are the most likely of all psychiatric disorders to be explained by psychological constructs, with specific reference to learning and conditioning processes and changes in behavior as a result of experience. Although there may be biological and perhaps dispositional vulnerabilities and contributors to these disorders, highlighting the role of the trauma in marking disorder onset necessitates exploring both the stimulus and response aspects of the disorder, as well as the affected person.

The following brief case study is one that involves a natural disaster. The mother and her 7-year-old daughter were seen at a local crisis center.

Case Study   *Posttraumatic Stress Disorder*

Ann and her 7-year-old daughter, Tiffany, were asleep when the January 17, 1994 earthquake began. Her husband, Neal, was out of town. Neal was a native Californian, but Ann had always lived in the Midwest. She moved to California 8 years before, when she and Neal married.

Although they did not live close to the epicenter, there was considerable shaking. Ann woke abruptly, confused. She realized that it was probably an earthquake and jumped out of bed, grabbed her robe, and ran out the front door. She was terrified. Their alarm system was on, and she could hear water running down the street.

Ann's neighbors were milling around, talking about what to do since all the lights were out. Several of the men were going from house to house, shutting off the gas lines. Suddenly, one of the women turned to Ann and said, "Where is Tiffany?" Ann stared at her in horror and said, "Oh, my God. I left her in the house!" As Ann turned to run back to her home, a neighbor, Jim, seeing her confusion, took her arm.

"I have a flashlight, I'll go with you," offered Jim. Trying to calm her he added, "Your daughter probably slept right through it."

When they got to the front door, which Ann had left open, they heard Tiffany crying and screaming, "Mommy! Mommy!" Ann almost collapsed.

Jim asked where Tiffany's room was. Ann pointed toward the left, down a hall. Jim yelled, "Tiffany, Mommy is coming." He practically had to hold Ann up, as he pulled her down the hall to Tiffany's room. Very firmly he said to Ann, "Straighten up. You have to be calm for her sake. Tell her you are coming."

Ann, still shaking said, "Tiffany, Mommy is coming." Jim shined the light on Tiffany, and they could see blood running down her face. Apparently a small picture on the wall above her junior bed had fallen, and a corner of the frame had hit her on the head. Jim picked her up and said, "You are fine. Mommy is right here. See!" He shined the light on Ann and started to give her Tiffany, but Ann was so weak she almost dropped her. Jim, with his arm around both of them, said, "Let's go outside with everyone else." Tiffany was still sobbing.

As they went outside, the street and other lights that had been on before the earthquake once again illuminated the area, and everyone cheered—except Ann. She still appeared to be in a state of shock. Everyone was looking at her rather strangely, and Jim was still carrying Tiffany and holding Ann up.

Jim's wife, Linda, said very soothingly, "Tiffany, you and your Mommy come to my house. I baked cookies yesterday, and you can have some with milk while your Mommy and I have some coffee." She added very firmly, "You are alright! Everyone is alright." Tiffany stuck her thumb in her mouth and stopped crying. Ann followed them into the house.

Linda got out cookies and milk for Tiffany and put on the coffee, keeping up a cheery chatter to distract Tiffany. As Linda cleaned the blood off of Tiffany's face, she said to both of them, "It's just a tiny cut. I'll put on a cute bandage."

Ann had asked Tiffany to come and sit on her lap while she ate her cookies. While sitting on Ann's lap, Tiffany looked up at her mother and said, "Where did you go, Mommy? It was dark and I couldn't see."

"I went outside. I thought you would be alright," said Ann. Linda didn't say anything.

When Ann finished her coffee and Tiffany her cookies, they thanked Linda and went home to find the telephone ringing as they walked in. Ann answered. It was Neal, and he wanted to know if they had felt the earthquake. Ann said that they had and asked when he would be home because she needed him. Neal said he would leave immediately and should be home in a couple of hours.

When Neal arrived, he could see that neither Ann nor Tiffany were injured, except for a small cut on Tiffany's head. When Ann saw Neal, she started crying and said, "I *needed you* . . . you are never here when I need you!" She was pale, trembling, and wringing her hands.

Neal tried to calm her down. He held her in his arms and told her that everything was alright and that he would take care of everything. He asked Tiffany if she had felt the "ground shake." She answered that she had felt it but didn't get scared until she called her mother and she didn't answer.

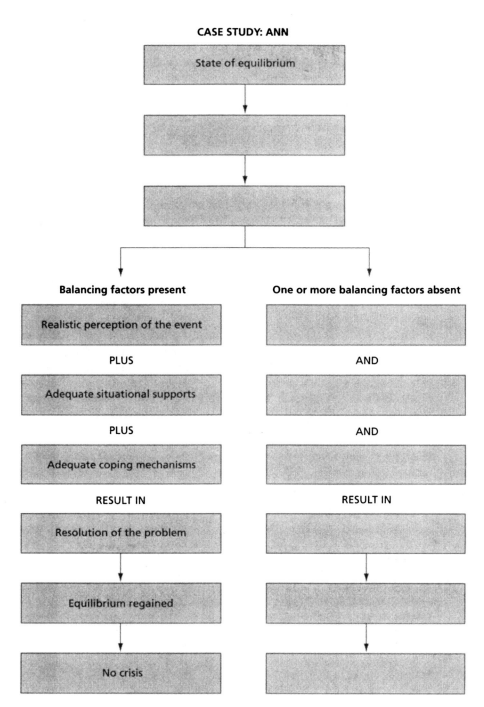

Figure 5-1

Her answer only increased Ann's guilt feelings. Neal felt that he should get her some immediate help. He asked their neighbors, Jim and Linda, if Tiffany could stay with them while he took Ann to the nearest crisis center. They said of course; Tiffany could have breakfast with them, and then she could stay and play with their two daughters.

Neal thanked them and asked Ann to get her coat. She just looked at him like she was in a daze. He took her hand and said, "Never mind, I'll get your coat." Neal realized that Ann was in a state of shock. He put her coat on and led her to his car. When they arrived at the crisis center, it was very busy. Neal asked one of the volunteers if someone could see his wife because he was very concerned about her. The volunteer took them to an office to wait. Ann had not said a word; she just acted like she was numb.

A therapist came in and asked Neal what the problem was. He told her that Ann left their daughter in the house during the earthquake and that she was probably feeling very guilty. The therapist agreed and tried to talk to Ann. Ann sat and cried and tried to tell the therapist how she felt. It was obvious that Ann felt under a great deal of stress and terribly guilty about leaving Tiffany in the house alone. The therapist told Neal that Ann was in all probability suffering from posttraumatic stress disorder. The therapist said that she would get Ann some medication so she could get some rest.

The therapist told Neal that Ann should be seen for crisis therapy and then probably for longer term therapy. She also recommended that Tiffany be included in a peer support group as soon as possible. She told Neal that the support groups would be available at all of the schools.

The therapist asked Neal if he would be able to stay in town until Ann and Tiffany were stabilized. He replied, "Wild horses couldn't get me away." He, too, felt guilty because he had not been available for Ann and Tiffany during the earthquake.

Of all the passions, fear weakens judgement the most.

–Cardinal de Retz

Complete the paradigm in Figure 5-1 for this case study, then compare it with the completed one in Appendix D. Refer to the paradigms in Chapter 3 as needed.

REFERENCES

American Psychiatric Association: *Diagnostic and statistical manual of mental disorders,* ed 4, Washington, DC, 1994, The Association.

Bile DA: Road to recovery: post-traumatic stress disorder: the hidden victim, *J Psychosoc Nurs Ment Health Serv* 31(9):19, 1993.

Blake DD, Cook JD, Keane TM: Post-traumatic stress disorder and coping in veterans who are seeking medical treatment, *J Clin Psychol* 48:695, 1992.

Davidson J: Drug therapy in post-traumatic stress disorder, *Br J Psychiatry* 160:309, 1992.

Fortinash KM, Holoday-Worret PA: *Psychiatric-mental health nursing,* St. Louis, 1996, Mosby.

Glynn SM and others: Behavioral family therapy for Vietnam combat veterans with posttraumatic stress disorder, *J Psychother Pract Res* 4(3):214, 1995.

Haber J and others: *Comprehensive psychiatric nursing,* ed 5, St. Louis, 1997, Mosby.

Henry JP: Psychological and physiological responses to stress: the right hemisphere and the hypothalamopituitary-adrenal axis, an inquiry into problems of human bonding, *Physiol Behav Science* 28:369, 1993.

Herman JL: *Trauma and recovery,* New York, 1992, Basic Books.

Kolb, LC: A neuropsychological hypothesis explaining post traumatic stress disorder, *Am J Psychiatry* 144:989, 1987.

Milgram NA: Social support versus self-sufficiency in traumatic and posttraumatic stress reactions. In Lerner B, Gershon S, editors: *New directions in affective disorders,* New York, 1989, Springer-Verlag.

Shelby JS, Tredinnick MC: Crisis intervention with survivors of natural disasters: lessons from Hurricane Andrew, *J Counsel Dev* 73(5):491, 1995.

Symes L: Posttraumatic stress disorder: evolving concepts, *Arch Psychiatr Nurs* 69(4):195, 1995.

ADDITIONAL READING

Breslau N and others: Traumatic events and posttraumatic stress disorder in an urban population of young adults, *Arch Gen Psychiatry,* 48:216, 1991.

Davidson J and others: A diagnostic and family study of posttraumatic stress disorders, *Am J Psychiatry* 142:90, 1985.

Kleber RJ, Brom D, Defares PB: *Coping with trauma: theory prevention and treatment,* Amsterdam/Berwyn, Penn, 1992, Swets & Zeitlinger.

van der Kolk BA: Group therapy with traumatic stress disorder. In Kaplan HI, Sadock BJ, editors: *Comprehensive textbook of group psychotherapy,* New York, 1993, Williams & Wilkins.

Kulka RA and others: *Trauma and the Vietnam War generation,* New York, 1990, Brunner & Mazel.

Nader K and others: Children's PTSD reactions one year after a sniper attack at their school, *Am J Psychiatry* 147:1526, 1990.

Stewart AL and others: Psychological distress/well-being and cognitive functioning measures. In Stewart AL, Ware JE, editors: *Measuring functional status and well-being: the medical outcomes study approach,* Durham, NC, 1992, Duke University Press.

Terr LC: Childhood traumas: an outline and overview, *Am J Psychiatry* 147:1526, 1990.

Ursano RJ, McCaughey B, Fullerton CS: *Individual and community responses to trauma and disaster: the structure of human chaos,* Cambridge, England, 1993, The Cambridge University Press.

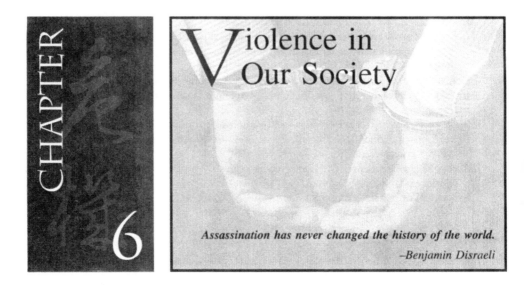

CHAPTER 6

Violence in Our Society

Assassination has never changed the history of the world.

—Benjamin Disraeli

The twentieth century has not been very tranquil or serene. Seldom does a week go by that we are not confronted by the news of violent acts of apparent random killing, rape, kidnapping, spousal abuse, abuse of the elderly, child abuse and neglect, or murder. There have been a multitude of traumatic events. It appears that violence is escalating in our lives and in the lives of those we love. Perhaps the violence we encounter in our lives does not always appear in banner headlines. Sometimes it does appear as a headline for a brief period, but it neither affects as many people nor receives the same notoriety over a lengthy period.

This chapter presents some of the events that occur daily, maybe not to us personally, but they still affect us. How can we as individuals *not* care when we read about children being neglected, sexually abused, or murdered by their family members or caretakers. Do we not identify with the wife or husband when we read that a husband has killed his wife and their three children because she has been unable to contend with his verbal and physical abuse and leaves him, seeking a divorce? Aren't we concerned about our children's exposure to drugs and violence in schools and with their peers? We are, of course, very concerned when we read of "gangs" who shoot and kill innocent young boys and girls because they were *thought* to be members of a "rival" gang. The police in most metropolitan cities are understaffed, overworked, and underpaid. They try to do the best they can, but they can only do so much.

In the November 6, 1996, *Los Angeles Times,* Boyer wrote, "A former city electrician was found guilty of slaying four city workers. He faces the death penalty after being convicted of killing four of his supervisors at the city's downtown technical center. Police said that he went to the communications area, where he worked as a radio repairman. He had an angry discussion there with someone about his performance and left, returning shortly with a Glock semiautomatic pistol. He then methodically searched out his victims and shot them." This is just *one* incident on *one* day in *one* city. Multiply this incident by the hundreds—because it does happen somewhere every day.

Child Abuse and Neglect

For decades Americans have been pelted with images of disadvantaged children. Though these images come from many sources, they reflect common assumptions. Disadvantaged children, stereotypically, come from poor and broken homes. They are commonly neglected or abused, and they (or their parents) often abuse drugs. Most are African-American and live in ghetto neighborhoods. The future for these children is dark and virtually sealed: it is widely assumed that most disadvantaged children are destined to fail in school, become parents too early, land in jail, neglect or abuse their own children, and drift in and out of employment and never earn a decent wage. Most will be poor their entire lives, and their children will be cemented into poverty (Cowen, 1994).

Many of these stereotypes are rooted in certain truths. Growing up poor can make childhood miserable, and the climb into adulthood is stressful and steep. To be protected from destruction all children, minimally, should live in an environment that provides some order and meets their basic physical and material needs. All children should have a continuous relationship with a consistently attentive and caring adult who treats them as special (not as just another inhabitant of this world), who is able to stimulate and engage them, who provides appropriate responsibilities and challenges, and who passes on important social and moral exceptions. Some strong friends and the affirmation and affection of community adults are often critical to children, especially those who are deprived of the consistent presence of a parent or guardian. All children should have freedom from exploitation and discrimination in their communities, some sense of the justice of their world, and opportunities in school and in the communities for constructive achievement. Many children also need special health, social, and educational services to deal with inherited and acquired ailments and disabilities. When children have these ingredients, they are likely to have trust in themselves and in the world, inner vitality and resourcefulness, and the capacity in adulthood for zestful play and gratifying work and love, even if they suffer hardships and abrasions.

Clearly not only African-American children, underclass children, or children in single-parent families grow up without these ingredients. Looking at children in terms of these ingredients forces policymakers and the public to widen their fields of vision to encompass all poor children, including poor white children and children from diverse ethnic groups. Looking at children in this way forces policymakers and the public to see the many vulnerable children in this country who are not poor. Stresses on parents, limited opportunities for accomplishment, peer problems, the absence of adults in the community, and learning and other disabilities are among the pervasive problems that hurt children in every race and class (Weissbourd, 1996).

When it comes to the deaths of infants and children at the hands of parents or caretakers, society has responded in a strangely muffled, seemingly disinterested way. Little money has been spent to comprehend this tragic phenomenon. The true numbers and exact nature of the problem remain unknown, and the troubling fact of abuse or neglect often remains a terrible secret that is buried with the child.

INCIDENCE AND PREVALENCE OF CHILD ABUSE AND NEGLECT

In 1988 a 15-member panel was established by the U.S. Congress to evaluate the scope of child abuse in the United States and recommend ways to improve the child protective system. Their report, titled "A Nation's Shame: Fatal Child Abuse and Neglect in the United States," (1995) represents the most comprehensive study yet of children's deaths at the hands of parents or caretakers in America.

Although it emphasizes that no single profile fits every case, the report attempts, for the first time, to fill in some of the *who, how,* and *why* of children's deaths. It found, for example, that most physical abuse fatalities are caused by angry, extremely stressed-out fathers, stepfathers, or boyfriends who unleash a torrent of rage on infants over such "triggers" as a baby's crying, feeding difficulties, or failed toilet training.

Likewise, studies suggest that mothers are most often held responsible for deaths resulting from bathtub drowning, starvation, or other neglect. Other major findings include the following:

- *Head trauma* is the leading cause of child abuse deaths. So-called *shaken baby syndrome* is so lethal that up to 25% of its victims die, and most survivors suffer brain damage.
- Domestic violence is strongly linked to child abuse deaths. An estimated 50% of homes with adult violence also involve child abuse or neglect.
- Many states lack adequate legal sanctions. Only 21 states have statutes that allow parents to be prosecuted for killing their children under "felony murder" or "homicide by child abuse" laws.

In describing the scope and patterns of the problem, the report details the particular susceptibility of very young children to fatal abuse. These victims are deemed the "invisible kids" because their youth leaves them largely out of sight of the community at large and the welfare system, but their young bodies are most vulnerable to the hitting, shaking, or other punishments that might not injure an older child as seriously.

The path to adulthood is stressful and steep. Weissbourd (1996) states that there is a good deal of evidence that most vulnerable children are *not* poor. Although the national debate on improving children's prospects is now focused on poverty and single-parent families, poverty and single parenthood are only two of many hardships that undercut our children. Whether parents are chronically stressed or depressed often more powerfully influences a child's fate than whether there are two parents in the home or whether the family is poor.

Perhaps the most serious misconception is the concept of the underclass that makes no allowance for variation in the nature of the poor children and forces attention away from problems that typically deprive poor children of basic needs. The underclass and similar concepts promote another dangerous myth about poor children—that they are doomed to a life of waste and failure, largely because poor parents are incapable of raising their children properly. Such images of poor families are not new. Although there has also always been a tendency to romanticize poverty—to find grace, purity, and innocence in the poor—these sentiments have long been buried in an avalanche of images of uncared for, poor children. Child abuse and neglect are neither the provinces of the poor nor the propensities of African-American, disadvantaged, or single-parent homes. Child abuse and neglect are found in every race, color and creed—they have no boundary or territory.

The level of violence aimed at young children in America has reached public health crisis proportions, claiming the lives of at least 2000 children annually and seriously injuring more than 140,000 others (Rivera, 1995). The U.S. Advisory Board on Child Abuse and Neglect (1995), concluding a 2½-year nationwide study, found a level of fatal abuse and neglect that is far greater than even experts in the field had realized. Abuse and neglect in the home is a leading cause of death for young children, as the majority of abused and neglected children are under 4 years of age. In fact, the homicide rate among children in this age group has hit a 40-year high, a chilling trend similar in scope to the violence directed at teenagers from street gunfire. Equally grim is the finding that the child protective system has largely failed to shelter our nation's children. The report describes an alarming national environment of underreported child abuse fatalities; inadequately trained investigators, prosecutors, and medical professionals; inconsistent autopsy practices; and an American public who continues to regard child deaths as "rare curiosities."

The congressionally established panel refers to research that concludes that 85% of child deaths from abuse or neglect are systematically misidentified as accidents or are the result of natural causes because police, physicians, and coroners are largely untrained in identifying evidence of intentional trauma and severe neglect in children. In addition, 69% of professionals (doctors, teachers, and social workers) who suspect child abuse do not report the incidents to the proper authorities. There are even cases when professionals have sought to *protect* child abusers. Many prosecutors concede that child homicides are reduced to lesser crimes because most prosecutors have little or no experience with abuse and neglect cases.

Also documented in this report is the emergence and success of child death review teams composed of members of local law enforcement and social welfare agencies who review cases of child death and offer appropriate follow-up. The report's other recommendations include state legislation that establishes regulations for child autopsies, a national effort to increase research on and reporting of child abuse fatalities, multidisciplinary training on child deaths, ensuring that children's safety is a priority in all family and child service programs, and increased funding for family support services (Rivera, 1995).

In her very widely read newspaper column, Abigail Van Buren, "Dear Abby," wrote recently, "The National Committee to Prevent Child Abuse . . . encourages everyone to become involved in preventing child abuse before it occurs. If every adult did just a little, fewer children would suffer pain, injury or death due to abuse" (Box 6-1).

DYNAMICS OF CHILD ABUSE AND NEGLECT

Child abuse occurs in a wide variety of ways. Recent trends have moved toward greatly expanding its definition from physical abuse alone to also include emotional and sexual abuse, as well as physical and emotional neglect. In general, however,

---

Box 6-1

SEVEN STEPS TO STAMP OUT CHILD ABUSE

1. *Report* suspected abuse or neglect. Inform authorities if you suspect that children are being harmed. Your concern may result in children being protected from an abusive environment.
2. *Advocate* services to help families. Communities need comprehensive services that address issues affecting families. Parenting programs, healthcare, and housing needs are vital to maintaining healthy children and families.
3. *Volunteer* at a child abuse program. Parent support groups, crisis centers, and hot lines are typical programs that often welcome volunteers. Check your telephone directory for the names of agencies in your area.
4. *Help a friend,* neighbor, or relative. Someone you know may be struggling with parenting responsibilities. Offer a sympathetic ear or a helping hand. Assisting occasionally with child care or offering to locate sources of community help can be a tremendous boost to someone under stress.
5. *Help yourself.* Recognize the signs that indicate outside help is needed. If you feel overwhelmed, constantly sad, or angry and out of control, get help. Remember, asking for help is a sign of strength not weakness.
6. *Support and suggest local programs* on child abuse prevention for community organizations. Kiwanis Clubs, Exchange Clubs, PTAs, church groups, and women's and men's clubs all offer excellent opportunities for raising public awareness in the community.
7. *Promote programs in schools.* Teaching prevention strategies can help to keep children safe from those who would abuse them. This is a national problem. It takes individuals who care, as well as organizations.

---

consensus is lacking among professionals for any single definition of the terms *child abuse* or *child neglect.* Definitions vary greatly because there is much diversity in sociocultural values and practices associated with child rearing, some of which may result in physical and psychological harm to the child.

People who abuse children are not limited to any one well-defined group. They can be found among widely differing socioeconomic, racial, cultural, age, and other socially defined groups. Specific differences, however, have been identified among factors related to specific forms of abuse. For example, the physical size, strength, and power of the abuser obviously do not play as great a role in child abuse as in the abuse of adults. Obviously, few are as physically powerless as the infant or small child.

The abuse and neglect of children have been recorded throughout the centuries. It has been suggested that these are by no means new problems, but rather ones that only now are being socially recognized and legally addressed. Not until 1871 was the first child protective agency, *The Society for the Prevention of Cruelty to Children,* established in New York. Nearly a century passed before all 50 states finally enacted legal mandates to report child abuse in 1968.

In 1962 Kempe originated the phrase *battered child syndrome,* which dramatically focused professional and public attention on the abusive actions by parents and other adults on select groups of children (Kempe, 1962). The phrase provided a base for the specific labeling and identification of the severest forms of child abuse, for which there is clinically verifiable evidence. Clinical signs include bruises, abrasions, lacerations, broken bones, burns, abdominal and chest injuries, and eye damage. Frequently, examination of new injuries yields clinical evidence of past injuries. Some children experience a single violent abusive event, others experience a long series of violent episodes. This label was later superseded by the more comprehensive term *child abuse and neglect* (Helfer and Kempe, 1976).

The federal Child Abuse Prevention and Treatment Act was recently reauthorized and otherwise amended by the Child Abuse, Domestic Violence, Adoption, and Family Services Act of 1992. In it "the term *child abuse and neglect* means the physical or mental injury, sexual abuse or exploitation, negligent treatment, or maltreatment of a child by a person who is responsible for the child's welfare, under circumstances that indicate that the child's health or welfare is harmed or threatened thereby" (Public Law 102-255, June 18, 1992).

Although the battered child syndrome may be among the easiest forms of child abuse to prove legally, it has been found to be only a part of the overall problem of abuse of children. Incidence reports on incest and sexual exploitation of children are admittedly incomplete and, at the most, educated estimates. Case finding is quite difficult, most often coming to the attention of healthcare agencies when the child is seen for other healthcare problems such as venereal disease or pregnancy. According to Justice and Justice (1979), sexual abuse, like child abuse, most often involves more than just the victim and the abuser. It also involves another family member or responsible adult who allows the victimization to continue.

In general, incestuous offenders do not exhibit any overtly psychotic or deviant behaviors (Giarretto, 1976). Generally, the perpetrator is between 30 and 50 years old, male, and, more than 75% of the time, the victim's father. Reported female victims outnumber male victims by a wide margin. Investigations of adults who were abused as children reveal that 20% of girls and 10% of boys had experienced some type of sexual molestation, abuse, or exploitation (Rubinelli, 1980; Salholz and others, 1982).

People who sexually exploit children are usually men who are emotionally dependent with feelings of inferiority and whose lives have been dominated by a significant woman. A significantly high correlation between sexual abusers and a history of parental abuse in childhood has also been found. The abused child frequently knows the abuser and may become involved solely to meet nonsexual needs for attention and affection. Children are particularly vulnerable because of ignorance; fear of losing the caring relationship; or ambivalence, shame, guilt, and the fear of not being believed as the "innocent" victim. All these factors contribute to an ongoing conspiracy of silence on the part of the child.

Documentation of the psychological and sociological damage resulting from abusive child-rearing patterns has been increasing. This damage, in turn, may lead to intergenerational patterns of abnormal parenting and increased numbers of violent crimes perpetrated by those with histories of child abuse. Violence as the norm is an expectation passed on from victims to the next generation (Silver, 1968; Gelles, 1972).

Three factors intrinsic to child abuse have been identified by the National Center for Child Abuse and Neglect (U.S. Department of Health and Human Services, 1993).
1. A capacity for abuse exists within the parent.
2. One child is perceived as special in some manner by the parents.
3. One or more crisis events occur before the abusive act is committed.

It is of great importance to recognize that what may appear to an observer as intentional abuse may be perceived by the victim merely as a normal way of life. Perhaps the only attention that some children can obtain from a parent or other significant person in their lives is abusive. To a child, love may be inextricably linked with violence. Unfortunately, those with whom they are closest also hold the power to punish, either physically or psychologically (Bandura, 1973). Indicators of a child's potential need for protection are defined in Box 6-2.

Several theories have attempted to explain why some parents abuse their children. Individually, none provides a comprehensive explanation for child abuse, yet each has contributed significantly to the overall base of information needed to explain this multidimensional problem. A broad scope of causal factors, none of which operates in isolation, is becoming increasingly evident. Each theoretical model proposes causal relationships to common problem areas. Collectively, this rapidly expanding base of knowledge supports the need for a holistic approach to intervention.

Several efforts have been made to categorize the personality traits and characteristics of child abusers in an effort to help explain their behaviors. A major problem has been that, for the most part, data for these studies have been empirical and drawn from clinical practice with identified child abusers. As such, they fail to explain why other persons with similar personality characteristics and traits and under similar circumstances do not abuse their children.

Personality or character traits that have been suggested as likely to lead to abusive behavior by parents include emotional immaturity, inability to cope with stress, chronic suspicion and hostility, and poor impulse control. Any of these could precipitate rage reactions in the parent who is confronted with frustration or undue stress. When parents with a requisite psychological profile come into confrontation with the demands of a child, an inner-directed rage reaction may be precipitated. As anger and frustration build, such parents suddenly erupt, striking out physically or psychologically at the most vulnerable person within their environment, the child (Halper, 1979; Walker-Hooper, 1981).

It is not uncommon to find the family scapegoat as the recipient of such parental acting out behavior. *Scapegoating* is an excellent example of psychological abuse. To survive as a unit, some families allocate the role of scapegoat to one member. Most frequently, the most vulnerable person is a child because a child is dependent and unable to retaliate against the parent's power (Vogel and Bell, 1960).

Based on the mechanisms of projection and displacement, scapegoating is often used to divert conflicts between parents. Undesirable traits or feelings are displaced or projected from the parent to the child when tensions become unbearable and parents lack the ability to discuss openly their reactions to stressful situations.

The abusive-dynamic model constructed by Kempe and Helfer (1972) is based on the presence and interaction of multiple dynamics. Kempe postulates that there are seven dynamics that interact and affect the parent's perception of the child:

Box 6-2

INDICATORS OF A CHILD'S POTENTIAL NEED
FOR PROTECTION

Physical abuse

Physical indicators

Unexplained bruises (in various stages of healing); welts; human bite marks; bald spots; unexplained burns, especially cigarette burns or immersion burns (glovelike); unexplained fractures, lacerations, or abrasions

Behavioral indicators

Self-destructive, withdrawn, and aggressive; behavioral extremes; uncomfortable with physical contact, arrives at school early or stays late, as if afraid to be at home; chronic runaway (adolescents); complains of soreness or moves uncomfortably; wears clothing inappropriate to weather to hide body

Physical neglect

Abandonment, unattended medical needs, consistent lack of supervision, consistent hunger, inappropriate dress, poor hygiene, lice, distended stomach, emaciated, regularly displays fatigue or listlessness, falls asleep in class, steals food, begs from classmates, reports that no caretaker is at home, frequently absent or tardy, self-destructive or school dropout (adolescents)

Sexual abuse

Torn, stained, or bloody underclothing; pain or itching in genital area; difficulty walking or sitting; bruises or bleeding in external genitalia; venereal disease; frequent urinary or yeast infections; withdrawal; chronic depression; excessive seductiveness; role reversal; overly concerned for siblings; poor self-esteem, self-devaluation, and lack of confidence; peer problems; lack of involvement; massive weight change; suicide attempts (especially adolescents); hysteria; lack of emotional control; sudden school difficulties; inappropriate sex play or premature understanding of sex; threatened by physical contact or closeness; promiscuity

Emotional maltreatment

Speech disorders, delayed physical development, substance abuse, ulcers, asthma, severe allergies, habit disorders (sucking, rocking), antisocial, destructive, neurotic traits (sleep disorders, inhibition of play), passive and aggressive behavioral extremes, delinquent behavior (especially adolescents), or developmentally delayed

---

mothering imprint, isolation, self-esteem, role reversal, spouse support, perception of the child, and crisis events.

Mothering imprint is the capacity to nurture and is learned only through one's own childhood experiences. Parents whose needs were not met in a loving, nurturing manner in their infancy tend to lack the capacity for providing nurturance in the care of their children. Overwhelmed by their own unmet dependency needs, they misperceive the dependency needs of their children. Lacking childhood memories of dependency gratification, they are unable to sense their child's needs or to respond empathetically. Rather than feeling sympathy and concern when a helpless infant or child continues to fuss and cry despite their caring efforts, the parents perceive the behavior as criticism. Feelings of failure and powerlessness arise, leading to lowered self-esteem and increased frustration and anger. Unable to redirect these feelings constructively, the parents project blame for the feelings of discomfort toward the cause—the "bad child."

Sometimes an abused child may be seen as special or unique by a parent. This uniqueness may be real, such as a physical or emotional problem. It may also be imagined, or the child may be perceived as quite similar to someone disliked or feared in the parent's past memories. In either case, when such a child behaves undesirably or does not live up to the parent's needs and expectations, he creates a negative reflection on parental abilities and causes the threat of loss of self-esteem or self-control to the parent. This child becomes the "bad child," the one who needs to be corrected, to be "straightened out" (Broadhurst and others, 1992).

Disciplinary actions taken by the parents are perceived as positive and corrective rather than abusive behavior. Parents who were raised by similarly abusing parents may see nothing abnormal in their abusive behaviors.

A common victim response to such abuse is to feel at fault and to feel that trying harder to be a "good child" in the future will stop further abusive episodes. This illogical response is supported by the abuser, and further blame is projected onto the victim. This vicious cycle continues until broken by circumstances that may be drastic enough to require medical-legal intervention. Examples of such could be the death of a child or injuries requiring professional care; sudden overt, socially deviant behavior by the child; or a child runaway.

Role reversal is another dynamic. In this situation the parent attributes adult powers to the child and comes to depend on the child for emotional sustenance and gratification of the parent's dependency needs. Such persons are seldom able to engage in any meaningful adult relationships or to intuit the needs of others. When this parent is confronted with the need to provide nurturance to another and is unable to meet his own emotional needs, conflict arises.

Other studies have suggested that abuse may occur when a child is perceived by one parent as winning in a competition for love and caring from the other parent. In this concept the parents are perceived as having developed a strong symbiotic relationship based on caring and love, with the advent of a child being a threat to the continuation of that relationship. Abuse is for the primary purpose of physically or psychologically eliminating the competition (Justice and Justice, 1976).

Social isolation has been identified as a contributing factor in all theoretical models of child abuse. Persons with low self-esteem and mistrust of others are unable to develop positive interpersonal relationships or to request, accept, or use help from others. Isolation may also be a learned behavior that parents actively teach their children by socializing them to distance themselves from experiences that might promote learning how to establish positive social relationships. It may also be due to environmental factors such as socioeconomic deprivation, living in an isolated area, moving into a new neighborhood, or a combination of any such related factors.

People who abuse have a strong tendency to be suspicious of others, most likely because of fear of exposure. Quite frequently, such persons make a great effort to isolate their families socially and to enforce maintenance of a minimum social network. Their goal is to present the appearance of a "normally" functioning family to their community, thereby reducing chances for disclosure and outside intervention (Bohn, 1990). Whichever the cause, social isolation has been found to reduce a person's access to situational supports and tangible resources. Without these, parents experience increased stress in child rearing and are unable to optimize their coping abilities to deal with the resulting feelings of powerlessness, frustration, and anger in their parental roles.

The following case study involves a young divorced woman who is socially isolated from her family and friends. She is the mother of two children and has physically abused her 6-year-old son. After she was seen in the emergency room with her son and daughter, it was recommended that she meet with a therapist on the hospital's crisis team.

Case Study   *Child Abuse*

Alice, a 24-year-old divorced mother of two small children, was referred to the therapist by the hospital's emergency room physician. Earlier that evening, she had brought her 1-year-old daughter, Joan, to the emergency room. The little girl was bleeding profusely from a deep laceration on her forehead. Alice explained that, less than an hour before, Joan had climbed over the rails of her crib and fallen, striking her head on the edge of the crib as she fell. Alice said that she hadn't heard Joan fall because she had fallen asleep on the living room couch. They had just moved into the house 2 days ago, and she was exhausted from unpacking all day. Her 6-year-old son, Mike, had awakened her by calling loudly for her to help his sister. She had rushed to the bedroom and found Joan lying on the floor, crying loudly, and bleeding heavily from the cut on her head. Mike was vainly trying to pick her up but had only succeeded in dropping her back on the floor. When Alice arrived, he too began to cry loudly and cling to her.

Alice said that suddenly all she wanted to do was sit down and cry, too. "I just wanted this all to go away. I wanted all of these problems out of my life. I have never felt so angry and helpless."

She tried to stop the bleeding. When she couldn't, she decided to take Joan to the nearby hospital. She said that she quickly told Mike to put on his bathrobe and get out to the car, but "he began to argue with me—something about getting dressed first—and then started to run out of the room. I suddenly had all I could take! I blew up and slapped him so hard that he flew across the hallway and hit the wall. I was still so angry with him that I just picked up Joan and grabbed him by the arm and dragged him along out to the car. As soon as we all got into the car, though, I began to shake all over. I was horrified at what I'd done to Mike. Sure, I've spanked him before, but I was so frightened and felt so alone right then. Right now I'm afraid to be alone with either of them again!"

After the doctor examined Joan and sutured the laceration on her head, he asked to have Mike brought into the room. An examination revealed evidence of new abrasions on the right side of his face and shoulder. Mike responded quietly to the doctor's questions about the injuries and said, "Mommy spanked me because I was a bad boy." He was no longer crying and clung tightly to his mother's hand as he spoke. There was no recent evidence of any other injuries.

In view of Alice's obvious emotional state, the doctor decided to admit the children to the hospital for overnight observation and further examination for signs of past physical injuries indicative of abuse. He strongly advised Alice to meet with a therapist on the hospital's crisis team before going home. She agreed, and a call was placed for the therapist to meet her at the hospital within an hour.

When the therapist arrived, Alice was waiting, slumped down in a chair in his office. She appeared disheveled, tearful, and physically exhausted. Her tone of voice sounded very depressed, yet defensive, as she began to speak about the incident that evening.

She said that she and the children had just moved to this city a few days ago from a small town in the northern part of the state. She was to start her new job as a receptionist in a large law firm the next week. Divorced for almost a year, she had no family or friends nearby.

When asked about her former marriage, she said that she had married when she was an 18-year-old college sophomore and that the marriage had lasted for 5 years. She added that her son Mike had been born only 5 months after the marriage. "That," she said rather cynically, "was definitely a case of 'marry in haste, repent at leisure.' We had 5 long years of trying to make a go of it. Having Joan last year was probably our last big mistake." She said that she became pregnant with Joan soon after Bob, her ex-husband, had finished his schooling and started his law practice. It was a planned pregnancy because they both believed that things in their lives would take a turn for the better as soon as Bob began to build a practice. As it turned out, his practice was slow in building, and it began to seem to her that the need for her additional income would never end. Arguments between them increased until, she said, "One day, heaven help me, I found myself agreeing with Bob when he told me that he wanted a divorce." She added that she had been given full custody of the children.

Bob had remarried less than a year ago, the day after the divorce became final, and, just 2 days before moving to this city, Alice had learned that a son had been born to Bob's new wife.

When asked about her childhood, she stated that she had been an only child and that her parents had divorced when she was 12 years of age. She had remained with her mother. Her father, an attorney, soon moved to a different state and remarried about a year later. She never saw him again but recalled him as a strict disciplinarian, someone to avoid in stressful situations because "he'd always blow up at me if I were around." He died in an auto accident when she was 15 years of age. She recalled that her life with her mother after the divorce had been "rather dull and uneventful." Alice met Bob during her freshman year at college; they soon became engaged and planned to be married after Bob's graduation from law school in about 4 years. She had planned to obtain a law degree, finishing about a year after Bob.

Alice described Bob as being everything then that she thought she would ever want a man to be. She doubted that she could ever love anyone else as much and assumed that he had felt the same way about her.

After she returned to school in the fall of her second year, she discovered she was more than 4 months pregnant, too late for her to consider an abortion. She recalled that neither she nor Bob was "exactly thrilled by this news" because neither had income to support a child. They were even more concerned about their parents' reaction to the news. At the time, the only solution that seemed feasible to both of them was to get married immediately and then tell their parents that they had been secretly married the past spring.

As expected, neither family was pleased to hear about the "secret marriage" and the impending birth of a grandchild. Their general attitude was that Alice and Bob were still too young and in no financial position to support a family and continue in college. Neither set of parents was financially able to help them any more than they were at present. After much discussion, Bob finally gave in to Alice's decision that she would drop out of school and find a job to help support them both until Bob graduated. Then she would return to school and complete requirements for her degree.

She quickly obtained a part-time job as a receptionist at a law firm and worked for a few months before Mike was born. After his birth, she was asked to return full time and had remained until just before her recent move to this city. Her new job here was similar and had been obtained through contacts made by her former employers.

As Alice described her relationships with her former husband and their children, the therapist noted that a pattern of scapegoating behavior by the parents seemed to evolve whenever she described Mike's role in the family. She frequently described Mike as a child who had "created problems for them from the day he was born." As she recalled, she and Bob began to have their first "real" arguments about the need to place Mike in a day nursery when she returned to work. Whenever she expressed concern about leaving Mike with "strangers," Bob would get very defensive and angry with her. She remembered him once saying, "It wasn't my idea alone to get married and start raising a family so soon. You're the one who got pregnant! If you'd been careful, you could have been going to school right now. That baby's causing problems, too, not just me!"

She said that Mike never was a "cuddly" baby, often bullied the other children at nursery school, and continued to create problems for her and Bob as he grew older.

Their arguments increasingly seemed to center on Mike as he grew older. Bob constantly criticized Alice's decisions about Mike's care yet never offered any suggestions of his own. When asked how she and Bob handled this, she responded that Bob always refused to get involved in any disciplinary problems; he always left that to her. She had never seen anything wrong with either spanking Mike or sending him to his room for a while. She added that spankings from her mother and father had never hurt her when she was young so, "whenever Mike deserved one, he got one, too."

She described her daughter, Joan, as being just the opposite of Mike, a child who was warm, loving, and very cooperative. With a sharp laugh, she added, "But Mike—heaven help me because he seems to be getting more like his father every day. He's always demanding attention and wanting to have his way about everything."

The therapist then asked her why she had decided to leave her old job and move away from her friends to this city. She responded that since the divorce, the town had just seemed too small for her to avoid meetings with Bob and his new family.

After the divorce, she had encouraged Bob to keep in close contact with their children and, through them, with her. This continued even after his remarriage. She frequently found herself calling him for advice. In fact, she was surprised to find herself depending on him for advice much more than before their divorce.

Earlier this year, she had heard that Bob's new wife was pregnant. She said that her immediate reaction was concern for the children, wondering if Bob would continue to visit with them as much after his new child was born or if he would focus all his attention on his new family and rarely visit them anymore. The more she thought about this, the more she felt an urgent need to get away from the whole situation before it even happened. As she recalled, "I suddenly felt that I couldn't stand even being in the same town with him when the new baby arrived."

She showed signs of increasing tension and anxiety as she discussed this with the therapist. Suddenly she began to pound her fists on the arms of the chair and sob loudly. "That woman! She'll get to live the sort of life with Bob that I'd always dreamed of. But me, I'm going to have to work the rest of my life and send my children off to strangers because of it. I'll never be able to get back to college, and it's just not fair! I have no one anymore to help me. I'm all alone and it's Bob's fault. I hate him! Why did he leave me to handle all these problems alone?"

The therapist felt that Alice had never fully accepted the divorce as final or dealt with her unrecognized feelings toward Bob. This was evidenced by her continued efforts to draw him back home through repeated requests for his advice in caring for the children and by encouraging his frequent contacts with her through the children. She was in crisis, precipitated by the news of the birth of Bob's son and the failure of her usual method of coping with her feelings toward Bob (flight from the situation). This was compounded by the stresses of moving to a new job in a new city far from her usual situational supports. She felt isolated and trapped in a situation not entirely of her own making.

Joan's sudden, unexpected injury was for Alice "the last straw." It served as a catalyst for the eruption of a rage reaction to her overwhelming feelings of frustration and anger about her current life situation. Her comment to the therapist that Mike "was getting more like his father every day" strongly suggested that her assault upon Mike was, in fact, displacement of her feelings of rage toward Bob.

The goals of intervention were to encourage Alice to explore and ventilate her unrecognized feelings about Bob and the divorce, to help her perceive the birth of Bob's new son realistically in relation to her own and her children's future, to provide her with an intellectual understanding of her psychological abuse of Mike caused by her displacement of her anger toward Bob on Mike, and to provide situational support as she learned new coping skills to deal with her new roles and responsibilities as a single parent.

Before the end of the first session, the therapist was notified that a more complete examination of Mike revealed two healed fractured ribs and a healed fracture, with no displacement, of his right shoulder. The x-ray technician told the physician that the injuries apparently had occurred at different times within the past 3 years. Alice was informed that the children would have to stay at the hospital for a few days.

Alice turned pale and began to cry. She asked the therapist, "Why? They are going to be all right, aren't they?" The therapist informed her of Mike's old injuries and asked if she knew how he had received them. She got up and began to pace the floor saying, "You don't know how difficult it is to control Mike—and Bob was never there!" The therapist asked Alice if she had beaten Mike. She looked up and replied softly, "Yes, I didn't mean to—honest—I just got so frustrated with him." It was decided that an immediate priority for her and for the children would be to provide her with situational support in her home as soon as possible. The purpose was to ensure protection of the children against any possible further physical abuse and to provide Alice with emotional support until she was better able to cope with the stresses of developing new social networks and adjusting to her new environment. She was given the telephone number and name of a woman who held weekly self-help support group meetings for parents who abuse their children. She was strongly encouraged to call as soon as she returned home, and she stated that she would.

The therapist explored with Alice the possibility of her having a friend or relative visit for a few weeks. Alice strongly agreed with this idea, admitting that she was fearful of being alone with the children because "I might blow up again if they make me angry. I'm just not sure how much more I can handle right now."

She decided to telephone her mother and added in a very depressed tone of voice: "It's for sure there is no point in calling Bob. He'll be much too busy with his new family to help me now." She called her mother from the therapist's office, briefly explained her need for help, and asked her to come for a few weeks. Her mother agreed immediately and promised to be there the next afternoon. Before leaving for home, Alice commented, "You know, suddenly I don't feel quite so alone. Maybe after I call that lady when I get home, I can just fall into bed and get some sleep for a change."

When Alice returned for her second session a week later, she appeared much more relaxed and less depressed. She said her mother had arrived just as the children came home from the hospital. "Never in my life have I been so glad to see my mother! She has been very helpful, and I never expected her to be so understanding." She had also attended one of the self-help group meetings.

Alice was particularly surprised by her mother's empathy when they discussed Alice's many problems since the divorce. Until then she hadn't realized that her mother, too, had had many of the same feelings and problems after she and Alice's father had divorced. She added that the children really enjoyed having their grandmother around and "have been behaving just like angels—I can't believe that Mike has quit bugging me all of the time."

During this session and the next two, through direct questioning and reflection, Alice began to recognize her present crisis as a reflection of her past unrealistic perception of her divorce and Bob's subsequent marriage. Throughout her marriage, she had always seen herself as being expected to assume the role of a strong, independent decision maker so Bob could be free of family problems to devote his full attention to his law studies. She recalled that he had often commented to her and to their friends that his law degree should really have both their names on it.

When asked if she had ever discussed these feelings with Bob, she said that she had tried to at first, but he would get so angry with her and "shout and storm out of the house" that she soon learned that it was easier for her not to argue back. With continued questioning and reflection, Alice gradually began to recognize how, unable to confront Bob directly with her feelings of frustration and anger, she had made Mike a scapegoat for her unhappiness. She had perceived Mike as the cause of arguments with Bob, and therefore it was Mike who she felt deserved to be punished. She seemed surprised with the realization that his behavior problems with other children possibly were his reaction to being scapegoated and abused at home. On further reflection, she expressed concern for its effect on his future relationships with her and with others. At the therapist's suggestion, she agreed to consider seeking a psychological evaluation and, if necessary, counseling for Mike.

She recalled that the year after Bob's graduation had been an unusually happy one for them. They had felt so optimistic about their future that they decided it would be a good time to have another child.

As things turned out, however, Bob's practice didn't do as well as anticipated, and Alice had to continue to work throughout her pregnancy. By the time Joan was born, their marriage had greatly deteriorated. They no longer seemed able to communicate anything but their anger and frustration toward each other. Bob began to spend most of his time away from home, and, when he finally suggested that they divorce, it seemed the only solution left for their problems.

When questioned directly, Alice admitted to the therapist how much she now regretted the divorce. She added that she always believed that Bob felt the same way, too. It was apparent to the therapist that Alice had still held hopes that Bob would return to her some day, despite his remarriage. His frequent visits with the children, even after his remarriage, had served to reinforce this belief in her mind. It was only when she heard that his new wife was pregnant that she began to experience some doubts and anxiety.

During the third session, through direct confrontation and reflection on her feelings about this news, she suddenly exclaimed, "Betrayed! That's how I felt when I heard the news. I felt like a betrayed wife, angry that he had done such a thing to me and our children. All of a sudden it came to me that, now, he couldn't just pack up and come back to us, even if he wanted to. Some way, I felt, I just had to get away. I just didn't want to be there to see him with a new family. If I stayed, I was sure that my life could never be peaceful again." As soon as she made that last comment, she gave a surprised laugh and said, "Did you hear what I just said? I was acting just like I did during our marriage. I was trying to keep peace by getting out of the situation—by taking a walk, or something like that. Well, I certainly took a walk, didn't I? All the way down to this city!"

She now realized that her choice of flight as a means of coping had indeed proved ineffective in that Bob's new son was born 2 days before she moved. At that time, she had regarded her overwhelming feelings of tension and anxiety as normal for anyone moving away from familiar friends and places. She had avoided any discussion of her feelings with anyone, afraid that she might have to discuss how she felt about Bob's new baby. She behaved as though she was much too busy with packing and moving arrangements to visit with friends.

After the move, she found herself isolated from any situational supports. She avoided telephoning Bob or friends, again using the excuse that she was too busy.

As her tension and anxiety increased, she soon felt too physically and emotionally exhausted to do more than feed the children their meals and try to keep them from interfering with the unpacking. After a deep pause, she said, "You know, when I look back, I must have been like a time bomb waiting to explode. I realize now that this wasn't the first time I'd ever felt that way. Perhaps it was easier, then, to just take a walk and get away for a while. That way it was easy to avoid dealing with the real cause of my anger—Bob. It was always much easier to talk *at Bob through Mike's problems than to* Bob about our problems!"

Providing immediate situational support while encouraging Alice to identify and ventilate her unrecognized feelings about Bob had assisted her in viewing the recent events in her life more realistically.

By the fourth week, Alice had made a good adjustment to her new job and was enjoying it very much. She had made several new friends and said that she was really enjoying time spent with her children at home. She said that she had even called Bob and congratulated him on the birth of his new son. An excellent day nursery had been found for Joan, and she had also located an after-school play group for Mike where he could be supervised until she got home from work in the evening.

As suggested by the therapist, she and Mike had visited the guidance counselor at Mike's new school and planned to meet with him regularly until Mike adjusted to the many new changes in his life. Even more important, and on her own, she had decided to attend meetings for divorced single parents that were held regularly at a nearby YMCA, as well as continuing with the self-help group.

Reflecting back on her marriage in the final session, Alice summed it up by saying, "Maybe we'd have never married if I hadn't become pregnant. But that was never Mike's fault, and I never should have blamed him when things went wrong. It's Bob and I who are to blame. I'll never know if things might have been different if we had been able to wait longer, but I guess I always will believe that I gave up much more of my life than Bob did to keep it going as well as it did. My anger is with Bob, though. It's not with Mike. I realize now why I felt so angry and frustrated when we divorced. All that I could see was Bob being completely free to start a new life all over again. He never seemed to show any regrets about leaving me and the kids behind. I guess I'd hoped that he would feel guilty, or something, and come back to us."

Most important, Alice was able to obtain an intellectual understanding of the relationship between her pent-up feelings and her displaced rage reaction toward Mike. She told the therapist that, if nothing else, she would always remember those moments and was quite positive it would never happen again, "even if I have to stand out in the street and scream until I feel better!"

Before termination, Alice and the therapist reviewed and assessed the adjustments that she had made and the insights that she had gained into her behavior. Alice was very optimistic about the future, both for herself and for the children. She was assured

CASE STUDY: ALICE

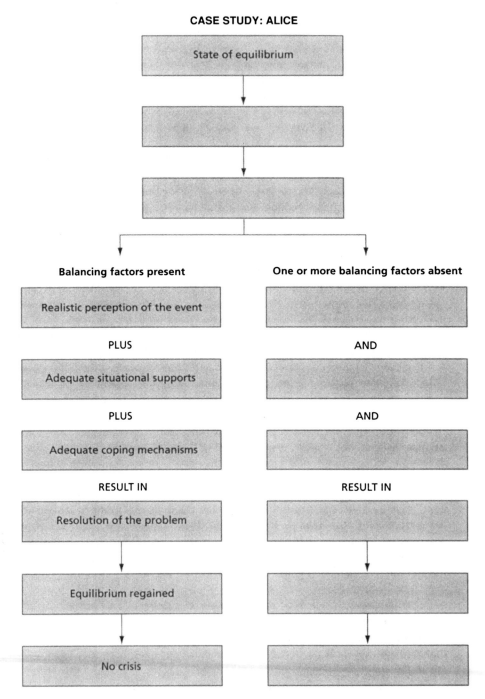

Figure 6-1

that she could always contact the therapist if she ever began to feel overwhelmed by problems again.

A simple child,
That lightly draws its breath
And feels its life in every limb,
What should it know of death?

—William Wordsworth

Complete the paradigm in Figure 6-1 for this case study, then compare it with the completed one in Appendix D. Refer to the paradigms in Chapter 3 as needed.

Violence in the Home

This may seem to be a very broad term—"violence in the home." The word *home* encompasses not only the nuclear family, but also those who *live* there. What is the interaction and action that occurs between them, and what are their responses?

Children may live in the home. The first part of this chapter was devoted to the staggering facts and figures on child abuse and neglect. Parents live in the home. How do they interact with each other *and* with their children?

Are there other members outside of the nuclear family living in the home, for example, a relative, perhaps an aunt or uncle? How do they fit in the family constellation? Are they members who give help and support to other family members? Do they create stress in the basic family unit by intruding (unintentionally) into the family's private territorial "space"?

Is there a grandmother and/or grandfather living with the family? Are they healthy, supportive, and helpful? Do they have physical or psychological problems and create more of a burden than a help?

Let's consider just a nuclear family. Is it stable or are there problems that create instability? Every family has occasional disagreements; no one is perfect. If communication is open and a husband and wife are able to sit down and discuss what is creating stress between them and if both are willing to listen and compromise, then they should be able to reach an understanding and solve their problem. Unfortunately this does not always happen.

Until approximately 25 years ago there was no such term as *battered women.* Men were expected to keep women in their place by whatever means necessary, and if it took battering, she had better shape up. In recent years, however, physical abuse has been dragged from the closet with books, television films, and well-publicized court cases like Hedda Nussbaum's, whose spouse Joel Steinberg, an attorney, not only brutally battered her but also killed their daughter in 1989. Research findings have also given women new awareness and, as a result, new strength to resist battering (Miller, 1995).

- According to former Surgeon General C. Everett Koop, battering is the single major cause of injury to women and is greater than accidents, rape, and muggings combined.

Box 6-3
DOES YOUR PARTNER ...

Hit, punch, slap, shove, or bite you?
Threaten to hurt you or your children?
Threaten to hurt friends or family members?
Have sudden outbursts of anger or rage?
Behave in an overprotective manner?
Become jealous without reason?
Prevent you from seeing family or friends?
Prevent you from going where you want, when you want?
Prevent you from working or attending school?
Destroy personal property or sentimental items?
Deny you access to family assets such as bank accounts, credit cards, or the car?
Control all finances and force you to account for what you spend?
Force you to engage in sexual acts you do not enjoy?
Insult you or call you derogatory names?
Use intimidation or manipulation to control you or your children?
Humiliate you in front of your children?
Turn minor incidents into major arguments?
Abuse or threaten to abuse pets?

- FBI figures indicate that a woman is beaten every 15 seconds.
- Twenty-one percent of the women who use hospital emergency surgical services are battered.
- As many as 4000 women are beaten to death annually by a family member—about one third of all female homicide victims.
- Fifty-nine percent of the women who killed a so-called loved one were abused at the time.
- In one half of all marriages there is at least one violent incident; in almost one third the violence is severe (Dutton, 1995).

Physical battering in all its enormity and horror is no longer a secret. Nonphysical battering, however, remains in the dark closet where few want to look. The Battered Women's Task Force of the New York State Coalition Against Domestic Violence, along with organizations in other states, has made great strides in helping women identify nonphysical abuse so as to offer support and guidance. The first step is to ask women to answer the questions that identify abusive behaviors (Box 6-3).

If they answered *yes to one or more* of these questions, they might be abused. Note that only *one* of the nineteen behaviors is physical. The other eighteen identify four different kinds of nonphysical battering (Miller, 1995).

Abuse seldom, if ever, goes away of its own accord; it escalates. Name-calling grows into public humiliation, isolation, and eventually threats, at which level a union may continue "until death do us part," or the threats may become the reality of beatings and eventually murder.

VIOLENCE IN "NEW" FAMILIES

Until fairly recently, the term "battered wife" has been the operative term. But life is a continuous process of change. When gays and lesbians came out of the closet, slowly, and then more rapidly (due to some degree to HIV and other sexually transmitted diseases), the concept of "family" changed. Gays living together for years were a family. Lesbians living together were a family. Their living together and rearing children constituted a cohesive family unit. The children may be theirs from a previous commitment, through adoption, or by artificial insemination.

Before continuing with the theoretical concepts of the current thinking of family violence, these "new" families should be considered. How are they functioning as a family? If errors are made when using the term "battered wife," patience and understanding is requested. There is so little research literature available at this time. It is certain that this field of research is fertile land for those who understand, accept, and realize that gays and lesbians, and their families, are here to stay.

Unfortunately the traditional nuclear family has no monopoly on violence. In 1996 Hawaii became the first state to grant permission for gay and lesbian couples to marry, legally. Although sexual orientation has little impact on the frequency of domestic violence, it can strongly affect how and when society intervenes. The Los Angeles Gay and Lesbian Center has embarked on an expanded program to publicize and help prevent gay domestic violence (Hanania, 1996). New terminology is now required. Instead of "battered wife," the terms that are more accurate and appropriate are *spousal abuse,* or *domestic abuse,* thus eliminating any gender bias.

A straight woman fleeing domestic violence may seek a women-only shelter that bars her batterer. A lesbian fleeing domestic violence may seek the same shelter only to find her batterer there, too. A straight man trying to escape his wife's explosive temper can usually walk away safely. A gay male trying to walk away from his partner may find himself physically threatened. Should he manage to leave and ask to be placed in a shelter, he might, instead, be referred to a mental hospital or to a homeless shelter, where his lover could seek him out.

Although a straight woman fleeing her batterer can reasonably count on police protection, a gay person often cannot. Rather, police often view same-sex domestic violence as either a manifestation of "boys will be boys" or a "cat fight" and sometimes do little to ensure the victim's safety. Police protection for battered victims remains separate and unequal, depending on sexual orientation.

This is the hidden world of gay domestic violence, a world all the more dangerous because many people, both straight and gay, would rather ignore it. And yet among both groups, 25% to 33% of all relationships may be marred by sometimes lethal physical violence. Susan Holt, program coordinator of the Los Angeles Gay and Lesbian Center, states that there are an estimated 1 million gay and lesbian battered victims nationwide.

To combat this violence, Holt has expanded the center's program, which counsels 250 people a month. Most important, the center offers a counseling program staffed by seventy-five volunteers, both men and women, trained in how the dynamics of domestic violence are intensified by homophobia.

Batterers may threaten to "out" their victims to family and friends, preventing escape. They may threaten to reveal victims' HIV status to employers, jeopardizing their jobs, or they may threaten to cut their victims off financially, leaving them penniless. Batterers also seek both to intimidate their partners and to undermine their emotional and spiritual well-being. Their goal is control, virtually telling their partners, "I can make you do anything I want."

Because victims frequently fail in their attempts to escape, Holt frequently advises victims that their safest short-term course may be to stay with the abuser, albeit with protective measures. These measures include keeping an extra car key and spare change in a jacket pocket by the door. They also include leaving a bag of emergency supplies at a friend's home, scouting out the closest pay phone or all-night convenience store, and putting sharp objects in hard-to-reach places.

The center's program also helps batterers—who are referred by the courts or join on their own—to explore how their conduct pushes away their lovers, adding to batterers' isolation and self-hatred. Participating in therapy groups, abusers explore the causes of their behavior and develop alternative ways of acting out their anger.

Finally, the center is reaching out to traditional anti-domestic violence programs, with volunteers informing their mainstream counterparts of the often unique circumstances faced by gay victims.

DYNAMICS OF VIOLENCE IN THE HOME

Battering involves a pattern of escalating abuse in a situation from which the victim believes he cannot escape. Because they are usually physically stronger than their spouse, men are less likely to be battered. Often a battered spouse has grown up with violence and accepts it as a pitiful form of caring or at least as something inevitable in a relationship. She may believe that the world is a dangerous place and that she needs a protector, even a spouse who beats her. Ashamed, terrified that any resistance will provoke greater violence, isolated from her family and friends, often without any means of support other than her spouse, many a battered spouse sinks into despairing submission from which the only escape is eventual widowhood, her own murder (or her husband's), or suicide.

Doctors, social workers, and psychiatrists have frequently been less helpful than the police. Straus (1980), in a study of family violence, concluded that the medical profession and social agencies are an essential part of the battered syndrome. They often treat the spouses like they are "crazy"; physicians fail to note signs of abuse, label battered spouses as psychotic or hypochondriacal, prescribe tranquilizers, and tell them to go home. They make battered spouses doubt their own sanity by sending them to a family therapist for psychotherapy.

What kind of person would hit a spouse—not only hit her but also blacken her eyes, break the bones in her face, beat her breasts, kick her abdomen, and menace her with a gun? There is a very good chance that he was beaten as a child. Perhaps because of his early trauma, he is often emotionally stunted. An interesting analogy exists between a male batterer and a 2- or 3-year-old child; their tantrums are very similar. Like a narcissistic child, the batterer bites when throwing a tantrum.

The spouse beater probably drinks, but he does not beat because he drinks; rather, he drinks to beat. Unemployment does not cause battering, but hard times make it worse. The typical spouse beater is unable to cope with the traditional notion of masculinity, or the male role, which requires men to be stoic. It requires men not to need intimacy, to be in control, to be the "big wheel," and when there is a problem, to "give 'em hell." The difficulty is that nine of ten men fail at that list, at least in their own judgment. The batterer is often afflicted with extreme insecurity. The man's spouse is the emotional glue that holds him together, and, as a consequence, he is desperately afraid of losing her. The husband is trying to make her be closer to him by controlling her physically, but he does not realize that he is driving her away (O'Reilly, 1983).

Batterers can be very calculating in how they deal with their spouses and with the authorities once they are caught. They are frequently charming to a fault. They can play therapy off against the court system and not have to be responsible.

The first self-help group for abusive men was formed in Boston in 1977. There are now about 85 such groups. Very few men go to such centers on their own. Either their partner has left or is threatening to, or they are attending under court order. By and large, they do not believe they have done anything wrong, sometimes insisting they are not batterers at all. Those who own up to being violent frequently believe their partners are at fault.

Historically, batterers have fallen between the cracks and were considered neither crazy nor criminal, at least by the standards of the day. A man beats up his spouse because he can. He usually does not beat up his boss or male acquaintances; the consequences—loss of job, a charge of criminal assault, immediate physical retaliation—are simply too great. Now, the consequences are rising for violence against one's spouse. Shelters for abused women have created a safety net for spouses who previously would have been afraid to take their husbands to court. Newspapers, judges, hospitals, neighbors, and even a growing number of once exasperated police officers are beginning to understand the dimensions of the problem. More important, states and municipalities are enacting laws that give women a realistic chance of getting protection and redress through the courts.

The tightening of laws against spouse beating has resulted in higher conviction rates. Still, only a fraction of abusive husbands are even reported to the authorities, much less arrested and convicted. For the glib, angry men who pummel their spouses, a brush with the law sometimes has a sobering effect. In general, arrests work because they show the man that such behavior is inappropriate. They also show the spouse that somebody will help her.

The following case study of a battered spouse illustrates how women who have been repeatedly beaten by their husbands assume, although incorrectly, that they "deserve it." The crisis represented below was precipitated when a young woman was hospitalized with serious injuries.

Case Study   *Battered Spouse*

Suzan, a 39-year-old housewife and mother of two daughters (Karen, age 15, and Leslie, age 12), was admitted to a large metropolitan hospital. Her husband, Ron, age 43, drove her to the emergency room and stated that she had "fallen down the stairs at home." When asked by the resident the name of their family physician, Ron casually shrugged his shoulders and said, "We don't have one." The resident asked permission to call in an internist and an orthopedic specialist because he believed that Suzan was badly injured.

The resident ordered x-rays for Suzan "from head to toe" and then contacted an internist and orthopedist and told them he suspected a possible case of spouse beating. Both physicians stated they would be at the hospital within 30 minutes to see the x-rays and Suzan. Suzan went through the series of x-rays and was admitted to the hospital.

The internist, Dr. W, and the orthopedist, Dr. V, looked at the x-rays with a sense of shock and disbelief. Suzan's current injuries included two black eyes, two fractures in the pelvic girdle, and two fractured ribs. The x-rays also revealed past injuries: four fractured ribs, fractures of the left wrist and left arm in two places, and fractures of the right ankle.

The two physicians went to Suzan's room, introduced themselves, and asked Suzan if they could sit down. Suzan's blackened eyes were almost swollen shut, but both physicians could see the fear in her eyes as she looked past them to see if her husband was with them. Dr. W ordered no visitors for Suzan, including family, unless they had the permission of one of the doctors. Suzan appeared to relax slightly.

During the taking of her medical history, Suzan stated that she had no previous injuries. Dr. W then casually asked Suzan how she had sustained her present injuries. Suzan responded quickly, "I tripped and fell down the stairs at home."

Dr. V told her about her current injuries, stating that they were quite extensive for a fall down a flight of stairs. Dr. V then told Suzan that she would have to stay in the hospital from 4 to 6 weeks for the fractures in her pelvic girdle to heal. Suzan gasped and repeated, "Four to six weeks! What about my daughters? They need me!" Dr. V asked, "Don't you have family that could stay with them?" Suzan replied, "My mother would love to come out and take care of them, but Ron doesn't get along with her."

The doctors explained the extent of Suzan's injuries to Ron, and then Dr. W told him that Suzan's mother would be called to take care of their daughters. Dr. W called Suzan's mother, who, when told of her daughter's injuries, commented that Ron had probably beaten her again. Her mother made arrangements to be at the hospital the next morning.

Dr. W then faced Suzan with her mother's accusation that Ron had beaten her in the past; Suzan denied this. After discussing the case, Dr. W and Dr. V decided to call in a psychotherapist with experience in dealing with battered wives.

The clinical psychologist called in to assist believed that he would have to work with Suzan's mother and her two daughters to break through Suzan's denial. The first step would be to confront Suzan with the x-rays that clearly showed the previous injuries and to demand an explanation. He would use Suzan's mother's statement that Ron had "beaten her many times before" as leverage against Suzan's denial. He would plan to see the daughters alone to see if they would admit that their father had abused their mother in the past, as well as in the most recent "accident." The second step would be to get Suzan to realize that other women had been battered by their spouses and that it was not her fault that she had been beaten. She had to be made to view the events in a realistic manner. The third step was to get situational support for Suzan and have her talk with other wives who had been battered and hear how they had coped with their situations. The fourth step would be to tell Suzan about the facilities that were available for battered spouses and about the therapeutic groups her husband could attend with other men who had battered their spouses.

The next morning Suzan was introduced to the psychotherapist and told that one of his areas of expertise was working with battered spouses. The therapist showed Suzan all her old fractures on the x-rays. He asked her when and how she had received them and told Suzan that he would ask her mother and her daughters if she did not answer. Then, the therapist sat back in his chair and waited in silence as Suzan began to cry. As Suzan continued to cry, occasionally he handed her more tissues but said nothing. Finally Suzan asked, "Aren't you going to say something?" The therapist replied, "No. It's time for you to answer my questions." (Because most individuals have difficulty coping with silence, it can be a very effective technique in psychotherapy—if the therapist can handle it.)

Suzan finally commented that none of the other doctors had ever asked her any questions, and the therapist asked her to start at the beginning. Suzan began by saying, "I know Ron loves me and I love him. You'll see, I'll probably receive a dozen yellow roses today with a card asking me to forgive him. And I will, I always do. I probably deserve to be beaten. I am not a good wife or mother."

Suzan continued, "It really is my fault. Ron didn't want to get married, but I got careless and ended up pregnant. Ron wanted me to have an abortion, but I refused. I just couldn't. I'm Catholic, but Ron isn't, so we got married. Karen was born 7 months after we were married. I loved him so much, and I really believed that he loved me." She said he was a good husband and a very good father. "I had no experience in taking care of a house, husband, or a baby. I didn't even know how to cook—thank heavens, someone gave me a good cookbook when we got married. I still can't iron his shirts to suit him. I have truly been a failure. You see, I was an only child and my mother and father spoiled me rotten. I never had to do anything around the house."

The first time Ron had hit her was after they had been married about 2 years because she had burned the dinner. She said she had been taking care of Karen, who had a fever, and completely forgot the roast in the oven. When Ron came home, she was rocking Karen trying to get her to sleep. He walked into Karen's room and said very coldly, "Put the baby in her crib and come with me." Suzan put Karen down, and Ron grabbed her by the arm and pulled her into the kitchen. He had taken the roast out of the oven. It was burned to a crisp, and the kitchen was filled with smoke. Ron said, "Do you think money grows on trees?" and he slapped her. Then he just kept hitting her. She said, "I begged him not to, but he just kept punching me. Finally, he stopped, probably because he was tired, but that is when I received my first black eye. So, you see, I did deserve it. It was my fault." The therapist told Suzan she did *not* deserve that beating and asked if the beatings continued. Suzan said that she "just couldn't seem to please him. He didn't like the way I ironed his shirts—that's when he broke my ribs. If I didn't season the food to his liking, another beating. Almost anything I did wrong ended up with his beating me. That's why we have never had just one doctor, he would take me to a different one or to a different emergency room every time."

The therapist asked Suzan if Ron drank much. She said that he usually had a couple of beers, maybe more occasionally. The therapist asked her if she could remember if he usually had been drinking when he beat her. She replied, "Yes, yes, I remember; every time he beat me, he had been drinking. He wasn't drunk, you understand. Even last night he had been drinking!" She asked, "Do you think his drinking makes him beat me?" The therapist answered, "Not really. Although he drinks to beat you, he doesn't beat you because he drinks."

The therapist asked about Ron's family. Suzan said that she really did not know them, and Ron wasn't very close to them. His father was apparently a violent man who had beaten his three sons and his wife. She continued, saying that Ron's father was an alcoholic and that his mother had died 5 years ago. The therapist told Suzan that because Ron's father had beaten him and his mother, he considered this acceptable behavior between a husband and wife.

The therapist explained to Suzan that shelters had been established for battered women and their children and that therapy groups had been formed for men who battered their spouses. The therapist then asked if he could have a woman who lived in one of the facilities come and talk to her. Suzan said that she would like very much to talk to someone who had been through what she had been through. The therapist told Suzan he would arrange it as soon as possible. He reminded her that she was safe in the hospital, but she must seriously think about whether she wanted to return home to more beatings or go with her daughters to one of the facilities.

As Suzan had predicted, Ron sent her roses and asked for her forgiveness. At the same time the flowers came, Suzan's mother arrived at the hospital, and the therapist left so that Suzan and her mother could talk. When he returned, they had decided that Suzan would divorce Ron and she and her daughters would move to Chicago and live with Suzan's parents. Suzan called Ron to come to the hospital so she could tell him of her decisions.

When Ron arrived, Suzan very quickly told him that she wanted a divorce and that she and the girls would be moving. At first, Ron was shocked and briefly tried to change her mind. He became angry with Suzan's mother, who he assumed was responsible for Suzan's unexpected actions. At this point, the therapist ushered Ron from the room and offered to talk with him later about his problems concerning his beating Suzan. Ron said he would call in a few days and then left the hospital.

Ron never called, but the therapist continued to see Suzan every few days until she was discharged in the fifth week. She fairly blossomed under the loving care of her mother. She filed for divorce, with no protest from Ron. Her daughters were delighted at the thought of moving to Chicago to live with their grandparents. They admitted they were terrified of their father and had been afraid of saying anything to anyone. They said he had moved out of the house because he could not stand being around their grandmother.

Suzan had been made to feel totally inadequate as a wife and mother. She had led a very sheltered life until her marriage and had no experience in keeping a home or caring for children. She felt that she deserved the beatings by her husband, and she was too embarrassed and ashamed to let anyone know that she was a battered spouse. She had an unrealistic perception of the event. Her only situational supports were her family, who lived in another state. She had no adequate coping mechanisms. Her

CASE STUDY: SUZAN

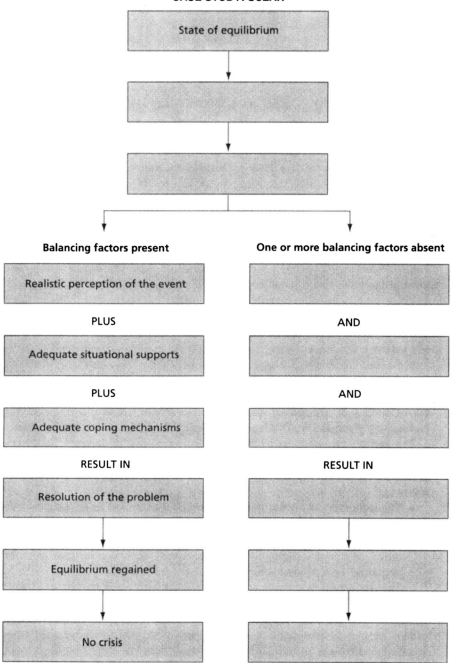

State of equilibrium

Balancing factors present

Realistic perception of the event

PLUS

Adequate situational supports

PLUS

Adequate coping mechanisms

RESULT IN

Resolution of the problem

Equilibrium regained

No crisis

One or more balancing factors absent

AND

AND

RESULT IN

Figure 6-2

injuries from the last beating were so extensive that she was unable to deny her fear of her husband and thus entered a state of crisis.

Nothing vivifies,
and nothing kills
like emotions.

–Joseph Roux

Complete the paradigm in Figure 6-2 for this case study, then compare it with the completed one in Appendix D. Refer to the paradigms in Chapter 3 as needed.

Violence in the Schools

The problem of violence in schools, which is part of the overall problem of violence in society, has become one of the most pressing issues in the United States. In many school districts, concerns about violence have even surpassed academic achievement—traditionally the most persistent theme on the nation's educational agenda—as the high-test priority for reform and intervention (Noguera, 1995). Public clamorings over the need to do something about violence in schools has brought the issue to a critical juncture; if schools fail to respond decisively to this problem, popular support for public education may be endangered. The escalation of violent incidents and the apparent inadequacy of traditional methods to curtail them has led to a search for new strategies to ensure the safety and security of children and teachers in schools (Toby, 1993/1994).

Accepting the fact that it may not be realistic to expect that schools can ever be completely immune from the violence that plagues society, this section seeks to understand why schools may be especially vulnerable to its occurrence. Current efforts aimed at combating violence may, in fact, have the opposite effect, particularly given the weakening of the moral authority schools once enjoyed.

The search for solutions to the problem of violence in schools has generated measures that closely resemble those used to combat the threat of violence and crime in U.S. society (Currie, 1994). Some of the more popular measures include the following:

- The installation of metal detectors at school entrances to prevent students from bringing weapons onto school grounds.
- The enactment of "zero tolerance" policies that guarantee the automatic removal of students (through either suspension, expulsion, or transfer) who perpetrate acts of violence.
- The use of police officers and security guards to patrol and monitor student behavior while school is in session (Kemper, 1993).

Accompanying such measures has been an increased tendency of school officials to treat violent incidents (and sometimes nonviolent incidents) involving students as criminal offenses to be handled by law enforcement officials and the courts, rather than by school personnel. In their desire to demonstrate toughness and reassure the public that they are in control, school officials have become increasingly rigid and inflexible when meting out punishment on students who violate school rules, even when the infractions are not of a violent nature (Davila, 1995; Freed, 1994).

Other less punitive approaches have been introduced to reduce the incidence of violence in schools. Conflict resolution programs have been promoted as a way of teaching children to settle disputes nonviolently. Mentoring programs that pair students with adult role models have also become popular in school districts across the country, serving to reduce violence by proving students perceived to be at risk with the attention, support, and counseling of an adult (McPartland and Nettles, 1991). Teachers have been encouraged to design curricula that teach children how to avoid violent situations and to explore in their classrooms the ethical and moral issues related to violent behavior. Finally, a variety of counseling programs has been implemented by establishing partnerships between schools and social service agencies to provide direct services to students.

Though some of these less coercive strategies for reducing violence have proven relatively successful in particular schools, the overall momentum of school policy has been biased in favor of the "get-tough" approach.

The phrase "fighting violence" might seem to be an oxymoron. For those concerned with finding ways to prevent or reduce the occurrence of violence, "fighting" it might seem to be the wrong way to describe or to engage in the effort to address the problem. The choice of terms, however, is not accidental. The prevailing wisdom among policymakers and school officials is that violence must be countered with force; that schools can be made safe by converting them into prisonlike facilities, and that the best way to curtail violence is to identify, apprehend, and exclude students who have the potential for committing acts of violence from the rest of the population (Noguera, 1995).

Within the context of the fight against violence, symbols such as crime statistics take on great significance, although they have little bearing on how people actually feel about the occurrence of violence. Pressed to demonstrate to the public that the efforts to reduce violence are effective, school districts often pursue one of two strategies: either they present statistics quantifying the results of their efforts or they go to great lengths to suppress information altogether, hoping that the community will perceive no news is good news (Nemeth, 1993). Metal detectors, barbed wire fences, armed guards and policemen, and principals wielding baseball bats as they patrol the halls are all symbols of tough action. A student who wants to bring a weapon to school can get it into a building without being discovered by a metal detector, and it is highly unlikely that any principal will hit a student with a baseball bat; the symbols persist, masking the truth that those responsible for school safety really don't have a clue about what to do to stem the tide of violence. Rather than looking to solve this problem through increased security or improved technology, school administrators must begin to ask more fundamental questions as to why these institutions have become so vulnerable to violence.

DISCIPLINE AS AN EXERCISE OF POWER

With concerns about order, efficiency, and control dominating the thinking that guided the early development of schools in the United States, we must ask ourselves how this legacy has influenced the current character of public schools. As the demographics of cities began to change in the 1950s and 1960s with the arrival of new immigrants (e.g., West Indians and Puerto Ricans), and the migration of African-Americans from the South (Moynihan and Glaser, 1987) and as social and economic conditions within urban areas began to deteriorate, the character and conditions of schools also began to change. However, this shift did not produce immediate changes, for although the student population changed, in many cases the teachers remained the same, with most still relying on methods of control that had proven successful in the past (Conant, 1961). Writing about the conditions of schools in what he described as "slum areas," James B. Conant (former President of Harvard University) (1961) spoke of the need to impose a harsher standard of discipline to ensure that discipline and order prevailed:

Many educators would doubtless be shocked by the practice of on-the-spot demotion of one full academic year, with no questions asked, for all participants in fights. In one junior high school I know of, a very able principal found so intolerable a situation that very rule. As a consequence, there are fewer fights in his school among boys, many whom at one time or another have been in trouble with the police. The school must attempt to bring some kind of order to their chaotic lives. . . . This formal atmosphere appears to work. School spirit has developed. . . . Children must stay in school till they are sixteen or till graduation to prevent unemployed, out-of-school youth from roaming the streets (Conant, 1961, p. 22).

By the mid 1960s, however, the situation had changed. Students' insubordination and aggression toward teachers were becoming increasingly common, and violence within schools, especially among students, was widely seen as the norm (Metz, 1978). Some educators made the connection between the difficulty schools were having in maintaining control over students and the political turmoil that accompanied the civil rights movement and the riots that took place in many cities across the country. Describing the political dimension of this problem and advising teachers about how to respond to it, Allan Ornstein (1972) wrote:

Some Negro children have newly gained confidence, as expressed in the social revolution sweeping across the country. Some see themselves as leaders, and not helpless, inferior youngsters. This new pride is evidenced by their tendency to challenge authority. The teacher should expect, encourage and channel this energy toward constructive goals.

With control and compliance increasingly difficult to obtain, many urban schools lowered their expectations with respect to student behavior. The preoccupation with enforcing rules was gradually replaced with a desire to maintain average daily attendance, since this was the key funding formula for schools. As teachers have come to realize that they cannot elicit obedience through the "terror of degradation," concerns about safety have led more of them to think twice about how to reprimand a student, lest their attempt at chastisement be taken as a challenge for a physical confrontation, for which most are unprepared.

Still, schools have not given up entirely on the goal of exercising control over students; though the task may be far more difficult now than it ever was, schools are still expected to maintain some form of order. Beyond being a threat to the personal safety of students and teachers, violence in schools challenges the authority and power of school officials. In carrying out their duties as caretakers of youth, school officials serve as both legal and symbolic representatives of state authority. With the power vested in their position, they are expected to control the behavior of those in their charge. When violence occurs with impunity, a loss of authority is exposed. Therefore the issue of violence is seldom discussed in isolation from other control issues. More often, violence is equated with insubordination, student misconduct, and the general problem of maintaining order in school. The way the issues become melded together is indicative of how schools perceive their role in relation to the social control function that schools have historically performed in the United States.

ALTERNATIVE APPROACHES TO SCHOOL VIOLENCE PREVENTION

The approach to discipline that is most widely practiced in the United States today is due to the fact that many teachers and students have been victims of violence and deserve the right to work at and attend safe schools. In many schools, violence is real, and the fear that it produces is understandable. In some classrooms teachers are working effectively with their students, and fear is not an obstacle to dialogue or even friendship; however, other teachers in the school may be preoccupied with managing their students' behavior, an endeavor at which they are seldom successful. The same students may enter other classrooms willing to learn and comply with their teacher's instructions.

Many of these "exceptional" teachers have to "cross borders" and negotiate differences of race, class, or experience to establish rapport with their students (Giroux, 1992). "Border crossing" is a phrase coined by Henry Giroux to describe the personal transformation experienced by teachers and students engaged in critical discourse and pedagogy. He writes (Giroux, 1992, p. 169):

Critical educators take up culture as a vital source for developing a politics of identity, community and pedagogy. Culture is not monolithic or unchanging, but is a site of multiple and heterogeneous borders where different histories, languages, experiences, and voices intermingle amidst diverse relations of power and privilege. Within this pedagogical borderland known as school, subordinate cultures push against and permeate the alleged nonproblematic and homogeneous borders of the dominant cultural forms and practices. . . . Radical educators must provide conditions for students to speak so that their narratives can be affirmed.

When students are asked what makes a particular teacher "special" and worthy of respect, students consistently cite three characteristics: firmness; compassion; and an interesting, engaging, and challenging teaching style. Of course, even a teacher who is perceived as exceptional by students can be a victim of violence, particularly because of its increasingly random occurrence. Some teachers confront student institutions that others would not dare to engage, boldly breaking up fights or dice games, or confronting a rude and disrespectful student, without showing the slightest bit of apprehension or fear (Noguera, 1995).

There are a variety of ways in which to humanize school environments and thereby reduce the potential for violence. Improving the aesthetic character of schools by including art in the design of schools or by making space available within schools for students to create gardens or greenhouses can make schools more pleasant and attractive. Similarly, by overcoming the divide that separates urban schools from the communities in which schools are located, the lack of adults who have authority and respect in the eyes of children can be addressed. Adults who live within the community can be encouraged to volunteer or, if possible, be paid to tutor, teach, mentor, perform, or just plain help out with a variety of school activities. These examples are meant to begin a discussion of alternative practices for building humane school communities. There are undoubtedly a variety of ways this can be done, and although such efforts may not eliminate the threat of random violence, they can help to make schools safer, less impersonal, and better able to provide students with a sense of stability in their lives.

The goal of maintaining social control through the use of force and discipline has persisted for too long. Although past generations could be made to accept the passivity and constraint such practices engender, present generations will not. Most urban youth today are neither passive nor compliant. The rewards that are dangled before them, such as a decent job and material wealth for those who do well in school, are seen by too many as either undesirable or unattainable. New strategies for proving an education that is perceived as meaningful, and relevant, and that begins to tap into the intrinsic desire of all individuals to obtain greater personal fulfillment must be devised and supported. Anything short of this will leave us mired in a situation that grows increasingly depressing and dangerous every day.

The urban schools that feel safe to those who spend their time there don't have metal detectors or armed security guards, and their principals don't carry baseball bats. What these schools do have is a strong sense of community and collective responsibility. Such schools are seen by students as sacred territory, too special to be spoiled by crime and violence and too important to risk being excluded. Such schools are few, but their existence serves as tangible proof that there are alternatives to chaotic schools plagued by violence and controlled institutions that aim at producing docile bodies (Noguera, 1995).

The following case study illustrates how a psychotherapist of one culture can work effectively with a patient of a different culture. Not only do they have different cultures, but they also have different backgrounds, values, and ideals.

Case Study   Violence at School

Ricardo was assigned to a particular therapist at the Crisis Center because the volunteer assumed (incorrectly) that she was also Latino. The therapist met Ricardo and introduced herself and asked him to come to her office. When they reached her office, she asked him to have a seat while she looked briefly at the chart that he had completed. He had stated that his problems were "problems at school."

The therapist asked Ricardo what school he was attending. He answered with the name of an intercity school that was notorious as being the "hub" of two well-known rival gangs. The therapist asked Ricardo if he was an active member of one of the gangs. He was quiet for a few minutes, and then asked the therapist, "You aren't Latino are you?" The therapist answered, "No, but my husband is from Spain—that is why everyone assumes that I am Latino. Why do you ask Ricardo?" He answered,

"Maybe you won't be able to understand my problem." The therapist smiled, "Well, we won't know until you tell me what the problem is, will we?"

Ricardo returned her smile, "I haven't talked to anyone about this—I just don't know what to do." She replied, "Ricardo please tell me what you are so concerned about, maybe I can help and maybe I can't." He looked at the therapist intently and said, "Okay, I've got to trust someone."

Ricardo began by asking the therapist if she knew anything about the two rival gangs at his school. The therapist told him that almost everyone had heard about them. One gang was Latino, and the other was African-American. The rivalry frequently erupted into violence with fights between the two with guns and knives. Not only had some of the members been killed but also innocent bystanders. Some had been shot and killed or severely injured from cars because one of the gangs assumed, wrongly, that those in the car were members of the rival gang. She related this to Ricardo.

The therapists asked Ricardo if he was a member of the Latino gang. He answered, "No, and that is the problem!" He continued, saying that he had a friend in the gang and had overheard him talking about one of members of the other gang. He heard him say that this member was on a "hit" list and that "it" was planned for the next evening, and even where they were planning to do the "hit." He said that he had refused to become a member of the Latino gang because he did not believe that violence achieved anything. He continued by saying that he didn't want to get his friend in trouble, so he couldn't say anything to anyone at school. There were too many "snitches," so if he went to the police, someone would find out that he was the one who leaked the information of the "hit."

The therapist asked Ricardo if he had told anyone that he was coming to the Crisis Center. He answered in the negative, saying, "God no! No one must know that I've been here."

The therapist asked him if he *wanted* to let the police know about the "hit." He looked at the therapist and said, "Yes, I just don't know how I can without someone finding out." The therapist said, "Ricardo, what if I just accidently, of course, left the telephone number of a 'hot line' on my desk that would not ask you anything about yourself but that handles problems like the one you are faced with? I, of course, will not be in my office with you." She paused, "I am going to get some coffee. Would you like me to bring you some, or perhaps a soft drink?" In almost a whisper she added, "In case you want to make a telephone call while I am gone, just dial '9' for an outside line." Ricardo hesitated, "Can they trace this number?" "No, they never have in the past." He looked at her knowingly and said, "You have done this before, haven't you?" "Done what?" They exchanged glances. "Did you decide if you wanted coffee or a soft drink?" Ricardo followed her lead, "I would like a coke, if you have one." The therapist put a card from her Rolodex in the center of her desk and placed the telephone next to it. "I'll be back with my coffee and your coke in about 10 minutes, okay?" Ricardo smiled, "Thanks." She returned the smile, walked out her office, and closed the door firmly behind her.

When the therapist returned, the card had been replaced in the Rolodex and Ricardo had left her a note, "Thanks, friend. Your pal, R." He had left "no clues."

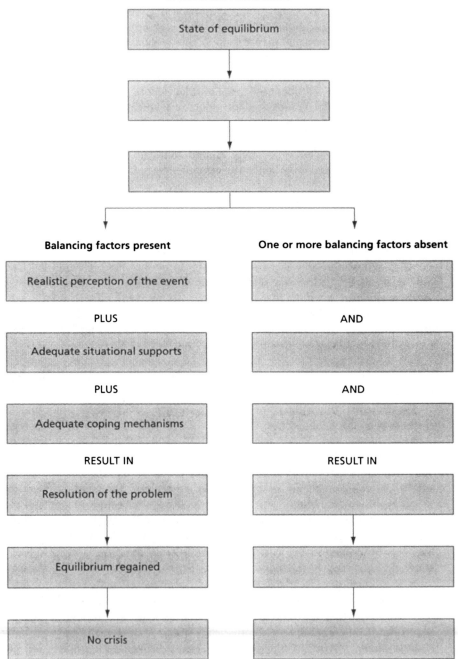

CASE STUDY: RICARDO

Figure 6-3

Ricardo was not her first experience with gangs, and she doubted it would be her last.

Violence is essentially wordless, and it can begin only where thought and rational communication have broken down.

–Mohandas K. Gandhi

Complete the paradigm in Figure 6-3 for this case study, then compare it with the completed one in Appendix D. Refer to the paradigms in Chapter 3 as needed.

Elder Abuse and Neglect

How many older people in the United States suffer in silence . . . abused, neglected, exploited and isolated, or trapped in nonfunctional bodies or by poorly functioning minds? Despite reports of "granny bashing" in the literature some 20 years ago and the fact that abuse and neglect of older people will be an increasing problem in the next century, we remain unsure of many aspects of this complex phenomenon, including its true incidence. Although frightening evidence exists that older individuals in institutions are more likely to be at risk than those living in the community, data regarding institutional abuse and neglect are so scarce that it would be impossible to make national estimates of the extent of the phenomenon. We do know, based on reports of advocacy groups, media, and a few random studies, that it exists and is not uncommon.

TYPES OF ELDER ABUSE AND NEGLECT

Abuse and neglect of older people are not uncommon. Problems of such abuse and neglect are estimated to be as widespread as child abuse and affect about 2 million older persons each year, many of whom suffer repeated episodes. Identification of abuse and neglect requires an awareness of its existence and knowledge of risk factors and signs.

Despite the fact that case reports of abused older adults appeared in the literature 20 years ago, there is still no clear and consistent definition of what constitutes abuse and neglect of older adults in the literature or the law. The term *elder mistreatment* is used by some to describe acts of commission or omission that result in harm or threatened harm to the health and welfare of older adults and refers to the suffering imposed as a result of abuse and neglect.

The manner in which mistreatment of older people is categorized varies in the literature. Categories commonly include physical abuse, physical neglect, psychological abuse, psychological neglect, financial/material abuse or exploitation, and violation of personal rights.

Physical abuse.   Physical abuse describes acts that include pushing, shaking, slapping, punching, kicking, biting, choking, using physical or chemical restraints in an inappropriate manner, force feeding, burning, or attacking with objects or weapons. Sexual abuse/exploitation is sometimes included within this category and consists of any nonconsensual sexual activity, including situations in which another is physically forced, pressured, or manipulated into sexual contact or is unable to grant informed consent. Forms of sexual abuse include verbal abuse (suggestive talk, jokes, and labeling); unwanted touching; rape; fondling; inappropriate sexual relations such as with a child or one's professional caregiver; or any other sexual activity with an older person when that person is unable to understand, unwilling to consent, physically forced, or threatened.

Psychological abuse.   Psychological abuse is an act that results in psychological distress or emotional anguish. Examples include threats, intimidation, provocation, harassment, ridicule, withholding security and affection, isolation from others, infantalization, and violation of rights.

Physical neglect.   Neglect can be defined as the failure or omission on the part of a caregiver or of oneself to provide the care and services necessary to maintain physical and mental health, including, but not limited to, food, clothing, medicine, shelter, supervision, and medical services that a prudent person would deem essential for the well-being of another. Neglect may represent repeated conduct or a single incident of carelessness that produces or could reasonably be expected to result in serious physical or mental harm or a substantial risk of death.

Neglect may be intentional or unintentional. Categories of neglect include physical neglect in which the caregiver fails to provide services and goods necessary for optimal functioning and avoidance of harm. Examples include the following:

- Failure to provide adequate nutrition and hydration
- Failure to provide physical assistance such as help with toileting or hygiene
- Withholding of medications or medical care
- Failure to provide for safety

Passive neglect is defined as the failure or refusal to fulfill a caretaker's role, excluding a conscious or intentional attempt to inflict physical or emotional distress on the elder person. Self-neglect is a controversial category recognized by some state laws and refers to the failure of an individual to provide oneself with the care and services necessary to maintain physical and mental health.

Psychological neglect.   Psychological neglect is often difficult to substantiate. Psychological neglect is defined as the failure to provide a dependent older person with social stimulation and includes leaving the person alone for long periods, failing to provide socialization or companionship, restricting access to community events, and socially or physically isolating an individual.

Financial abuse or exploitation.   Financial or material abuse, sometimes termed *exploitation,* involves the unauthorized use of an older person's money, property, or other resources for personal gain. Deceit, treachery, coercion, or intimidation may be knowingly used by a person in a position of trust and confidence to gain access to an older person's funds, assets, or property. Examples include stealing money or goods, coercing another to obtain goods or property or to change legal documents, and using another's guardianship or power of attorney for one's personal advantage. Some indicators of exploitation follow.

Unusual activity in bank accounts, such as unexplained withdrawals
Disparity between income and lifestyle
Excessive payments for services
Unusual interest by others in the older person's assets

A power of attorney given when the person is unable to understand the financial situation and in reality is unable to give valid power of attorney

Numerous unpaid bills, especially overdue rent, when someone is supposed to be paying the bills

Recent acquaintances expressing gushy, undying affection for a wealthy older person

A friend or housekeeper trying to isolate the older adult from family or friends

Violation of rights.   Violation of rights of an otherwise able older person include the following:

Failure to allow decision making

Deprivation of the right to privacy, self-determination, or to worship and vote

Verbal, sexual, physical, or mental abuse

Failure to allow participation in healthcare decisions, including refusal of treatment

Involuntary seclusion

Failure to allow full access to advocates

Inappropriate physical or chemical restraints

Physical findings indicative of possible abuse and neglect include patterns of bruising or of injuries that are morphologically similar to an object (e.g., belt marks, hand marks, lesions at the corners of the mouth indicating use of a gag, and marks left by restraints, ropes, or cords), burns, immersion injuries of extremities in a stocking/glove distribution, and unexplained fractures and falls. Sexual abuse should be suspected when findings include trauma or tenderness of genital, rectal, or mouth areas; bruising in areas of thighs, buttocks, face, and chest; gait abnormalities related to genital/anal trauma; the presence of sexually transmitted diseases in adults unable to consent to sexual activity; or fear, shame, anxiety, or other nonverbal signs of distress when receiving personal care. Other general indicators of abuse and neglect are listed in Box 6-4.

DOCUMENTATION OF ELDER ABUSE AND NEGLECT

Accurate documentation in cases of suspected abuse and neglect is crucial. Information obtained from interviews of the alleged victim, perpetrator, and witnesses should be recorded verbatim, if possible, and a detailed description of the physical examination, including injuries, functional status, and cognitive status, should be documented. Injuries must be described in detail, including size and location and, if possible, photographs of the injuries obtained. These may be invaluable in proving cases of abuse or neglect.

CHARACTERISTICS OF ABUSIVE CAREGIVERS

Characteristics of the caregiver are more predictive of an abusive situation than are victim characteristics. Johnson (1986) indicates that perpetrators of abuse commonly display psychopathology. They are dependent persons who often rely on the elderly for housing and financial and emotional support. Abusive caregivers often have had difficulties with the law, hospitalizations for psychiatric illnesses, and problems with alcohol and other drugs. They tend to have poor social and communication skills,

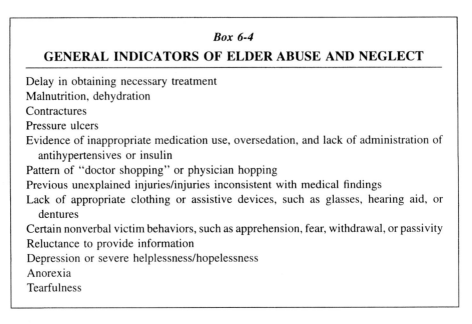

Box 6-4

GENERAL INDICATORS OF ELDER ABUSE AND NEGLECT

Delay in obtaining necessary treatment

Malnutrition, dehydration

Contractures

Pressure ulcers

Evidence of inappropriate medication use, oversedation, and lack of administration of antihypertensives or insulin

Pattern of "doctor shopping" or physician hopping

Previous unexplained injuries/injuries inconsistent with medical findings

Lack of appropriate clothing or assistive devices, such as glasses, hearing aid, or dentures

Certain nonverbal victim behaviors, such as apprehension, fear, withdrawal, or passivity

Reluctance to provide information

Depression or severe helplessness/hopelessness

Anorexia

Tearfulness

which are often reflected in their interpersonal relationships and employment histories, and may demonstrate poor emotional reserve and coping skills. Pillemer and Finkelhor (1988) summarize the profile of the abusive caregiver when they indicate that abusers do not tend to be well-meaning persons driven to abuse by the demands of another but are severely troubled individuals with histories of antisocial behaviors or instability.

Assessment protocols have been developed that concentrate on physical and behavioral symptoms of elder abuse. These protocols are focused on identifying abuse but were developed with the assumption that problems can be identified after abuse has occurred. Protective services and mandatory reporting of elder abuse resulted in the identification of potential problems (Faulkner, 1982; Salend and others, 1984). Despite these measures, elder abuse is an invisible problem. In *Elder Abuse: The Hidden Problem* (U.S. Congress, House Select Committee on Aging, 1980), it was estimated that one of every three cases of child abuse is reported, but only one of every six cases of elder abuse is reported. Several explanations for the invisibility of elder abuse reflect factors that affect both research and applied efforts.

The family is sacred, and interference with family life by outsiders is not tolerated, even when professionals believe they are justified in intervening when there are family dysfunctions. Family members may engage in a conspiracy of silence and reject attempts by outsiders to explore or intervene in their lives.

The American Medical Association (AMA) has issued its first guidelines on elder abuse, urging physicians and other healthcare professionals to be more alert to signs of mistreatment or neglect of older patients by their families or caregivers (Formica, 1992). The 42-page guidelines, part of a new AMA campaign against family violence, come amid growing national concern about a long-hidden problem in which as many as 2 million elderly Americans are believed to be victims of abuse or neglect

(Formica, 1992). Because abuse occurs within the confines of a private dwelling, it is hidden from outside scrutiny. Unlike the circumstances of children, whose abuse can be detected outside the home, there are no requirements such as school attendance and health checkups for the elderly. They do not need to leave their homes and risk being seen by non-family members.

The elderly are reluctant to report abuse by relatives. Lau and Kosberg (1979) found that one third of the elderly who were judged to have been abused denied any problem. It is not difficult to understand the reasons the elderly do not report abuse. They may believe that the problem is a family affair. They may fear reprisals by the abuser or may be embarrassed or ashamed of the behavior of the abuser. The elderly may be reluctant to initiate legal or criminal action against a relative for fear that the solution will be worse than the problem itself—institutionalization. They may believe that they are being paid back for their earlier abusive behavior toward others, such as a child or spouse.

The invisibility of elder abuse can result from the failure of professionals to detect or report the problem, even in states having mandatory reporting legislation. Although empirical verification is lacking, the reluctance on the part of professionals to report child abuse may also be a characteristic of the professional responses to mandatory reporting laws for elder abuse. It is suspected that not all professionals in states with mandatory reporting legislation are aware of their responsibility (O'Brien, 1986).

For these reasons, elder abuse often remains invisible. Community efforts, protective services, and mandatory reporting legislation affect only a fraction of the abused elderly and only after the abusive behavior has occurred. Accordingly, it is important to place frail and vulnerable elderly persons in the care of appropriate family members or other persons.

Family membership does not prevent people from engaging in abusive behavior; in fact, family members have been found to be the major perpetrators of elder abuse. The instinctive and uncritical use of family members as caregivers of vulnerable, elderly persons should not continue. A systematic assessment of the capacity of potential or present family caregivers to provide nonabusive care is needed (Kosberg, 1988).

The predominant image of elder abuse, which has been derived from earlier studies and reinforced by the popular media, is that abuse is primarily committed against the elderly by their children. The stereotype is that of a mentally and physically dependent elder who moves in with and becomes a difficult burden to a resentful daughter or son. The son or daughter, in response to frustration, lashes out or withholds certain necessities of life. Pillemer and Finkelhor (1988) found that 58% of elder abuse was committed by the victim's spouse; 24% of the abusers were the victim's children. Among elders who lived with their spouses alone, the rate of abuse was 41 per 1000. Among those who lived with their children alone, the rate was 44 per 1000. The percentage difference is because many more elderly live with their spouses than with their children. Actually, spouses do not seem inherently more violent toward their partners than children toward their parents, but spouses are more likely to be present in an elderly person's household, and thus their opportunities for abusive behavior are greater.

Elder abuse has been the most recent and most neglected form of family violence to vie for public attention. Those who have sought to gain this attention have cast the problem in its most compelling light. The image of one elderly person hitting or neglecting another does not convey the same pathos as an elderly person being abused by an adult child.

Although ample evidence of variables associated with elder abuse exists, inappropriate placements continue to result in problems for vulnerable, elderly persons. Most community programs and state legislation focus on the problem of elder abuse after it has occurred and necessitate the detection and reporting of abuse. Yet the problem is essentially invisible, and greater attention should be given to assessing the potential caregivers of impaired older persons. Assessment should include attention to high-risk indicators for the aged person, caregiver, and family system, along with the perceptions of family members. Such assessments will not eliminate the problem, but public education, professional awareness, detection protocols, alternatives for and support of family care, and social legislation may contribute to a comprehensive effort in preventing this form of abuse (AMA, 1992).

Collaboration between researchers, legislators, practitioners, professionals, and the general public needs to continue. Those working with the elderly should remember that no group of elderly persons is immune to the possibility of abusive behavior.

Elder abuse will continue as long as ageism and violence exist. The following characteristics appear to make the elderly especially vulnerable to elder abuse:

1. *Female.* Simply because there are more older women than there are older men, more of the abused elderly are women. Older women also are less likely to resist abusive behavior and are more vulnerable to sexual molestation.
2. *Advanced age.* The older the person, the higher the risk of abusive behavior. Advanced age is also associated with physical and mental impairments and an inability to resist adversities.
3. *Dependency.* Older persons who depend on others for their care are more vulnerable. Economic dependency can result in hostility by a caregiver and lead to abuse.
4. *Internalizing blame.* Older persons engaged in self-blame may be especially vulnerable to elder abuse through self-deprecating behavior. They may fail to acknowledge the abuse as the fault of the abuser.
5. *Excessive loyalty.* An older person who has a strong sense of loyalty to an abusive caregiver will probably not seek to report the problem.
6. *Past abuse.* Older persons who have been subjected to abusive behavior by a family member in the past are candidates for similar treatment when they display increasing impairments and dependency.
7. *Isolation.* An older person isolated from others may be especially vulnerable to abusive behavior because of the lack of detection and intervention by neighbors, friends, other relatives, or service providers.

People who provide services to the elderly need to be educated about the problem of spouse abuse. If their image of elder abuse is limited to the current stereotype of elderly persons mistreated by their adult children, they are not likely to properly identify situations where the aged are being abused by their spouses.

The elderly themselves need to be educated about spouse abuse. They grew up in an era when spouse abuse was tolerated more and when information on the subject was not available. Elderly victims may be vulnerable to spouse abuse because they believe it to be acceptable. They need to be encouraged not to accept it and to see it as a serious problem. Education can reduce the feelings of embarrassment and shame at being a victim and make it easier to take actions to stop the abuse.

Services need to be provided that are tailored to the problem of spouse abuse among the elderly. Nursing homes, which are used as a solution to elder abuse in a substantial number of cases, are often inappropriate because they are designed for persons much less capable of taking care of themselves. Shelters for battered women may be better solutions, but many of these shelters are not suited to the needs of the older woman. Furthermore, the presence of young women and children may intimidate older women and prevent them from seeking assistance. It would be more appropriate to establish safe apartments in congregate housing units where abused elders can take refuge. The types of self-help groups that have been effective with younger abused wives should be offered to groups of abused elderly women. Perhaps they can help the elderly stop the abuse, escape from it, or get other kinds of assistance (Pillemer and Finkelhor, 1988).

The following case study concerns the abuse of a 72-year-old woman by her 76-year-old husband.

Case Study   *Elder Abuse*

A young boy visiting friends in the neighborhood where Hattie and Max lived accidentally threw his ball into their backyard. He climbed the fence to get his ball and heard Hattie crying for help. The boy looked in the window and saw that Hattie had bruises on her face, a black eye, and blood pouring from her nose. He ran to the house he was visiting and reported what he had observed; the neighbors then called the police and paramedics.

The paramedics took Hattie to a local hospital. She was seen in the emergency room immediately. The physician discovered that she had a broken nose, a concussion, and a compound fracture of the right forearm, in addition to multiple facial bruises and a black eye. She was emaciated and confused, and when she was asked what had happened, she said, "I must have fallen." When asked if she was married, Hattie said, "Yes. Max went to the market."

The police had left a note on the door saying that Hattie had been taken to the local hospital. After about an hour, Max showed up at the hospital and was met by the police. He was very angry and wanted to know where his wife was and what she was doing at the hospital. It was apparent to the police that he had been drinking. They asked him where he had been and he said, "I went to the market; I was out of beer." He was told of Hattie's injuries and asked if he had beaten her. He responded, "Hell, no! All I did was give her a shove. She didn't have dinner ready on time—she never does!" They told him that his wife would have to be hospitalized and that they were taking him into custody until his wife could tell them how she had been injured.

Hattie was hospitalized and most of her injuries were treated; her arm would require surgery. The physician requested a consultation with members of the hospital's Elder Assessment Team (EAT). The team consists of nurses, social workers, physicians, psychologists, and an ethics specialist. He met briefly with representatives of the EAT and told them of Hattie's injuries and his belief that her husband, Max, had beaten her. Ellen, a nurse, and James, a psychologist, would interview Hattie. Bill, a social worker, and Alan, the ethics specialist, agreed to interview Max at the city jail the next day.

Ellen and James went to Hattie's room. She was drowsy from the pain medication but did not appear confused. They introduced themselves and explained that they were members of the EAT. They asked Hattie if she felt like talking. She hesitated with tears in her eyes and said, "Yes, I do. Max is a good man and he really doesn't mean to hurt me. I just can't seem to please him. It really is my fault, I know he likes his dinner at 6 PM every night—not 5 minutes earlier or 5 minutes later. It's my fault, it always is. Can we talk tomorrow? I'm getting sleepy. Can we call our daughter, Angela, tomorrow?" Ellen and James agreed to meet with Hattie the following day and to help her call her daughter.

The first priority was to get help for Hattie. The second priority was to find out from Hattie and Max how long he had been abusing her. The third priority was to talk with their daughter, Angela, to determine if she was aware of the abuse and what she could do to help her mother and father.

The morning following Hattie's admission, the EAT members met to discuss the information received from their interviews with Hattie and Max. Bill and Alan, who had visited Max at the jail, told the team what they had learned from Max. Max said that he had retired late (at age 70) and that he had been an engineer— "a damn good one." He and Hattie had been married for 52 years and had one daughter, Angela, age 49. Angela was divorced and lived in another state approximately 2500 miles away. Max said that they rarely saw her because she was a "big-shot career woman." Hattie had worked as a "dumb cashier" until they had married. He had made her quit. "I made *good* money—no wife of mine was going to work." When asked what Hattie did all day when he was working, he said, "What a wife is *supposed* to do, take care of the house. You know, clean, cook, wash and iron clothes, and mow and water the lawn. She had enough to keep her busy!" He was then asked what Hattie and he did after he retired. He looked confused and said, "What do you mean? Nothing *changed*. She took care of the house, and I watched television." When asked if they ever went out with friends or traveled, he responded, "What for? I don't need to waste my money on things like *that*, and believe me, I have enough to take care of *me* for as long as I live. I've never been sick a day in my life."

Bill and Alan admitted that they were very frustrated with Max. When Alan asked Max, "Why did you hit Hattie?" Max answered angrily, "She asked for it! Always with her nose stuck in a book or knitting. She knows I always want my dinner on the table at 6:00 sharp! She hadn't even started dinner, and it was 5:45!"

Alan asked, "Do you beat her often when your dinner is late?" Max replied, "I don't call it beating, I just knock her around a bit." Bill said, "We *do* call it beating. Do you know the extent of her injuries?" Max looked a little guilty and said, "Well, I probably had one or two beers too many." Bill replied, "How many beers do you usually have during the day?" "Maybe a six-pack," said Max, "sometimes more." "You always have at least six beers a day and sometimes more?" asked Alan. "Yeah," replied Max. "So what? I buy it!"

Bill and Alan told the EAT members that they strongly believed that Max was a chronic abuser. They asked Ellen and James what they had learned about Hattie. Ellen said that after talking with Hattie, they had met with the radiologist. He showed them the x-rays he had taken. They disclosed previous multiple fractures of her ribs, fingers, toes, and the bones in her face. They also agreed that Hattie had been abused over many years by Max.

James had called Angela and told her of Hattie's injuries. Her response was, "I'm amazed he didn't kill her. He has always slapped or knocked her around for as long as I can remember. I left home as soon as I could. He hit me one time when I was 13. I told him I would kill him if he ever touched me again. Mom just never had the guts to stand up to him. I have begged her to leave him and move here, but she wouldn't leave him. I'll fly out there this weekend and *make* her come back with me."

The team agreed that they would do everything they could to persuade Hattie to leave Max and live with or near her daughter.

The orthopedic surgeon was asked to treat Hattie's arm as soon as possible. He agreed. Hattie came through the surgery quite well and was getting stronger every day. She was eating and sleeping well. Angela arrived and talked with her mother at length. Hattie agreed to return with her but stated she didn't want to live with her. Angela told her mother that there was an excellent retirement home close to where she lived. Hattie agreed to try it but was worried that Max wouldn't agree to pay for her leaving him and moving away. Angela told her mother, "He'll pay or I'll see that he never gets out of jail. I've already talked with an attorney here, and you will get half of everything Dad has, *and* more!" Hattie said, "Well, in that case, I won't worry. I just didn't want to be a burden to you. You work so hard." Hattie asked when they could leave. She was reassured by Angela and the EAT members that she could leave the next day. Hattie and Angela were both very pleased.

Hattie has been abused repeatedly by her spouse, Max. She always believed the beatings to be her fault. Max kept her isolated, and she was not permitted to have friends. Their only daughter lived out of state. Hattie had never stood up to her husband or defied him. After a severe beating, she was hospitalized and her husband put in jail. Her daughter came and took her back with her to live in a nearby retirement home.

Last scene of all,
That ends this strange event in history,
Is second childness and mere oblivion,
Sans teeth, sans eyes, sans taste, sans everything.

–William Shakespeare

Complete the paradigm in Figure 6-4 for this case study, then compare it with the completed one in Appendix D. Refer to the paradigms in Chapter 3 as needed.

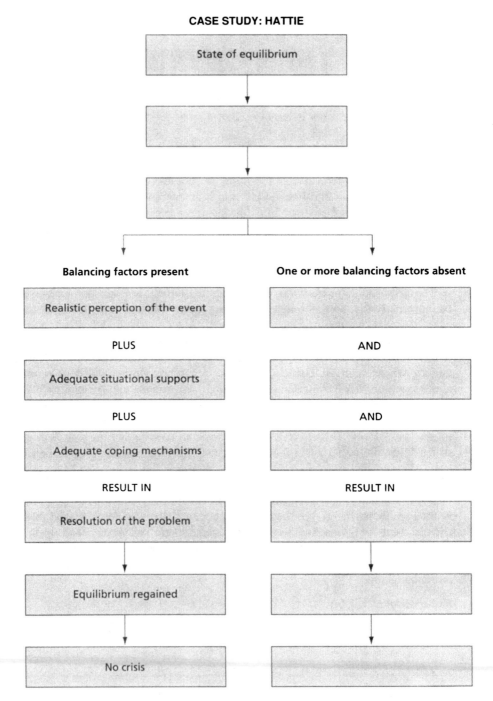

CASE STUDY: HATTIE

State of equilibrium

Balancing factors present

Realistic perception of the event

PLUS

Adequate situational supports

PLUS

Adequate coping mechanisms

RESULT IN

Resolution of the problem

Equilibrium regained

No crisis

One or more balancing factors absent

AND

AND

RESULT IN

Figure 6-4

REFERENCES

American Medical Association: *Panel to curb elderly abuse,* New York, 1992, The Association.

A nation's shame: fatal child abuse and neglect in the United States, U.S. Bureau of Census, Washington, DC, 1995.

Bandura A: *Aggression: a social learning analysis,* Englewood Cliffs, NJ, 1973, Prentice Hall.

Bohn D: Domestic violence and pregnancy implications for practice, *J Nurse Midwifery* 35:86, 1990.

Broadhurst DD and others: Early childhood programs and the prevention and the treatment of child abuse and neglect, *The Users Manual Service,* Washington, DC, 1992, U.S. Department of Health and Human Services.

Conant JB: *Slums and suburbs,* New York, 1961, McGraw Hill.

Conant, p. 22.

Cowen PS: *Child abuse: current issues in nursing,* ed 4, St. Louis, 1994, Mosby.

Currie E: What's wrong with the crime bill? *The Nation,* p. 4, January 31, 1994.

Davila F: Denver debates school ousters, *Washington Post,* p. 18, January 20, 1995.

Dutton DG: *The batterer: a psychological profile,* New York, 1995, Basic Books.

Faulkner LR: Mandating the reporting of suspected cases of elder abuse: an inappropriate, ineffective and ageist response to the abuse of older adults, *Fam Law Quart* 16:69, 1982.

Formica PE: AMA hopes to curb abuse of the elderly, *Washington Post,* December 3, 1992.

Freed K: Youth receives three years for stealing ice cream, *Los Angeles Times,* p. 23, September 30, 1994.

Gelles RJ: *The violent home,* Beverly Hills, Calif, 1972, Sage.

Giarretto H: Humanistic treatment of father-daughter incest. In Helfer RE and Kempe CH, editors: *Child abuse and neglect: the family and the community,* Cambridge, Mass, 1976, Ballinger.

Giroux H: *Border crossings,* New York, 1992, Routledge.

Halper M: *Helping maltreated children: school and community involvement,* St. Louis, 1979, Mosby.

Hanania J: A hidden world of violence, *Los Angeles Times,* November 19, 1996.

Helfer RD, Kempe CH, editors: *Child abuse and neglect: the family and the community,* Cambridge, Mass, 1976, Ballinger.

Johnson T: Critical issues in the definition of elder mistreatment. In Pilemar KA, Wolf RS, editors: *Elder abuse: conflict in the family,* Dover, Mass, 1986, Auburn House.

Justice B, Justice R: *The broken taboo,* New York, 1979, Human Sciences Press.

Kempe CH: The battered child syndrome, *JAMA* 181:17, 1962.

Kosberg J: Preventing elder abuse: identification of high risk factors prior to placement discussions, *Gerontologist* 28:43, 1988.

Lau EE, Kosberg JI: Abuse of the elderly by informal care providers, *Age Ageing,* September/October, 1979.

McPartland, Nettles SM: Using community adults as advocates or mentors for at-risk middle school students: a two-year evaluation of project RAISE, *Am J Education* 99(4):568, 1991.

Metz MH: *Classrooms and corridors: the crisis of authority in desegregated secondary schools,* Berkeley, 1978, University of California Press.

Miller MS: *No visible wounds,* Chicago, 1995, Contemporary Books.

Moynihan DP, Glazer: *Beyond the melting pot.* Cambridge, Mass, 1987, Joint Center for Urban Studies.

Nemeth P: Controlling school violence, Editorial, *New York Times,* p. A 24, May 3, 1993.

Noguera P: Preventing and producing violence: a critical analysis of response to school violence, *Harv Educ Rev,* vol 63, No. 2, Summer 1995.

O'Brien J: *Elder abuse: barriers to identification and intervention,* paper presented at the meeting of the Gerontological Society of America, Chicago, Ill, November 1986.

O'Reilly J: Battered wives, *Time,* September 5, 1983.

Ornstein A: Discipline: a major function in teaching the disadvantaged. In Heidenreich R, editor: *Urban education,* Arlington, Va, 1972, College Readings.

Ornstein, p. 8.

Pillemer K, Finkelhor D: The prevalence of elder abuse: a random sample survey, *Gerontologist* 28:51, 1988.

Rivera C: Child abuse rose 9.4% last year, *Los Angeles Times,* November 15, 1996.

Rivera C: Child abuse in U.S. is at crisis levels, panel says. *Los Angeles Times,* April 26, 1995.

Rubinelli J: Incest: it's time we faced reality, *J Psychiatr Nurs* 18:17, 1980.

Salend E and others: Elder abuse reporting: limitations of statutes, *Gerontologist* 24:61, 1984.

Salholz E and others: Beware of child molesters, *Newsweek,* p 45, August 9, 1982.

Silver LB: Psychological aspects of the battered child and his parents, *J Child Hosp Clin Proc* 24:355, 1968.

Straus MA and others: *Behind closed doors: violence in the American family,* Garden City, NY, 1980, Doubleday.

Toby J: Everyday school violence: how disorder fuels it, *Am Educator,* p. 4, Winter 1993/1994.

U.S. Department of Health and Human Services: *Study of national incidence and prevalence of child abuse and neglect,* DHHS Publ No. (OHDS) 105-85-1702, Hyattsville, Md, 1992, U.S. Government Printing Office.

Van Biema D: Abandoned to her fate, *Time* 146(24):32, 1995.

Vogel EF, Bell NW: The emotionally disturbed child as a family scapegoat, *J Psychoanal* 47:21, 1960.

Walker-Hooper A: Domestic violence: assessing the problem. In Warner CG, editor: *Conflict intervention in social and domestic violence,* Bowie, Md, 1981, Brady.

Weissbourd R: *The vulnerable child,* Reading, Mass, 1996, Addison-Wesley.

ADDITIONAL READING

Barnett OW, Kyson M, Thelen RE: *Women's violence as a response to male abuse,* Paper presented at the meeting of the American Psychological Association, Washington, DC, August 1992.

Bennett G, Kingston P: *Elder abuse,* London, 1993, Chapman & Hall.

Browne A: Violence against women by male partners: prevalence, outcomes and policy implications, *Am Psychol* 48:1077, 1993.

Byers J: Seven steps to stamp out child abuse, *Los Angeles Times,* 1996, National Committee to Prevent Child Abuse.

Coontz S: *The way we never were: American families and the nostalgia trap,* New York, 1992, Basic Books.

Cremin L: *American education: the metropolitan experience 1875-1980,* New York, 1988, Harper & Row.

Foner N: *The caregiving dilemma: work in an American nursing home,* Berkeley, 1994, University of California Press.

Garbarino J and others: *Children in danger,* San Francisco, 1992, Jossey-Bass.

Gleason WJ: Mental disorders in battered women: an empirical study, *Violence Vict* 8:53, 1993.

Hallisey E: Gang activity in state's prisons on the increase, *San Francisco Chronicle,* p 14, May 17, 1994.

Hamberger LK, Saunders DG, Hovey M: Prevalence of domestic violence in community and rate of physician inquiry, *Fam Med* 24:283, 1992.

Hendricks-Matthews M: Family physicians and violence: looking back, looking ahead, *Am Fam Physician* 45(5):2033, 1992.

Hewlett SA: *When the bough breaks: the cost of neglecting our children,* New York, 1991, HarperCollins.

Johnson J, Immerwahr J: *What Americans expect from the public schools* p. 4, Winter 1994/1995.

Kemper P: Disarming Youth. *Calif School Boards J,* p. 25, Fall 1993.

Kemper, p. 27.

Lach MS, Pilemer K: Abuse and neglect of elderly persons, *N Engl J Med* 332:437, 1995.

Morrison G, Furlong MJ, Morrison RL: School violence to school safety: reframing the issue for school psychologists, *School Psychol Rev* 23(2):236, 1994.

Nemeth P: Caught in the crossfire, *Am Teach* 77(2):6, 1994.

Potakow V: *Lives on the edge: single mothers and their children in the other America,* Chicago, 1993, University of Chicago Press.

Prothrow-Stith, Weissman D and M: *Deadly consequences: how violence is destroying our teenage population and a plan to begin solving the problem,* New York, 1991, HarperCollins.

Rothman D: *Discovery of the asylum,* Boston, 1971, Little, Brown.

Rothman, p. 15.

Rothman, p. 137.

Rothman, p. 235.

Sherman A: *Wasting America's future: the children's defense fund report on the cost of child poverty,* 1994, Beacon Press.

Wilson G: Abuse of elderly men and women among clients of a community psychogeriatric service, *Br J Soc Work* 124(6):681, 1994.

Wilson HE: School violence and campus security, *School Manage Advisor,* No. 20, 1993, North Carolina Department of Education.

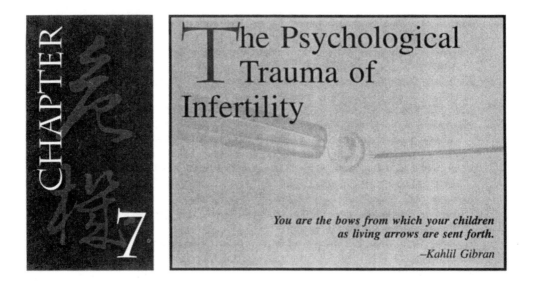

The Psychological Trauma of Infertility

You are the bows from which your children as living arrows are sent forth.

–*Kahlil Gibran*

CHAPTER 7

M any couples now plan their families as meticulously as they plan their education, choice of career, living situation, and other major financial investments. They measure all factors and wait for the opportune moment to start their family.

For one of every six couples of childbearing age, fertility is not a force that can be turned on at will. *Infertility,* the inability to achieve pregnancy after 1 year of regular sexual relations or the inability to carry pregnancy to a live birth, is experienced by 15% of the population of childbearing age. The U.S. Census Bureau (1993) states that there are now over 300 million Americans; of these, 66 million, or about 30%, are between the ages of 22 and 40 years. If the accepted rate of infertility (15%) is applied to this number, it is probable that there are more than 10 million who may, at some time, be unable to achieve or carry pregnancy. Of this number, about 40% have an infertility problem related solely to the female, another 40% have a problem related solely to the male, and the remaining 20% have a problem that either affects both members of the couple or is of unknown origin (Halpert, 1994).

Although the childless couple is more socially acceptable in modern society, there is a distinct group of infertile couples who feel what they consider to be social pressures to become parents. As a woman and her partner begin to realize that she may never bear a child, an emotional state develops that can be called the *crisis of infertility* (Bresnick and Taymor, 1979). Approximately 30 years ago, 40% to 50% of infertility cases were thought to be the result of emotional factors. Infertile couples were described as having typical personality traits that resulted in their inability to conceive. More recently our increased understanding of neuroendocrinology, as well as other advances in the field, has reduced emotional factors as a cause of infertility to less than 5%. Infertility itself is frequently a source of emotional trauma for couples, placing considerable stress on their relationship (Eisener, 1963).

Infertility as a Life Crisis

At some point during infertility investigation and attempted treatment, it is common for an infertile person to experience a state of crisis. Crisis in this situation can be succinctly defined as a disruption in the steady state, or a *period of disequilibrium.* Since there may be repeated crisis states during infertility investigation and treatment, there is a very real risk of maladaptive behavioral changes, just as there is the real chance for positive growth and increased insight. Crisis intervention by an understanding, knowledgeable, and caring professional may make all the difference (Menning, 1980).

It is naive for the physician who treats infertility to say that feelings are not within his province. Whether by acts of omission or commission, the physician very much affects the outcomes of the crisis state. The person in crisis is extremely vulnerable and can be gravely hurt by indifference, lay psychiatric advice, or comparisons with those who have suffered more. Members of a couple, as if by tacit agreement, do not usually get into crisis at the same time. This may lead the one who is dysfunctional to believe that the other cannot understand. The man and woman may have little to give each other, forcing the person in crisis to depend on outside help. The physician is immensely important at such a time, and if he does not possess the necessary counseling skills, at least he may be an important bridge to therapeutic intervention (Winkleman, 1995).

There is a very positive side to the disequilibrium and vulnerability of the crisis state. Since existing coping mechanisms have failed, the person is very open to change and growth. Old, defeated coping patterns are often discarded at times of crisis, and new and more appropriate methods may be learned. The anxiety that most people in crisis experience is actually a high-energy state. If this energy can be focused on a tangible problem by a skilled therapist, it can be useful in resolving the situation. The fundamental goal of crisis intervention should be *"primum noli nocere"*—above all do not harm. The therapeutic goal in crisis intervention is for the individual to achieve a level of equilibrium equal to or, preferably, better than the precrisis level.

The Emotional State of the Infertile Couple

The crisis of infertility evokes many feelings in the couple. Some feelings are rational and based on very real and correctly perceived insults that society or the infertility investigation and treatment have thrust on them. Other feelings may be more irrational and based in part on myths and superstitions or on magical childlike thinking. Feelings vary in order and intensity, but most individuals face a similar syndrome of feelings as they attempt to work through the infertility crisis. Regardless of the cause of infertility, both men and women feel "damaged" and "defective." Women have described themselves as feeling "hollow" or "empty," and men have spoken of intercourse as "shooting blanks." In addition, some couples begin to feel that they are "doing it wrong" or that there is something about sex that they do not know.

THE AFFECTIVE STAGES OF INFERTILITY

Rosenfeld and Mitchell (1979) emphasize that the infertile couple in a crisis situation experience tremendous stress as a couple, as well as individually. They view the stages of emotional response to infertility as surprise, grief, anger, isolation, denial, and acceptance. They feel that therapy can be very helpful in each of these areas and extremely helpful in the area of acceptance. According to Menning (1982), the following seven affective stages occur in a logical order:

Surprise. The first reaction most people have to the news of infertility is one of total shock and surprise. Most couples in their childbearing years are usually thinking in terms of *preventing* pregnancy. They naturally assume that they can have children if and when they desire them. It is ironic that most couples discover their infertility after having used some form of birth control, sometimes for many years. The discovery of an infertility problem is felt most keenly by those who are highly achievement oriented and who believe themselves capable of surmounting any obstacle if only enough effort and will are exerted.

Denial. "This can't happen to me" is often the reaction to infertility, especially if the initial tests reveal an absolute and untreatable problem in either partner. Denial serves a purpose. It allows the mind and body to adjust at their own rate to an overwhelming situation. Denial is dangerous *only* when it becomes a long-term or permanent coping mechanism, for example, when chronically depressed women staunchly maintain that they never really wanted a family and when both men and women refuse to apply the label "infertile" to themselves in spite of 5 to 10 years of involuntary childlessness. Psychotherapy of some duration is usually indicated for individuals who need this level of defense.

Anger. When a couple enter into an infertility investigation and attempt treatment, they surrender much of their control over their bodies. Even in the best physician-patient relationship, frustration, helplessness, and embarrassment may be present. Anger is a predictable response to loss of control. The anger may be quite rational and focused on real and correctly perceived insults, such as social pressuring from family and friends to "produce," and the pain and inconvenience of the tests and treatments themselves. Sometimes the anger is more irrational and is projected on targets, such as the physician or marriage partner, or even social issues, such as pro-choice abortion advocates or people who "breed like rabbits." This irrational anger is usually a front for more primary feelings, such as intense loss or grief that has not yet been acknowledged. Whatever the source or type of anger, it is necessary that the person be able to ventilate it. Anger tends to dissipate in the telling and retelling of the indignities that produce it. This can be done without detriment to the angry person or others in the milieu, such as a peer support group.

Isolation. It is common for infertile couples to state that they are the only people they know who cannot achieve a pregnancy. Infertility is a difficult subject for most people to discuss. It is very personal and inherently sexual.

Couples may keep their infertility a secret because they do not wish to be the objects of pity or because they fear unsolicited advice, such as "relax" or "why don't you take a second honeymoon." However, secrecy may have several negative effects. It usually increases the pressuring and needling from family and friends about the plans of the couple to start a family. More important, it cuts the couple off from potential sources of comfort and support in a time of great stress. In extreme cases infertile couples may be so sensitized to the sight of children or pregnant women that they withdraw from any social situations that might produce such contact. This may even involve a change of work or living situation.

Isolation may occur between the members of a couple as well. The woman may despair over her husband's inability to empathize with her feelings about menstruation, her fixation on her basal temperature chart around ovulation, or her nervous hopes if menstruation is overdue. The man may find it impossible to share his anxiety over being "counted and scored" in semen analysis or over having to perform sex on demand, whether he feels like it or not. The result may be a breakdown in communication and a loss of pleasure in the sexual relationship. Marital stress and tension over sex are commonly present in certain phases of infertility. Since the couple often have no others to validate their feelings, they may presume that not only are they infertile, but also their marriage and sex life are in jeopardy. It is always a relief when infertile couples find each other because they share the same frustrations and concerns. One of the most helpful ways to ease the isolation of infertility is to help couples find each other and join a support group.

Guilt. Another reason for the secrecy that so often surrounds infertility is the presence of guilt. People seem to need to construct a cause and effect relationship for events that happen to them. The infertile couple review their mutual and individual histories and search for a guilty deed for which they are being punished. Some common guilt producers are premarital sex, use of birth control, a previous abortion, venereal disease, extramarital sex or interest, masturbation, homosexual thoughts or acts, and even sexual pleasure. Once the guilty deed is discovered, the infertile person may go to great lengths to atone and achieve forgiveness. Atoning may take any form, from religious acts to personal denial or working in painful areas such as counseling unwed mothers or teaching other people's children. Guilt and atonement appear to have no relationship to one's educational level. Some of the most sophisticated people have applied a mystical belief in "God's punishment" to their own infertility, even in the absence of religious beliefs. Certainly the teachings of the Old Testament and folklore from early civilization can contribute to the view that the infertile person (particularly the woman) has fallen from grace and is being punished by higher powers. People who have poor self-esteem tend to be particularly vulnerable to guilty thoughts about infertility. Believing in their hearts that they really do not deserve a pregnancy and child, they may keep their infertility secret for fear how bad they really are might be discovered.

Grief. Without question the most compelling feeling of conclusive infertility is grief. This state may be preceded by a period of depression, as the final testing or treatments are pursued to no avail. Once all hope for pregnancy and live birth is abandoned, the appropriate and necessary response *should* be grieving. It is a strange and puzzling kind of grief, involving the loss of a potential, not actual, life. Society has elaborate rituals to comfort the bereavement in death. Infertility is different. There is no funeral, no wake, and no grave. Family and friends may never even know. The infertile couple often reach the point of grief alone. Stillbirth or miscarriage, although tragic, is more often perceived as an actual death. Family and friends are more often aware of the loss and offer solace and support.

Infertility that is conclusive represents many losses: the loss of children, the loss of genetic continuity, and the loss of fertility and all of its means to sexuality, including the loss of the pregnancy experience itself. For each individual, some aspects of loss are keener than others. When grieving over infertility does take place, it is quite focused. As painful as the initial grief work may be—accompanied by weeping; sobbing; and its physical symptoms; such as loss of appetite, exhaustion, and choking or tightness in the throat—it does run a predictable course and it does end. This is important to point out to the person who is afraid to express these feelings.

Resolution. The desired goal of any crisis, including infertility, is its successful resolution. The process of resolution requires that each of the difficult feelings detailed above be discovered, worked through, and overcome. Feelings are never laid away forever. They may be reactivated by special reminders, such as the anniversary of a loss, or by new and different crises. However, the feelings are never as difficult or as overwhelming as they initially were. Reactivation is usually brief and to be expected.

The state of resolution may be described as a return of energy, perhaps even a surge of zest and well-being; a sense of optimism and faith returns, a sense of humor returns, and some past absurdities may even become grist for storytelling. The concepts of sexuality, self-image, and self-esteem are reworked to become disconnected from childbearing but are nevertheless wholesome and complete. The couple plan for the future again, building a way around the obstacle of infertility. They are ready to act with confidence in selecting an alternative life plan. Once resolution is achieved, the couple are ready to proceed with their lives.

Miscarriage and Stillbirth

Infertility is a complex life crisis. It rarely proceeds as ideally as suggested in the preceding discussion, for example, from discovery of a problem to working through feelings to resolution and development of an alternative plan for building a family. One of the more complex issues involved in infertility is a couple's experience with miscarriage or stillbirth.

One aspect of infertility concerns itself not with the inability of a couple to achieve a pregnancy but with problems resulting from termination of a pregnancy before a live birth. Miscarriage is a more common occurrence than many people realize. It is estimated that one in six pregnancies ends in miscarriage. Seventy-five percent of all miscarriages occur in the first trimester and are the result of unavailable care and medically untreatable problems (e.g., lack of prenatal care, appropriate vitamins, and adequate diet). These random mistakes of nature rarely repeat themselves in the childbearing years of normal couples. Infertile couples may be defined as those who have repeated miscarriages possibly caused by structural, hormonal, or genetic problems. It also appears that couples who have had great difficulty in conceiving are at greater risk. It is thought that they run a 40% risk of miscarriage, often resulting from the very problem that made it difficult for them to conceive.

Medically, miscarriage is a potentially dangerous, even life-threatening, situation. When emotional aspects are added to the physical trauma, this may seem like a life event of critical importance. Miscarriage is almost always totally unexpected. It may be over within a matter of minutes, in early pregnancy, or it may drag on for days and even weeks. Occasionally, medical intervention is successful in preventing loss of pregnancy, and the couple may experience alternate states of hope and despair as they await the *final* outcome. Most often the onset of bleeding and cramping continues until the fetus is expulsed.

There are a number of issues that are unique to the experience of miscarriage. One that is most troublesome is the practice in many hospitals of admitting a person who threatens miscarriage into the obstetrical unit. There she may be in close proximity with laboring and newly delivered patients and also with the newborn nursery. Hospitals justify this policy by explaining that miscarriage is not a routine gynecological event and must be managed in the obstetrical area where the delivery room is available for surgical intervention. The emotional impact on the couple, however, may be profound. The couple who have experienced a miscarriage should, at the very least, be screened from laboring and newly delivered patients. A special indicator should be posted on the door so that hospital staff are aware of the situation. The husband should not be treated as a visitor but allowed unlimited access to his wife. Privacy from all but a few caretakers will facilitate the couple in experiencing their grief.

The need for grieving after a miscarriage—especially for the couple who had longed for a child—is obvious. Unfortunately, many hospital personnel are uncomfortable with this basic human emotion. They may interpret grieving as "suffering" or disturbing to the welfare of other patients. It is all too common for physicians to prescribe sedation, tranquilizers, or even mood-elevating drugs. Probably the best management for the grieving couple is the earliest possible discharge home, where both grief work and recovery can take place unimpeded in familiar surroundings.

The reaction of family and friends to news of a miscarriage is usually one of abbreviated support and assurances of successful pregnancy in the near future.

Platitudes and assurances are not only medically unsound, but they also invalidate the couple's right to grieve their particular loss.

In some cases couples have endured five, six, or more miscarriages before giving up hope. They received news of each subsequent pregnancy with dread and foreboding instead of with joy. They kept their pregnancy secret for fear of raising the hopes of family and friends, and they heavily practiced denial to prevent their own nervous hopes from mounting with each passing week. The emotional toll in such cases is exhausting. Some couples finally choose sterilization in preference to more attempts at pregnancy.

Stillbirth is technically the loss of a body that has reached sufficient gestation to be viable outside the womb (usually after 28 weeks). It is a much less common occurrence than miscarriage and usually is not a recurring event. There are several possible situations, each fraught with its own pain and turmoil. There may be cessation of fetal life, whereby the couple are admitted to the hospital and know before delivery that their baby is dead. There may be a viable baby who expires in the labor or delivery process or as a result of congenital abnormalities at birth when it is separated from its placental blood supply. In these cases the death is not anticipated. Finally, there may be a crisis for both mother and child such as premature separation of the placenta, in which bleeding may be profuse and oxygenation of the baby is interrupted. This latter example is a life-threatening situation, and the emotional issues become secondary.

Whatever the circumstance, several common issues arise. The couple are inevitably admitted to the labor and delivery area and afterward to the postpartum unit. Screening and privacy from normally laboring and delivering patients and those in the recovery phase is paramount. If the baby is known to be dead, delivery by the least hazardous means to the woman and attendance of the husband or another person to comfort her are recommended. It appears to be important to the grieving process for the couple to be able to view and handle the body of the baby. This option should be sensitively suggested and available on request. Since an autopsy is often done in these circumstances, it is best for the couple to view the body before it is sent to the pathology laboratory. The woman who has had a stillbirth is in a postpartum state of recovery, as well as in a state of grieving. She has all the needs of the usual postpartum patient in addition to her emotional needs. Sensitive caretaking and nurturing from hospital staff plus unlimited access to her husband will facilitate recovery. The couple who have been through a miscarriage or stillbirth need to know why. They may fantasize that they did something wrong, which resulted in this event. Any information of medical value that can be discovered by autopsy, especially if it has bearing on future pregnancies, should by all means be researched and shared (Menning, 1982).

Psychotherapy and Infertility

Frustration and anxiety over failure to achieve pregnancy must inevitably underlie the decision of all infertile couples to seek medical help. Sturgis and others (1957) suggest that it would be reasonable to include a screening psychiatric interview as part of the initial evaluation of *all* infertile couples. A psychotherapist is also suggested as an integral part of the routine evaluation of infertile couples. In a report by Karahasanglu and others (1972), the therapist functions in four major areas:

1. Screening and evaluating
2. Relationship improvement
3. Sexual compatibility guidance
4. Supportive counseling

Realizing that most infertile couples thought that children should inevitably result from marriage and that many infertile couples thought that failure to reproduce was synonymous with failure to fulfill one's biological role led others to use group therapy as a supportive adjunct in the treatment of the infertile couple. In this experience, marked improvement in the spontaneity and frequency of sexual intercourse occurred as the couples achieved deeper mutual understanding. Patients' attitudes became more positive, and tension diminished. In addition, the husband became more actively interested, and both partners decreased their sense of isolation.

Group sessions have also been used with the result that much of the pressure and marked sense of personal failure diminished when patients were able to share their feelings and anxieties with others who were experiencing infertility. The psychotherapist's role in infertility should include therapeutic techniques combined with education, encouragement, behavioral techniques, and situational support. Other areas where a therapist may be of assistance to a couple include helping them to mourn the fact that they have been unable to have children; helping in decisions involving artificial insemination and adoption; and helping couples deal with the uncertainty when no definite cause for the infertility is found.

Although it may be clear to the physician and therapist that for certain patients little hope exists, as long as a patient is receiving medication or undergoing laboratory tests, she is usually putting aside resolution of her infertility crisis by postponing decisions about career, life plans, and adoption and personal confrontation with her childlessness. At this crucial time the therapist may be of great assistance in helping patients recognize, work through, and overcome this situation. In particular, in cases of unexplained infertility it is imperative to exercise caution in inadvertently suggesting that the patient is "causing her own infertility" psychogenically unless the physician is absolutely certain of this fact. Quite to the contrary, Taymor and Bresnick (1978) state that in most cases it is the infertility that results in emotional tension. They describe the intense, emotionally charged "crisis of infertility" that affects every area of the couple's relationship and their employment. They suggest more widespread use of infertility counseling to diminish the various forms of anxiety, depression, frustration, guilt, isolation, and obsession that crisis exacts. In a subsequent study (1979) they demonstrate that infertility counseling enhances the quality of life in many patients who become victims of their "infertility crisis."

PSYCHOSOCIAL THERAPY

Many couples will need therapy during the psychological trauma of suffering one or more spontaneous abortions or having a stillborn child. This is a tremendous loss to them. They will need to go through the stages of grief and mourning, and they will need emotional support and a therapist who can listen to them, with an impartial, unbiased, and empathic approach. Menning (1980) suggests the following:

- **Treat infertility as a problem of the couple.** No matter whose body ultimately has the problem, the other partner has a very strong interest in investigation and treatment. Involving the partner in discussions and planning from the beginning is optimal. From the patient's perspective, to be seen as a couple allows several distinct advantages. When two people visit a physician, the power tends to be equalized. They gain courage and assertiveness from each other's presence and will often negotiate their needs more honestly right away. "Blame" seems to be dispelled; not just one person is involved. Each member of the couple will have twice the opportunity for hearing information at a time when they are anxious and twice the opportunity to ask questions and seek clarification.

- **Plan the investigation and treatment with the couple.** The physician is the only one who will know what tests or treatments are indicated for a given couple. These can be offered as recommendations not as mandates. There is room for negotiation in a number of areas: the *sequence* of tests or treatments can often be flexible if there is no detrimental effect; the pace of testing and treatment can always be slowed for those who are cautious or accelerated for those who are pushing an age deadline or are highly motivated; and the cost of tests and treatment and the patient's ability to pay or the insurance situation needs to be made clear at the onset.

- **Provide emotional support and education.** Emotional support and education should be the responsibility of the physician and his staff. A number of physicians now employ nurses or therapists to educate, for example, in charting basal body temperature and in fertility awareness, and to assist in offering emotional support and in screening couples for important decisions, such as donor insemination. A well-informed patient is much easier to deal with than a partially educated one. Literature by some respected infertility specialists should be provided at the very beginning. Recognizing that the physician has limited time for providing emotional support, the therapist's role should be a very important adjunct. There is not a complete dichotomy of the physical and emotional aspects of infertility; they are interwoven. The physician becomes an important and powerful figure to the infertile couple. It is very difficult for the couple with absolute infertility or with "normal infertility" to be sent away at the end of the period of contact because "there is no need to return." Offering such couples a chance to return for several therapy sessions to discuss their feelings can be very productive and can offer them a lifeline until they find new resources for emotional support.

- **Refer the couple to a qualified infertility specialist.** Physicians seldom agree among themselves about who is qualified to conduct the complete infertility investigation and treatment. It should come as no surprise that the infertile couple are often confused. Fortunately, physicians with specialized and additional training in reproductive endocrinology, obstetrics and gynecology, and urology are now available as qualified infertility specialists. Most university medical centers have a list of these specialists.

Determining the Cause of Infertility

The first step in infertility treatment is a diagnostic workup that is usually performed by a physician who specializes in infertility, such as a reproductive endocrinologist. The workup may include an internal pelvic examination; a postcoital test, in which cervical mucus is examined microscopically shortly after unprotected intercourse to determine the consistency of mucus and whether the sperm are swimming properly; and a hysterosalpingogram (HSG), in which radiopaque dye is injected into the uterus and viewed on x-ray films to see if the uterus and the fallopian tubes are clear. Blood and hormone tests, laparoscopy, and genetic counseling might also be recommended.

The male partner should have a semen analysis and a complete physical examination. According to estimates, 30% of infertility cases are due to male reproductive problems, 30% are the result of female reproductive problems, 20% are due to a combination of factors in both sexes, and 20% are unexplained.

Age can be a factor. A woman's fertility declines gradually every year past the age of 30 but especially after 40. The older the woman gets, the more likely she is to develop a purely mechanical cause of infertility. Endometriosis, for example, is a disorder in which fragments of the uterine lining migrate to other parts of the pelvic cavity and can cause obstructions in the fallopian tubes and other problems.

After a complete workup, the next step is treatment. This is true whether the cause of infertility is found. A physician will try to correct any obvious physical maladies, such as blocked fallopian tubes. Beyond that, treatment options range from low to high. Most physicians begin by trying the least invasive methods of aiding conception (Winkleman, 1995).

When Someone You Know Miscarries

Friends and family often try to reassure a woman who has had a miscarriage by offering well-intentioned platitudes, but often these only end up making her feel worse. To help someone through this difficult time, some things to say and not to say follow (Bennetts, 1994).

Don't tell her that the miscarriage was "nature's way" of getting rid of a defective fetus. Not only is this very insensitive but also may not be true.

Don't say, "It wasn't really a baby." To the woman who was busy knitting little booties, it was a baby, and denying her emotional reality will only make her feel desolate.

Don't say, "You'll get pregnant again soon." This is unknown, and although it might be true, right now the woman is afraid that she will never have a baby. False assurances are infuriating.

Don't say, "It won't happen again," because it might. This is grossly presumptuous.

Do remember that mourning is a process, and it takes time. Telling a woman to put the experience behind her can make her feel angry that you do not understand what she is going through. Emotions do not run on a set schedule. She will get there when she gets there.

Do say, "How do you feel? Do you want to talk about it?" Then just listen. Don't try to talk her out of her feelings or minimize them. Be sympathetic, but don't tell her you know how she feels unless you have experienced a similar trauma.

Do include the would-be-father. He is dealing with the same loss, and men's grief is often overlooked.

Do offer to help by getting the names of books or local support groups on pregnancy loss.

There are many organizations available as support groups for individuals and couples faced with a diagnosis of infertility. A list of some of these groups is found in Appendix C.

The following case involves a young woman and her husband. They were referred to the Crisis Clinic by the woman's obstetrician after she had experienced a second miscarriage.

Case Study   Infertility

Angela and Barry were assigned to a therapist who was experienced in working with patients who had suffered a recent loss, especially a child or someone who had suffered a miscarriage. She met them, introduced herself, and asked them to come to her office. She remarked that she had read what they had written on their chart. She expressed her deepest sympathy. She asked Angela if she would like to tell her what had happened or if she preferred Barry to tell her about the crisis. Angela looked at Barry, he took her hand and said, "Angela, let me tell her about us, not only about our crisis but also about us, you and I—everything. I think she can help us more if she knows all about us as individuals, as well as a married couple." Angela, with tears in her eyes, agreed. Barry held her hand tightly and began to tell the therapist "all."

Angela had a second spontaneous abortion (miscarriage) 6 days ago. She still was in a state of disbelief. She is 35 years of age and Barry is 39. They have been married for 5 years. Originally from the East Coast, they had moved to the West Coast 18 months ago. Barry's company had recommended him for a promotion in their corporate law firm on the West Coast. Angela and Barry were thrilled; they had always wanted to live "without all the humidity." Barry said that Angela's company had a branch on the West Coast and that she had no trouble transferring to that branch. He continued, saying that she would also be receiving a promotion because Angela was their top programmer.

Barry and Angela had bought a house that they both "loved" and spent their free time on weekends furnishing it, "just the way *they* had always talked about." They had discussed having children before they were married. Angela was the oldest from a family with four children, three girls and one boy. She had told Barry that she would be happy with two children, but no more.

Barry was an only child and agreed with Angela that two would be ideal. "I didn't enjoy being an only child." They enjoyed traveling and skiing, both water and snow. They always planned their vacations together and had decided that they wanted time "just" for themselves before they started a family.

After they had moved to the West Coast, bought their home, and kept busy getting it furnished, they discussed having children. They had agreed 9 months ago that "now" was the time to start a family. With both of them getting promotions, they felt financially secure. They had planned on getting a housekeeper when their children came so Angela could return to her job, which she loved. Angela went off the "pill" and became pregnant 8 months ago. They were both excited and thrilled.

Since they didn't know any physicians in the area, they asked a fellow employee who had a 2-year-old daughter for a recommendation. She recommended her own obstetrician and said that he was "great." Angela made an appointment to see him. She told Barry that he was older than she had expected (he reminded her of her father) but was very nice. He confirmed that she was pregnant, prescribed vitamins, and told Angela that she was "very healthy" and would probably have a healthy baby.

Other than about 3 weeks of morning nausea, Angela said that she felt fine. She admitted that she would become tired in the afternoon, but since she was working, she just ignored it.

When she was 3½ months pregnant, one evening after dinner she asked Barry if he would rub her lower back because she was very uncomfortable. Barry gave her a nice long back rub. Angela said that the back rub felt good but that it really didn't help. She got up and went to the bathroom and discovered that she was spotting blood. She called Barry, and when he came, she told him. He suggested that she go upstairs, undress, and get in bed while he called the doctor. Barry called the doctor and told him that Angela was spotting. The doctor said that it was "very common," that Angela should just stay in bed, and that the spotting would probably stop.

The bleeding became heavier, and Angela began to have cramps. Barry called the doctor again and told him what was happening. He told Barry to take her to the hospital and that he would meet them there. By the time they reached the hospital, Angela was having severe cramps and the bleeding was getting heavier by the minute. Both Barry and Angela were very frightened. When they got to the hospital, the doctor was waiting for them. He gave Angela a pelvic examination and said that she had probably already "lost the baby" and that he would have to do a D&C (dilatation and curettage) to stop the bleeding.

Angela was given a general anesthesia. When she woke up, she said that other than a few mild cramps, she felt *fine*. She stayed at the hospital with Barry at her side for 3 hours. She had no more bleeding, just some spotting, and the doctor said that she could go home but should stay home tomorrow and not go to work. He told her to make an appointment to see him in a week. If she had anymore bleeding, she was to call him.

The therapist asked Angela how she and Barry had felt about losing the baby. Barry answered, "We were upset, but I was more concerned about Angela. I wanted to be certain that she was alright physically and mentally. I figured we could always have other children, but I could only have one Angela."

Angela smiled at him and held his hand tighter. The therapist turned toward Angela and said, "How did you feel about losing the baby, Angela?" Angela looked at the therapist with tears in her eyes and answered, "Terrible. I didn't know how it happened . . . I don't really know why I lost this one 6 days ago . . . there must be something wrong with me." The therapist asked, "What did your doctor tell you? You have lost two babies now." Barry spoke up and said, "That is the problem . . . he hasn't told us anything . . . we don't know why. He just says stupid things like 'these things happen' and sometimes it just isn't meant to be!"

The therapist asked, "Has he recommended an infertility specialist to you?" Angela and Barry looked at each other and both said, "NO!" Barry said, "I didn't know there was such a specialty." The therapist told them that there were definitely infertility specialists and that she felt they should see one. She told Barry to contact the University Medical Center and get the names of the three top infertility specialists. She emphasized that they *both* should be seeing an infertility specialist. "It may not be anything wrong with you," she said to Angela. "It could be something wrong with Barry."

Barry turned pale. "ME?! What could be wrong with me?" The therapist smiled and replied, "There may not be anything wrong with you, Barry, but you should have tests conducted too. Any number of things could contribute to a miscarriage . . . it isn't always something wrong with the wife. That is what an infertility specialist could find out . . . that is his specialty."

"What do we tell the doctor Angela has been seeing?" Barry asked the therapist. "The truth," she replied. "You want to find out why Angela is having miscarriages and you are going to consult an infertility specialist."

The therapist took a list of support groups out of her desk and handed it to Angela. "In the meantime I think it would be to your advantage to contact one of these support groups. They have all been through the same thing you are going through—repeated miscarriages. They not only could be a valuable source of information, but they also could help you and Barry ventilate your feelings. They could help you get rid of some of the misconceptions, fears, and anxieties that you both are experiencing."

Both Angela and Barry looked more relaxed. The therapist asked if they would like to continue in crisis therapy for approximately 5 weeks. By that time they should have selected and seen a specialist in infertility and gone through some of the tests. They should also be attending one of the support groups.

Angela said, "We want to continue to see you, but why just 5 more times?" The therapist smiled and replied, "You should be over your crisis by that time, and you should have some answers from your infertility specialist. I want to know what he discovers. Shall we make an appointment for next week?" Barry answered firmly, "We will be here. For the first time I feel we are finally getting somewhere." Angela answered with a smile, "Me too!"

Angela and Barry kept all of their appointments. They were always eager to relate everything that was happening in their lives. Both said that the support group was incredible. They not only enjoyed meeting couples in their circumstances, but they also were learning so much from them. They said that they really liked their infertility specialist . . . that he was young and always explained every procedure and told them what to expect. Angela said that she and Barry respected him tremendously. She

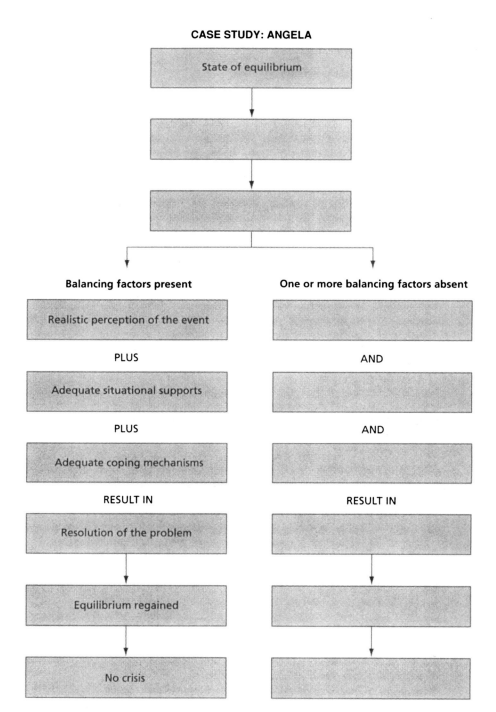

Figure 7-1

added that nothing had been found yet, but that they were just beginning all of the tests. They were terminated at the end of 6 weeks, and they promised to let the therapist know what they discovered. Both expressed their gratitude for her help in getting them "on the right track."

From fairest creatures we desire increase.

–William Shakespeare

Complete the paradigm in Figure 7-1 for this case study, then compare it with the completed one in Appendix D. Refer to the paradigms in Chapter 3 as needed.

REFERENCES

Bennetts L: Preventing miscarriages, *Parents* p. 64, February 1994.

Bresnick E, Taymor ML: The role of counseling in infertility, *Fertil Steril* 32:154, 1979.

Eisner BG: Some psychological differences between fertile and infertile women, *J Clin Psychol* 19:391, 1963.

Halpert FE: When you can't conceive again, *Parents* p. 29, September 1994.

Karahasanglu A, Barglow P, Growe G: Psychological aspects of infertility, *J Reprod Med* 9:241, 1972.

Menning BE: The emotional needs of infertile couples, *Fertil Steril* 34:313, 1980.

Menning BE: The psychosocial impact of infertility, *Nurs Clin North Am* 17(1):155, 1982.

Rosenfeld DL, Mitchell E: Treating the emotional aspects of infertility: counseling services in an infertility clinic, *Am J Obstet Gynecol* 135:177, 1979.

Sturgis SH, Taymor M, Morris T: Routing psychiatric interviews in a sterility investigation, *Fertil Steril* 8:521, 1957.

Taymor M, Bresnick E: Infertility counseling in infertility, 1978, Grune & Stratton.

U.S. Census Bureau: Estimates and projections, October 1993.

Winkleman M: The struggle for a second child, *Parenting* p. 64, June/July 1995.

ADDITIONAL READING

Allen M, Marks S: *Miscarriage: women sharing from the heart,* 1993, John Wiley & Sons.

Berg BJ, Wilson JF: Psychological functioning across stages of treatment for infertility, *J Behav Med* 14(9):11, 1991.

Borg S, Lasker J: *When pregnancy fails,* 1992, Bantam Press.

De Cherney AH: Male infertility. In Kase NG, Weingold AB, Gerson DM, editors: *Principles and practice of clinical gynecology,* New York, 1990, Churchill Livingstone.

Isle S: *Empty arms: coping with miscarriage, stillbirth & infant death,* 1982/1990, Wintergreen Press.

Isle S, Hammer Burns L: *Miscarriage: a shattered dream,* 1985, Wintergreen Press.

Keaggy B, Keaggy J: *A deeper shade of grace,* 1993, Sparrow Press.

Kedem P and others: Psychological aspects of male infertility, *Br J Med Psychol* 63(1):73, 1990.

Kohn I, Moffitt PL, Wilkins MD: *Silent sorrow: pregnancy loss,* 1992, Dell.

Meerabeau L: Husband's participation in fertility treatment: they also serve who only stand and wait, *Sociol Health Ill* 13(3):369, 1991.

Menning BE: Counseling infertile couples, *Contemp Obstet Gynecol* 13:101, 1979.

Menning BE: The emotional needs of infertile couples, *Fertil Steril* 34(4):313, 1980.

Menning BE: The infertile couple: a plea for advocacy, *Child Welfare* 54:454, 1975.

Oldereid NB, Rui H, Purvis K: Male partners in infertile couples, personal attitudes and contact with the Norwegian health service, *Scand J Soc Med* 18(3), 207, 1990.

Pines D: Emotional aspects of infertility and its remedies, *Intl J Psychoanal* 71:561, 1990.

Schiff HS: *The bereaved parent,* 1978, Penguin Books.

Seibel MM, Taymor ML: Emotional aspects of infertility, *Fertil Steril* 37(2):137, 1982.

Shapiro CH: The impact of infertility on the marital relationship, *Soc Casework* 67:387, 1982.

Taylor PJ: When is enough enough, *Fertil Steril* 54(5):772, 1990.

Williamson W: *Miscarriage: sharing the grief . . . facing the pain . . . healing the wounds,* 1987, Walker.

Wright J and others: Psychological distress and infertility: men and women respond differently, *Fertil Steril* 55(1):100, 1991.

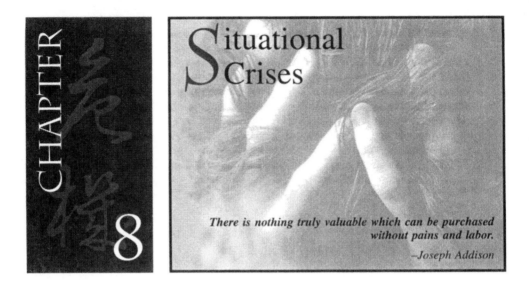

CHAPTER

8

Situational Crises

There is nothing truly valuable which can be purchased without pains and labor.

—Joseph Addison

Defining Situational Crises

Any situation that occurs in our milieu has an impact on us. It may be something that happens physiologically, psychologically, or sociologically. It may be something that is extremely pleasant or extremely unpleasant, depending on our individual mental attitude and our point of view. We will respond as *individuals*. What is stressful and traumatic to one person may be something another person has been eagerly anticipating. This is why crisis intervention techniques always ask the individual the vital question, "What does this mean to you; how is it going to affect your life?" It matters not that the therapist working with the client sees the precipitating event as "unimportant" or not, particularly pleasant or particularly stressful. The frame of reference is always from the patient's point of view.

It is vital that the therapist accepts the situation as a problem for the patient. Circumstances that may create only a feeling of mild concern in one individual may create a high level of anxiety, depression, or stress in another. The therapist must recognize the factors influencing a return to a balance of equilibrium or homeostasis. These factors are the perception of the event, available situational supports, and available coping mechanisms.

The perception of the event for each individual is a product of all his past experiences, his present expectations, and his future anticipations. There are two major ways in which the definition of life events can lead to confusion. The first is the distinction between subjective events and objective events.

Subjective events (e.g., sexual difficulty, a major change in the number of arguments with his spouse, and a major change in sleeping habits) are more likely to be manifestations of or responses to underlying pathology. The problem is also not limited to subjective events because many *objective* events, such as divorce or being fired from work, are as likely to be consequences as causes of pathology. The limitation on causal inference is especially severe in investigations of psychiatric disorders that are often of insidious onset and of long duration.

Most samples of events also include major physical illness or injury, which seems appropriate, since these are negative events that often entail serious disruption of usual activities. It is a basic proposition of psychosomatic medicine that physical disorders are accompanied by some degree of emotional disorder and that emotional disorders are accompanied by some degree of somatic disturbance.

There is clearly a close relationship between crisis theory and intervention and stressful life events. Both areas are concerned with the changes that occur within an individual's life and the impact of these changes on physical and mental health. Crisis theory is closely linked to practice, and its emphasis is on understanding what is likely to lead immediately to therapeutic intervention. Crisis theory investigates whether and to what extent significant associations between life events and illness exist. Those who work in crisis intervention begin, for the most part, with the assumptions that there is something about life events that makes a difference to well-being, whether these events be bereavement, premature births, or others.

It is important to recognize that the theoretical material preceding each case study in this chapter is presented as an overview that is relevant to the crisis situation. Therapists already trained in crisis intervention will recognize the need for much greater depth of theoretical knowledge than is presented in this and the following chapters. The intent is to provide only guidelines; further study of problem areas is suggested for more comprehensive knowledge.

To clarify the steps in crisis intervention, extraneous case study material has been eliminated. In crisis a person may be confronted with many stressful events occurring almost simultaneously. He may have no conscious awareness of *what* occurred, let alone which event requires priority in problem solving. These studies may seem oversimplified to anyone who has struggled through the phases of defining the problem and planning appropriate intervention.

The paradigm is a means devised to keep the reader focused on the problem area and on the balancing factors that influence the presence or absence of crisis. It is doubtful that it could be successfully used as a form that could be quickly completed after an initial interview; rarely are stressful events so easily defined. It is the very nature of a crisis that interrelated internal and external stresses compound the problem area and distort the causes of objective and subjective symptoms.

One responsibility essential in assuming the role of a therapist in this method of intervention is recognition of the need for knowledge of the generic development of crisis.

Status and Role Changes

From the time our life begins until it ends, we "play" many roles and change our status frequently, depending on our age and a multitude of circumstances. According to Chaplin (1985) *role* is defined as "the function or behavior expected of an individual or characteristic of him." Chaplin also defines *status* as "the position of an individual in a social group in terms of his relative standing in the class structure, the honors or awards accorded to him, and the formal or informal power accorded to his position." When we change our role and our status voluntarily and willingly, we are not in conflict. But if our role or status is changed by other forces, either internal or external, then we experience stress, low self-esteem, anger, depression, and in some individuals a state of grief and mourning.

New words and terminology appear with each new generation. The present generation's new word is "down-sizing." The prior generation would have stated that they had "lost their jobs" or had been "laid-off." Our work or profession is part of our identity. It lets others know what group we belong to; it becomes very important to us. If for some reason we lose our position, we lose more than just a job; we lose so much more.

Patterns of careers and job transitions are constantly changing as organizations attempt to respond to both short-term fluctuations and longer term cyclical developments in economic systems. The consequences for the lives of individuals at work can often be quite radical, demanding changes in job skills, self-concept, work hours, and even location of home. Relocation, or job transfer, in particular can have profound effects on the lives of individuals and families. It can require changes in children's school, partner's job, and also provoke difficulties associated with selling and buying property in changing markets (Munton and others, 1993).

A study conducted by Munton and West (1995) found that people are more likely to innovate in their new jobs if they perceive that they have the freedom to innovate. The association between job discretion and role innovation may simply be a result of an underlying operationalization of the two concepts. People may only discover the extent to which they can innovate by pushing at the limits of discretion.

What are clear, at least within the context of job relocation, relatively stable individual differences in symptom reporting, as monitored by self-esteem, are more likely role requirements, such as job novelty, to determine personal change and role innovation. This suggests a need to further develop the theory of work-role transitions, since relationships between role factors and adjustment strategies have been shown to be mediated by individual differences in effect.

If individual difference factors influence role adjustment, then one might expect that role innovation as an adjustment outcome could be facilitated by specifically supporting people's confidence in the new role. This could be achieved through training, coaching, and similar strategies. Also, this suggests that since esteem is an important variable in predicting the likelihood of personal adjustment orientation, social support and supportive supervision strategies might decrease the likelihood that individuals will attempt to adjust by using the elements of personal change strategies that have a negative impact on subjective well-being.

The relationship between role innovation and self-esteem could be a reflection of the impact that self-evaluation can have on choice of adjustment strategy. People whose self-esteem is low may believe that they lack the ability or confidence to innovate after a job change.

Understanding patterns of adjustment to job change and relocation is of enormous practical and theoretical importance, both because of the ubiquity of change in people's lives and because of the increasing requirement for employees to relocate both nationally and internationally. This suggests the need for practitioners to be aware of the dual dimensions of adjustment—personal change and role change—and the very different factors within individuals and their environments that may influence adjustment (Munton and West, 1995).

Case Study   *Status and Role Changes*

Mr. E requested help at the Crisis Center on the advice of his attorney. He was in a state of severe depression and anxiety. He described his symptoms as insomnia, inability to concentrate, and feelings of hopelessness and failure. He is a well-dressed 47-year-old man who looks older than his age because of his tense posture; dull, depressed facial expression; and rather flat, low tone of voice. He has been married for 22 years and has three children, a daughter 13 years of age and two sons whose ages are 8 and 10.

His symptoms began about 3 weeks previously when his company closed its West Coast branch and he lost his job. During the past 2 days, his symptoms increased in intensity to the point where he remained in his room, lay in bed, and did not eat. He became frightened of his depressed thoughts and feared losing complete control of his actions.

During the initial session, he stated to the therapist that he had never been without a job before. Immediately after graduation from college 22 years ago, he started his own advertising agency in New York City. It expanded over the years, and he incorporated, retaining controlling interest and the position of company president. On several occasions he was approached by larger companies with merger proposals. About a year ago, one of the "top three" advertising companies offered him the presidency of a new West Coast branch, which he could run with full autonomy, gaining a great increase in prestige and income. All expenses were to be paid for his family's move to the West Coast.

Mr. E saw this as a chance to "make it big"—an opportunity that might never come his way again. His wife and children, however, did not share his enthusiasm. Mrs. E had always lived in New York City and objected to his giving up his business, where he was "really the boss." She liked the structured security of their life and did not want to leave it for one that she thought would be alien to her. The children sided with her, adding personal objections of their own. They had known only city life, had always gone to the same schools, and did not want to move "way out West." Despite resistance from his family, he made the decision to accept the job offer. His business friends admired his decision to take the chance and expressed full confidence in his ability to succeed. Selling out his shares in his own company to his partner, he moved west with his family within a month.

In keeping with his new economic status and the prestige of his job, he leased a large home in an exclusive residential area. He left most of the responsibility for settling his family to his wife and became immediately involved in the organization of his new business. He described her reaction to the change as being "everything negative that she told me it would be." The children disliked their schools, made few friends, and did not seem to adjust to the pace of their peer group activities. His wife could not find housekeeping help to her liking and consequently felt tied down with work in the home. She missed her friends and clubs, was unable to find shops to satisfy her, and was constantly making negative comparisons between their present lifestyle and their previous one. He felt that there had been a loss of communication between them. His present work was foreign to her, and he could not understand why she was having so many problems just because they had moved to a new location. Her attitude was one of constantly blaming everything that went wrong on his decision to move west and into a new job.

About a month ago, the company suddenly lost four big accounts. Although none of these losses had been a result of his management, immediate retrenchment in nationwide operations was necessary to save the company as a whole. The decision was made to close the newest branch—his branch. There was no similar position available in the remaining offices, and he was offered a lesser position and salary in the Midwest. He was given 2 months in which to close out his office and to make a decision.

Mrs. E's attitude toward these sudden events was a quick "I told you so." She blamed him for their being "stranded out here without friends and a job." He said that he was not a bit surprised by her reaction and had expected it. He had been able to tune out her constant complaints in the past months because he had been so occupied by his job, but now he was forced to join her in making plans for his family's future and in considering their tenuous economic status. He felt that he had been able to hold up pretty well under the dual pressures of closing out the business and planning for his family's future security. A week ago his wife had found a smaller home that would easily fit into their projected budget during the interim until he decided on a new job. He had felt a sense of relief that she had calmed down and was "working *with* me for a change."

However, 2 days ago their present landlord sent an attorney, threatening a lawsuit if Mr. E broke the lease on their present home. His wife became hysterical, blaming him for signing such a lease and calling him a self-centered failure who had ruined his family's lives. "Suddenly I felt as though the bottom had fallen out of my world. I felt frozen and couldn't think what to do next, where to go, and who to ask for help. My family, my employees, everyone was blaming me for this mess. Maybe it *was* all my fault."

Until now Mr. E had always experienced a series of successes in his business and home life. Minor setbacks were usually anticipated and overcome with little need for him to seek outside guidance from others. Now, for the first time, he felt helpless to cope with a stressful situation alone. The threat of having to fulfill the lease on a house he could no longer afford not only destroyed his plans for his family but also broke off what little support he had been receiving from his wife. His feelings of guilt and hopelessness were reinforced by the reality of the threatened lawsuit and the loss of situational supports.

Because of his total involvement in his new work, Mr. E had withdrawn from his previous business and family supports. The sudden loss of his job threatened him with role change and loss of status, for which he had no previous coping experiences. Perceiving himself as a self-made success in the past, he now perceived himself as a self-made failure, both in business and in his parent and husband roles.

When asked by the therapist about his successful coping methods in the past, he said that he had always had recourse to discussions with his business friends. He now felt ashamed to contact them "to let them know he failed." He had always felt free to discuss home problems with his wife, and they usually had resolved them together. Now he seemed no longer able to communicate at home with his wife. When questioned if he was planning to kill himself, he said, "No, I could never take *that* way out. That never entered my mind." After determining that there was no immediate threat of suicide, the therapist initiated intervention.

One goal of intervention was to assist Mr. E in exploring unrecognized feelings about his change in role and status. His loss of situational supports and lack of available coping mechanisms for dealing with the present stressful situation were recognized as areas in need of attention.

In the next 4 weeks, through direct questioning, he began to see the present crisis as a reflection of his past business and family roles. Mr. E had perceived himself as being a strong, independent, self-made man in the past, feeling secure in his roles as boss, husband, and father. He now felt shame at having to depend on others for help in these roles. Coping experiences and skills learned in the past were proving to be inadequate in dealing with the sudden, unexpected, novel changes in his social orbit. The loss of situational support from his wife had added to his already high level of tension and anxiety, which resulted in the failure of what coping skills he had been using with marginal success and in precipitation of the crisis.

After the fourth session Mr. E's depression and feelings of hopelessness had diminished. His perception of the total situation had become more realistic, and he realized that the closing of the branch office was not the result of any failure on his part. It was, in fact, the same decision that he thought he would have made, had he been in charge of the overall operation. He further recognized what great importance he had placed on the possibility that this job would have been his "last chance to make it big." His available coping skills had not lessened in value but had, in fact, been increased by the experience of the situation.

By the fifth week, Mr. E had made significant changes in his situation, both in business and in his family life. He had been able to explore his attitudes about always feeling the need to be the boss and a sense of shame in being dependent on others for support in decision making. He was now able to perceive the stressful events realistically and to cope with his anxieties.

He met with his former landlord and resolved the impending lawsuit, breaking the lease with amicable agreement on both sides. His family had already decided to move into a smaller home, and his wife and children were actively involved with the planning. He had contacted business friends in the East and accepted one of several offers for a lesser position. He would return East alone, his family choosing to follow later when he had reestablished himself. His wife and children made this choice rather than repeat the sudden move into an unsettled situation as they had a year ago. He felt pride that his friends had competed for his services rather than giving him the "I told you so" that he had been dreading.

Before termination, Mr. E and the therapist reviewed the adjustments and the tremendous progress Mr. E had made in such a short period. It was emphasized that it had taken a great deal of strength for him to resolve such an ego-shattering experience. He was also complimented on his ability to recognize the factors he could change, those he would be unable to change, and his new status in life.

He viewed the experience as having been very disturbing at the time but believed he had gained a great deal of insight from it. He thought that he would be able to cope more realistically if a similar situation occurred in the future. He was quite pleased with his ability to extricate himself from a seemingly impossible situation. In discussing his plans for the future, he stated that he no longer believed he had lost his chance for future advancement. He was realistic about past happenings and the possibility that such a crisis could occur again. He was relieved about his family's rapid adjustment to the lesser status of his new position. They were happy to be returning to family and friends on the East Coast. He expressed optimism about again rising to a high position in business and concluded, "I wonder if I could ever really settle for less."

Mr. E's crisis was precipitated by a sudden change in role status (loss of his job) and threatened economic, social, and personal losses. Assessment of the crisis situation determined that he was depressed but not suicidal. Because he was overwhelmed by a sense of failure in both business and family roles, his perceptions of the events were distorted. Having no previous experience with personal failure of this scope, he was unable to cope with his feelings of guilt and depression. His wife's actions reinforced his low self-esteem, and she withdrew as a situational support.

Realistic perception of the event developed as the therapist assisted him in exploring and ventilating unrecognized feelings: he was able to gain insight into relationships between his symptoms of depression and the stressful events. Mrs. E resumed her role of situational support as his new coping skills were successfully implemented in resolving the crisis.

Work and acquire, and thou has chained the wheel of Chance.

–Ralph Waldo Emerson

Complete the paradigm in Figure 8-1 for this case study, then compare it with the completed one in Appendix D. Refer to the paradigms in Chapter 3 as needed.

Rape

The word *rape* arouses almost as much fear as the word *murder.* In a sense it kills both the rapist and his victim. The rapist dies emotionally because he can no longer express or feel tenderness or love, and his victim suffers severe emotional trauma.

Women have nightmares about being sexually assaulted; they anguish over what to do. Either they can resist, hoping to fend off the rapist, or they can obey his commands, hoping he will leave without seriously injuring or killing them. Unfortunately, in 1997 the multitude of sexually transmitted diseases (STDs) only compounds their fears; the reality of being raped is exacerbated knowing that they may have contracted human immunodeficiency virus, acquired immunodeficiency syndrome, herpes, venereal warts, chlamydia, or other sexually transmitted diseases.

CASE STUDY: MR. E

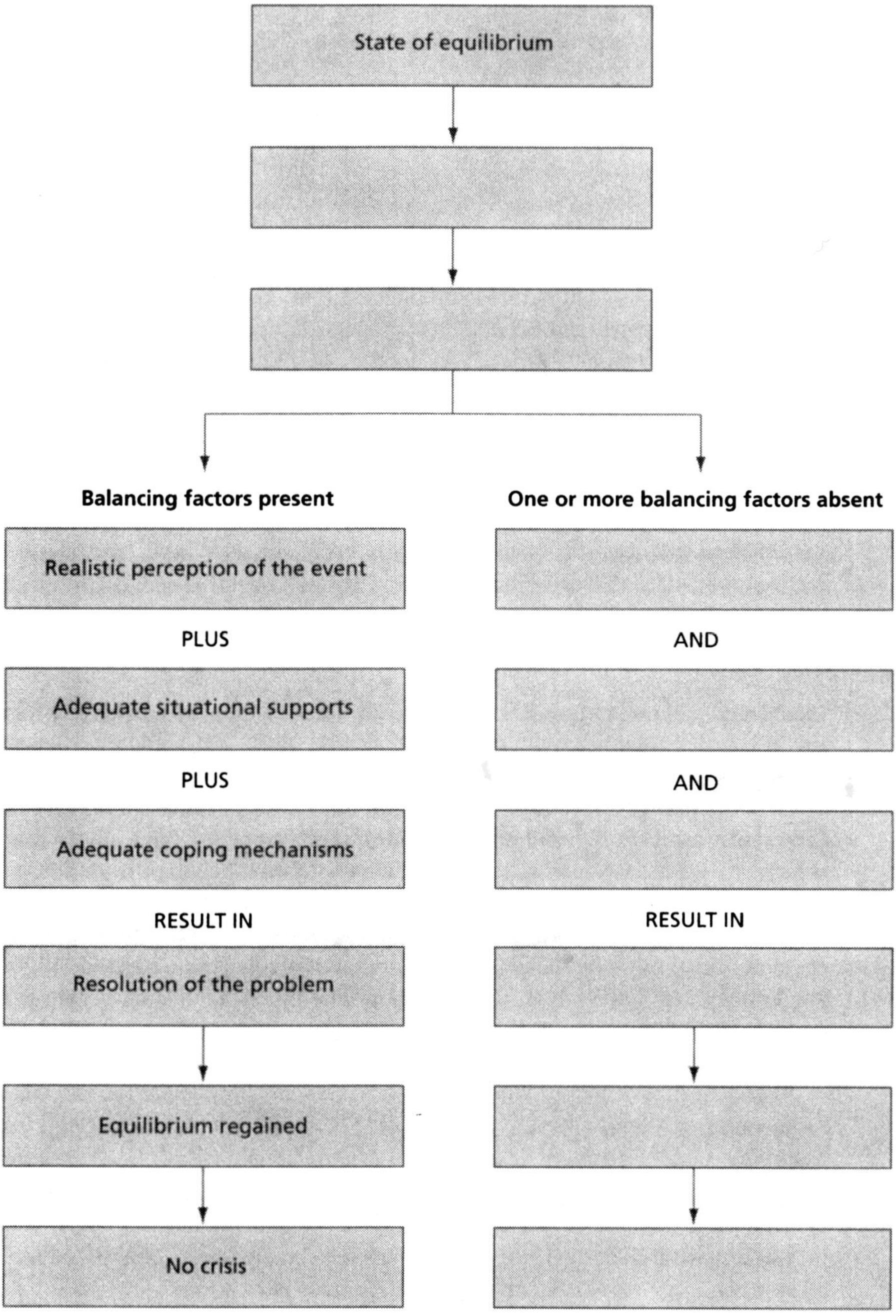

State of equilibrium

Balancing factors present

Realistic perception of the event

PLUS

Adequate situational supports

PLUS

Adequate coping mechanisms

RESULT IN

Resolution of the problem

Equilibrium regained

No crisis

One or more balancing factors absent

AND

AND

RESULT IN

Figure 8-1

The 1990s are also characterized by a phenomenon that has occurred for a long time but is now receiving a great deal of attention—date rape. In all probability, the increased recognition and publicity are due to the feminist movement. Women are more aware of their rights and are acting on them. They have been the silent majority for too long.

Over the past 20 years, there has been a significant increase in the publicity and media focus on rape. The feminist movement took the lead in calling society's attention to the problem of sexual violence directed against women and was instrumental in bringing about legal reform and the establishment of rape crisis centers throughout the country. Rape laws have been reformed, many police departments have instituted specially trained sex crime squads, and many hospitals have created special programs for the medical and psychological treatment of rape victims. Clinical research has been ongoing in developing and evaluating assessment and treatment strategies for both rape victims and sexual aggressors. However, the fear of rape remains a major issue for women in our society, and, in spite of all the attention and special programs, it does not appear that rape rates have declined significantly (Becker and Kaplan, 1991).

Stermac and others (1990) note that we must consider the context of sexual violence as a socially constructed and socially legitimized phenomenon. They also note the prevalence of sexual harassment, acquaintance rape, and abuse within families, and state that contributing factors include negative social attitudes toward women, sex role ideology restricting roles for women, and beliefs in rape myths.

RAPE DEFINED

Traditionally, the common law definition of rape is "carnal knowledge of a female forcibly and against her will" (Koss and Harvey, 1991). Carnal knowledge refers to penile-vaginal penetration only.

Over the past several years, rape statutes have been reformed in numerous states. These reforms have focused on substituting other terms for rapes, including sexual battery, sexual assault, and criminal sexual penetration; placing the emphases on the perpetrator's acts; and acknowledging the violent aspects of rape. In general, reform statutes define rape as nonconsenting penetration obtained by verbal threat or physical force. Individuals who are developmentally disabled, mentally ill, or under the influence of alcohol or drugs are considered incapable of giving informed consent. Reform statutes are not gender specific; both males and females can be victims or perpetrators.

Studies of rape should identify the various forms and types of rape. A rape may be perpetrated by one person, two persons, or more than two as in gang rape. An individual may be raped by a stranger, an acquaintance, a date, or by a spouse. The rape may involve oral, vaginal, or anal penetration. Rape may be planned or spontaneous. The victim may report the rape to the police, may tell family or friends, or may not inform anyone. Researchers need to be precise in defining rape, as well as assessing the various forms of sexual aggression.

Although there is considerable individual variability in response to a sexual assault, a number of commonalities of response have been observed. Koss and others (1991) described the three sequential phases that represent a victim's emotional response to rape as shock, outward adjustment, and integration. They described a cluster of symptoms consistently described by most rape victims. They defined these as *rape trauma syndrome.* The syndrome has two stages: the acute stage, during which the victim's life is completely disrupted by the rape, and the long-term process of recovery, during which the victim attempts to reorganize her life.

During the acute phase *(disorganization phase),* the victim may experience physical reactions including sleep disturbances; eating pattern disturbances; and physical symptoms, including mouth or throat irritation (if she was forced to perform oral sex), vaginal discharge or itching, urogenital problems, and rectal pain and bleeding or generalized pain.

Emotional reactions include fear (of death or physical injury), humiliation, degradation, guilt, shame, anger, self-blame, and embarrassment. Victims may be prone to mood swings during this period. Cognitively, victims may attempt to block thoughts of the rape or to ruminate on how they might have escaped or handled the situation differently.

The long-term process of recovery *(reorganization phase)* can last weeks, months, or years. Various factors can influence the long-term recovery factors. Women may experience changes in lifestyle, they may relocate, and they may terminate relationships or have relationships terminated. They may have difficulty functioning at work or school; they may curtail activities. Sleep disturbances and nightmares about the assault may continue. Victims may develop phobias or other forms of anxiety disorders.

FEAR AND ANXIETY

Perhaps one of the most frequent sequelae of a sexual assault is fear. During the assault, victims often fear for their lives. After the assault, victims have fears for their personal safety and of the assailant returning and attacking them again. Recently fear of HIV infection has become a major concern of those victims by perpetrators unknown to them. Some victims may become phobic as a result of the rape.

DEPRESSION

Depression is frequently noted in victims immediately after the rape. Rape victims describe mild to severe levels of depressive symptoms during the first month post-assault in 75% of the reported cases. By 4 months these levels decreased for most symptoms to within the normal range. Attempted suicide is also a sequela to rape.

Calhoun and Atkeson (1991) state that despite almost 3 decades of clinical observation and empirical research, we are only now beginning to understand the serious consequences that sexual assault can have for a woman and those close to her. Data indicate that a significant number of women are victims of rape. The impact of victimization can be both short term and long term. Rape can have an impact on the emotional, cognitive, social, and physical functioning of victims. Rape can also have an emotional impact on the victim's family and significant others.

Therapy outcome studies for rape victims should control time since the rape, and victims should be in active interventions within a support group. Factors such as social supports and ways of coping must also be included.

Unfortunately, most rapists can neither admit nor express the fact that they are a menace to society. Even convicted rapists who are serving long prison terms deny their culpability; they tenaciously insist that women encourage and enjoy sexual assault. These men tell others that they are the greatest lovers in the world.

The case study that follows concerns a legal secretary who was raped. After the rape, she went home to shower and change her clothes, and then she went to work. She was obviously in a state of shock and disbelief.

Case Study   Rape

Ann, an attractive 26-year-old legal secretary, was brought to the Crisis Center by her employer. That morning on her way to work, she had been raped. After being raped, she returned to her apartment, showered, changed her clothes, and calmly went to work.

At approximately 11:30 AM she matter-of-factly announced to her employer that she had been raped and told him the details. He was shocked and horrified. He asked her to go to the hospital for treatment and to notify the police. She stated very unemotionally that she was "fine" and had only numerous superficial cuts on her breasts and abdomen and would continue working. By midafternoon she appeared to her employer to be in a state of shock and was acting disoriented and confused. He drove her to the Crisis Center where she was seen immediately in the emergency room by a female therapist who had expertise in working with rape victims.

The therapist offered Ann a cup of coffee, and she accepted. While they were drinking their coffee, the therapist quietly asked Ann to tell her what had happened. Ann began to sob. The therapist handed her some tissues, put her arms around her shoulders, held her close, and told her that she understood how she was feeling. Gradually Ann calmed down and stopped crying. She then said, "I feel so filthy; I feel I should have resisted more; I am so confused." She was reassured that these feelings were normal and was asked to tell what happened.

Ann stated that she always got up early and took the bus to work because it was very convenient, and she arrived before anyone else was in the office. She liked to get her desk in order for the day and make the coffee so that she could serve coffee to the attorney she worked for when he arrived. She smiled slightly and said, "He isn't fit to talk to until he has finished his second cup of coffee in the morning. He commutes in from a suburb, and he has to battle the traffic for at least an hour or an hour and a half." The therapist smiled and asked her to continue. She took a deep breath and stated that this morning she had gotten up as usual and ridden the bus to work. As she was walking from the bus stop to her office building, approximately three blocks, a man walked toward her. He was tall, attractive, and well dressed. When he approached her, he smiled and said, "Can you tell me where Fifth Street is?" She returned his smile and said, "You are going the wrong way. It's the next street up" (pointing in the direction she was walking). He said, "Thank you" and, turning around, fell into step with her and started talking about the weather—"what a beautiful morning"—and other small talk. They had walked approximately 100 yards when he suddenly pulled out a knife, shoved her against a car, put the knife to her throat, and said, "Don't scream or I'll kill you. Get in the car." Ann began to tremble and tears rolled down her cheeks. The therapist said, "How frightening! What did you do?" Ann said, "I was so shocked and terrified; I thought he *would* kill me. So when he opened the car door, I got in."

Ann continued to tell what had happened. He made her slide over to the driver's seat, keeping the knife firmly at her waist, ordered her to start the car, and told her where to drive (an isolated area near the river). He then made her get in the back seat and undress. He started caressing her and talking obscenities to her, telling her how he was going to make love to her "like no other man could." Ann said that she began to cry and plead with him, but it only seemed to make him angry. He began making small cuts on her breasts and abdomen and kept saying he would kill her if she did not "cooperate." Ann said that he acted "spaced out" and had a glazed look in his eyes, as if he were not really raping her *personally*—just somebody.

Ann stated that after he raped her, he seemed to "come to" and started to cry, saying, "I'm so sorry. I didn't mean to hurt you. Please forgive me; I just can't help it. Please don't tell anyone." Ann got dressed, and he helped her into the front seat and kept asking her if she was alright and generally expressing concern for her well-being. He asked if he could drive her someplace, and Ann asked him to drop her off approximately four blocks from her apartment, telling him she was going to a girlfriend's to "clean up." He dropped her off and again begged her not to tell anyone and to please forgive him. Ann said that when she was certain he had driven away, she walked to her apartment in a daze. All she could think about was taking a shower to "get clean again" and to change her clothes completely to try to erase her feelings of degradation. She stated that she thought she should go to work "to keep her mind off it." Only later in the afternoon as she "relived" the events in her mind did she begin to feel terribly guilty over not "resisting" or "fighting back" when he first pulled the knife. She said (with a tone of great remorse), "I didn't even scream!"

The therapist felt that Ann should go to the hospital immediately for treatment of her numerous cuts and determination of the presence of spermatozoa in the vagina, and then she should report the incident to the police. After this was done, she should return to the center to meet with the therapist and continue her mental catharsis. The therapist explained to Ann that someone from the rape hot line would go with her to the hospital and remain with her there and while she gave her report to the police. She was assured that the therapist would contact the hospital to arrange that Ann be examined by a female physician and that she would be interrogated by a female police officer. Ann agreed to go, and a member of the rape team was called to be with her and then to return her to the center.

When Ann returned, she was pale and trembling but apparently in control of her emotions. Again she was offered coffee, which she accepted, and she and the therapist discussed how things had gone at the hospital and with the police interrogation. Ann stated it was definitely *not* pleasant, but that it was not as bad as she had thought it would be. She added, "Thank God I didn't take a douche!"

The therapist asked Ann if she had a friend or family member whom she would like to contact and possibly have spend the night with her because she was still very frightened by her experience. Ann turned even paler and explained, "Oh, my God—Charles!" She was asked, "Who is Charles?" She replied, hesitantly, "My fiancé." The therapist asked Ann if she could call Charles and tell him what happened. Ann began to cry and said, "I am so ashamed. He will probably hate me. He probably will never want to touch me again. What have I done?" She was comforted by the therapist and told that *she* had done nothing wrong. She continued to cry and berate herself. The therapist gave her a mild sedative and asked her to lie down and rest. Twenty minutes later, Ann asked the therapist if she would call Charles and tell him what had happened, but she said that she did not want to see him until she knew how he felt about her being raped. The therapist agreed and asked for Charles's telephone number.

The call was placed to Charles, and the therapist briefly explained that Ann was raped and that she was not severely injured but psychologically very traumatized. Charles responded with concern and anger and asked if he could see Ann. He was told to come to the center and to ask for the therapist.

Charles arrived and was extremely upset and angry. The therapist took him to her office and explained fully what had happened to Ann and what had been done for her. He started to cry and to curse, stating, "My God, poor Ann" and "I'll find that dirty bastard and kill him!" The therapist allowed him to ventilate his feelings of pity and anger, and he began to calm down. When he seemed calmer, he was asked, "Does this change your feelings for Ann?" He appeared startled and said, "No, I love her. We are getting married!" The therapist told him that Ann was afraid he would not love her anymore. He replied, "It wasn't her fault; of course I still love her!"

The therapist explained that after being raped, a woman usually feels "guilty," "unclean," and very fearful of intimacy with another man, even if she loves him very much. She added that Ann needed his strength, love, and constant reassurance that nothing has changed between them. He listened and said, "I'll do anything I can to help her forget this."

The therapist asked if he sometimes stayed overnight at Ann's apartment, and he answered, "Yes, often." He was asked if he would spend the night with her (if she agreed) and hold her (if she would let him), touch her, reaffirm his love for her, and speak about their coming marriage but not attempt sexual intercourse unless she asked him; he agreed and asked to see Ann. The therapist asked for a few minutes alone with Ann first.

When the therapist entered, Ann was lying on the couch staring at the ceiling. She turned her head and looked fearfully at the door. The therapist smiled, sat down by Ann, held her hand, and said, "I like your Charles. He is a fine young man. He will probably break down that door if I don't let him in to see you!" Ann asked, "What did he say?" The therapist told her that he had stated he loved her very much and that he would do anything to help her forget the rape, that it was not her fault, and that he would like to "kill the bastard who hurt *her*."

Ann said hesitantly, "Are you sure?" The therapist replied firmly, "Positive! Now comb your hair and put some makeup on, so I can let him in!" Ann smiled weakly and complied.

Charles entered the office, took Ann in his arms, and held her gently, stroking her hair and face, saying, "I'm so sorry, my love. Let me take care of you. Everything is going to be alright. I love you. You are the most precious thing in my life." Ann cried softly on his shoulder.

The therapist said, "Why don't you two go home and get some rest, and I'll see you both next week." Ann and Charles agreed and left with their arms around each other and Ann's head on his shoulder.

(*Note:* The therapist had listened to Ann's account of the rape and modus operandi with increasing feelings of helplessness and anger because in the past 3 months she had worked with two other rape victims who had described the same details but with one major difference: the first victim had only one minute cut on her throat, which she received when he pushed her against the car; the second had several small superficial cuts on her breasts; and now the third victim, Ann, had numerous cuts on her breasts and abdomen. The rapist was obviously becoming increasingly violent with each rape.)

The next sessions were spent in collateral therapy with Ann and Charles. The focus was on ventilation of their feelings and helping Ann begin to express anger toward her rapist. By the end of six sessions, they had resumed their normal sexual activities and had advanced their wedding date 3 months. Charles felt he was really living at Ann's apartment because he wanted to be with her as much as possible; therefore they agreed to get married sooner than they had planned.

Because rape is so emotionally traumatic, Ann was treated as an emergency patient by the therapist. The sooner intervention begins with a rape victim, the less psychological damage occurs.

Most women are totally unprepared for rape; therefore it is a new traumatic experience to cope with, and previous defense mechanisms are usually ineffective to resolve the crisis.

Ann greatly feared total rejection by her fiancé (a very real and common occurrence). This is why the therapist saw both Ann and Charles in collateral sessions; thus both would have a chance to explore and ventilate their feelings together.

Ann perceived that the rape was her fault because she did not resist immediately and did not scream. These feelings are common in women who have been raped. Usually everything occurs rapidly, and the ever-present fear of being killed or seriously injured tends to immobilize the victim.

ADDENDUM

Four months later a patient was referred to the center because he was on probation for rape, and he became the same therapist's patient. When he was questioned about how and why, as he described his modus operandi, the therapist *knew* that he was the one who had raped Ann and the two other victims. After the rapist discussed his feelings—guilt, shame, and helplessness in controlling his actions—the therapist asked about his background and family. This new patient, Phillip, described his childhood as one deprived of affection. His mother had left his father, and Phillip had been reared by an aunt who was very cold, undemonstrative, and—to him—uncaring and rigid.

When questioned about his present living circumstances, he stated that he was married (happily) and had three small children. When asked why he felt the need to rape, he stated, "I don't know." He began to cry and said, "Please help me. I can't help myself."

When the therapist asked if his wife knew that he was on probation for rape, he said, very hesitantly, "No, but I *know* she thinks something is wrong with me." The therapist told Phillip that she had worked with three of his victims, and she felt that he was becoming increasingly more violent, as evidenced by the increasing use of the knife and the sight of blood to stimulate him.

Phillip stared intently at the therapist and said with amazement in his voice, "My God, don't you hate me? I hate myself." The therapist was able to admit that her bias was toward his victims but that she felt he needed help because she was afraid he might kill his next victim. He admitted that he did not know whether he *would* or *would not* kill someone.

The therapist then asked him how his wife and children would feel if they found out that he was a potential murderer. He shuddered and said, "Help me! I don't know what to do!" The therapist stated that he should tell his wife about being on probation and about the rapes, and then the therapist would do all she could to get him help. He agreed and called his wife and asked her to come to the center.

His wife arrived, and Phillip, with the therapist present, told her what he had done and the possibility of what he could do in the future. She began to cry and said, "I've *known* something was wrong, but I didn't know what." She turned to the therapist and asked, "What can we do?" The therapist was very candid and stated that Phillip should be at a well-known maximum security prison where he could receive consistent, intensive psychiatric therapy in order to protect the reputation of their family and to protect the community.

They agreed with this decision. The therapist then called the judge and told him the facts. He agreed that maximum security was needed and said that he would send a car to transport Phillip to the facility.

It must be noted that *rarely* does a therapist work with rape victims and then with their offender. It was extremely difficult to remain "cool, calm, and collected" while Phillip related his modus operandi; however, he too was a "victim" who needed help, and he did receive it.

Vicious actions are not hurtful because they are forbidden, but forbidden because they are hurtful.

–*Benjamin Franklin*

Complete the paradigm in Figure 8-2 for this case study, then compare it with the completed one in Appendix D. Refer to the paradigms in Chapter 3 as needed.

Physical Illness

Diseases are known to have their places and their times (see Chapter 11). Primitive societies have been characterized by health problems related to recurrent famines, and urban societies have been characterized by epidemics of infectious disease. Modern industrial societies are characterized by a new set of diseases: obesity, arteriosclerosis, hypertension, diabetes, and widespread symptoms of anxiety. Arising from these are two of the three greatest disablers of our own place and time: coronary heart disease and stroke.

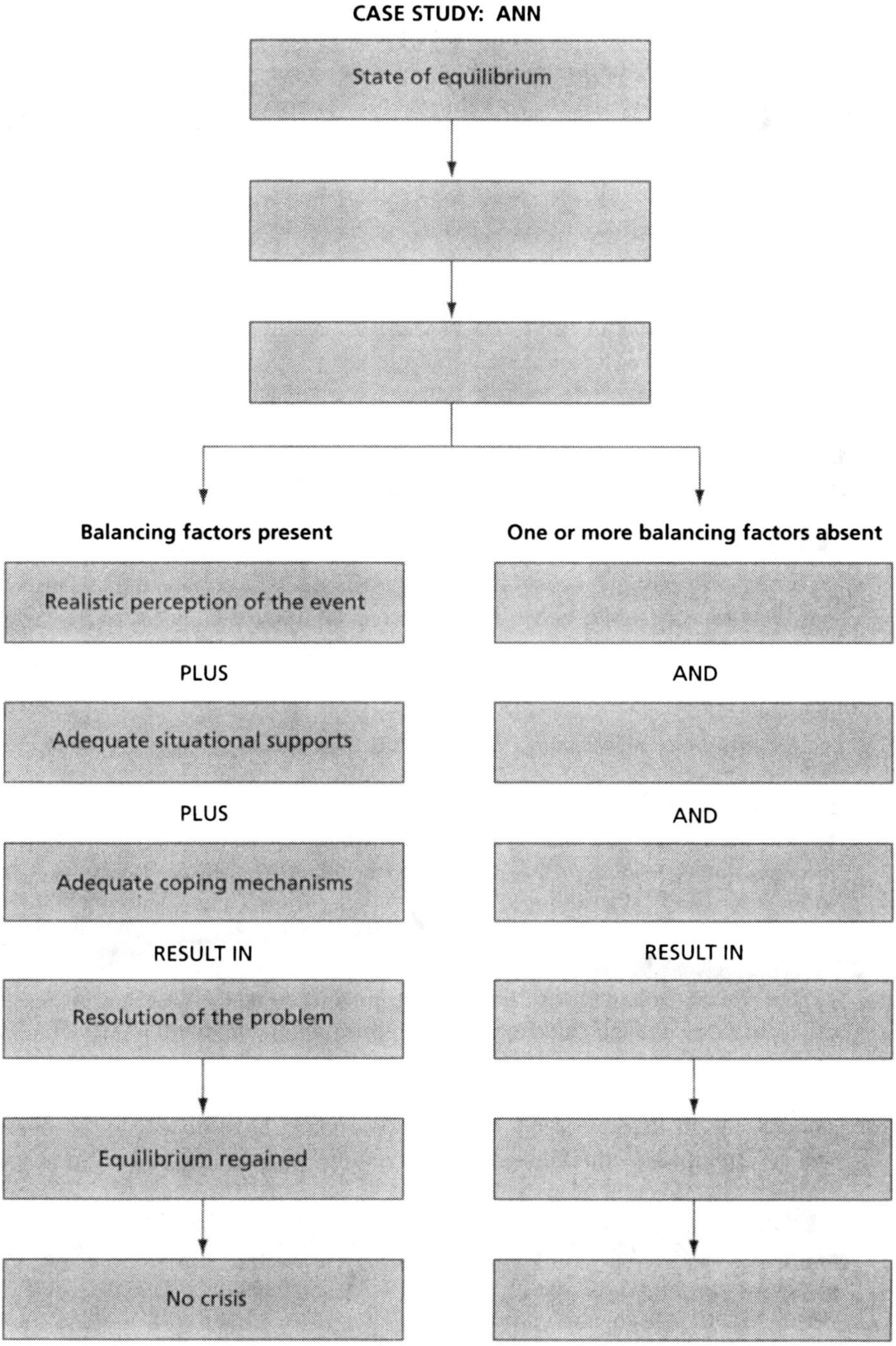

Figure 8-2

In recent years increasing concern has focused not only on the etiology and epidemiology of cardiac disease but also on factors affecting the process of recovery. Statistics indicate that approximately 35% of deaths among adults between 25 and 44 years of age result from chronic medical conditions such as heart disease, cancer, cerebrovascular, and pulmonary diseases (National Center for Health Statistics, 1994).

It is clear that chronic illness can be identified as a major stressor for all family members. Illness demands have been found to be related to higher levels of psychological distress in chronically ill adults (Kotchick and others, 1996). If one family member has an illness, its effects can create repercussions in all other family members. The family member who is ill does not live in isolation from the rest of the family. This creates stress and in many cases role changes, which creates more family stress.

A variable assumed to mediate between the impact of illness and psychological distress among family members is the use of effective coping strategies. Coping has been broadly defined as a constellation of responses that serve to control or reduce emotional stress in the face of some externally imposed life strain, such as chronic illness. Active coping consists of those strategies intended to directly affect the stressor, either behaviorally (such as doing something to eliminate the source of the problem) or cognitively (such as thinking about the stressor in a more positive light). Avoidant coping strategies are behaviors and cognitions intended to draw attention away from the stressful event; such avoidant strategies include doing something to keep from thinking about the problem or denying the presence or impact of the stressor.

Although the relationship between the use of certain coping strategies and individual outcome has been established, little is known about the effects of the maladaptive coping of one family member on significant others. Maladaptive coping by one family member may have adverse effects on the psychological functioning of other family members by increasing the level of distress experienced by the individual using such coping strategies, which, in turn, has negative effects on the functioning of other family members. A person's use of avoidant coping strategies has been associated with elevated levels of depression and anxiety.

The conceptualization of the recovery process in heart disease as a response to crisis provides strategic advantages in approaching the problem. It leads to focusing on the kinds of adaptive and maladaptive mechanisms that patients employ in coping with this illness, on the stages of recovery, and on the resources that patients use and require at each stage. Viewing response to coronary heart disease as a problem that can be approached through crisis intervention permits the use of concepts and formulations inherent in crisis theory.

In a discussion of the rehabilitation of patients with cardiac disease, a report by the World Health Organization in 1996 distinguished between phases of the recovery process in terms of time and coping tasks. The first phase is categorized as one in which the patient spends approximately 2 weeks in bed, with minimal physical activity. In the next phase the patient spends approximately 6 weeks at home, with a variety of sedentary activities. In the third phase, which lasts from 2 to 3 months, the patient makes a gradual reentry into the occupational world.

Lee and Bryner (1961) conceptualize phases according to the kinds of care the physician must provide for the patient at each point of the process. They specify (1) evaluation of the patient and his environment, (2) management of the patient, and (3) reestablishment of the patient in his community.

In other formulations of recovery phases, emphasis is on the kinds of therapeutic or rehabilitative relationships that predominate at each point. Hellerstein and Goldstone (1954) describe the first, or acute, phase as one in which the relationship between the physician and patient is of primary importance. The convalescent phase follows, and the relationship between the patient and family and friends becomes primary. During the recovery, or third, phase the employer or vocational counselor becomes the vital participant in the rehabilitation of the patient with cardiac disease.

Phases have also been viewed in terms of the emotional adaptation of the patient. Kubie (1955) suggests that the first phase is marked by initial shock, and the second phase is marked by appreciation of the full extent of the disability. In the third phase there is "recovery from the lure of hospital care"; in the fourth and final phase there is "a facing of independent, unsupported, and competitive life."

Among the most obvious and critical determinants of the outcome of the recovery process are the severity of heart damage, the degree of impairment, and the physiological resources of the patient. Although cardiac damage has much to do with setting limits on performance and affecting levels of adjustment, studies of physiological factors alone contribute only partially to understanding the recovery process. Research on the importance of the premorbid personality of the patient as a determinant of adjustment to illness suggests that it is a second important factor in the recovery process.

Other important factors bearing on the recovery process include the various psychological mechanisms that the patient uses in handling illness. If the recovery process is viewed as a response to a crisis situation, then the individual mechanisms used by patients appear particularly important in the resolution of the crisis. The significance of emotional response to disease has often been underlined in discussing the elements that determine recovery. McIver (1960) states, "The way in which a crisis is handled emotionally may significantly influence the eventual outcome of a case in terms of the extent of recovery and the degree of rehabilitation achieved." Reiser (1951) emphasizes that it is essential to deal with the anxieties associated with the diagnosis and symptoms of heart disease if the therapy of cardiac disease is to attain its optimal effect. A common view is that during the acute phase of any serious illness the patient's emotional state is characterized by fear because the illness threatens his total integrity, as well as his sense of personal adequacy and worth to others.

Compared with other serious illnesses, heart disease has several unique features. Associated as it is with sudden death, it is viewed by the patient and family as an immediate and severe threat to life. Hollender (1958) has written that even in the most stable patients the onset of heart disease is associated with an onslaught of anxiety. During the first days of illness, the patient with heart disease must assume a passive role, and some believe that this role tends to compound anxiety. Physical restriction usually increases feelings of helplessness, vulnerability, and depression. The patient is then handicapped in utilizing defense mechanisms that should ultimately help him to adjust to an altered status.

Although coping responses vary widely, there appears to be a core of relatively uniform responses of adjustment. For example, depression and regression have often been reported as the initial reaction to the illness. Some patients display aggression and hostility, placing the blame for the illness on external factors. Some deal with the threat to life by denial of the illness.

It has been suggested that certain coping responses are appropriate at one stage of recovery but are inappropriate at another. When patients at the same stage of recovery are compared, similar responses may function in different ways: constructively for some patients but hindering recovery for others. There is disagreement at present about the role denial plays in recovery. Some regard denial, which may lead to noncooperation with the physician, as a response of self-destruction. Others consider that denial arises from a belief in the integrity of the self and the invulnerability of the body and regard it as constructive and associated with the maintenance of health.

Because each patient reacts as an individual in this life-threatening situation, the therapist, in all probability, sees a variety of coping responses being utilized. It is not the therapist's role to change the patient's pattern of coping but to understand that his reaction to illness is part of the patient's defense.

King (1962) states: "Man's basis for action in health and disease is a composite of many things. One crucial variable is the way that he sees or perceives the situation . . . and all of the social ramifications that accompany it." These perceptions are conditioned by socialization in a sociocultural context. How the patient responds to the disease is influenced by what he has learned. The content of the learning is in turn determined by the norms and values of the society in which he lives. The meaning of the disease, attitude toward medical practitioners, willingness to comply with medical advice, and the patient's management of his life after a heart attack are all influenced by the attitudes and beliefs that he has learned.

Pertinent to the recovery process is the conceptualization of the "sick role," which Parson (1951) describes as a social role, with its own culturally defined rights and obligations. Although a person may be physiologically ill, he is not recognized as legitimately ill unless his illness fulfills the criteria or standards set by the society. Once defined as legitimately able to be in the "sick role," he is expected to meet certain expectations of others. The person is expected, for example, to make an effort toward becoming well and to seek help. In turn, he has the right to expect certain kinds of behavior from others toward him, including a willingness to permit him to relinquish his normal social role responsibilities.

Willingness to accept the sick role may mean that a patient with heart disease is likely to follow the regimen of his physician and to care for himself in ways that maximize his recovery. At the same time, reluctance to accept the sick role may also influence the recovery process favorably. Such a patient may be anxious to avoid being defined as sick. Like the willing patient, he too may follow the therapeutic regimen to shorten the period of incapacity. However, reluctance to view himself as sick may lead a patient to comply minimally with medical advice and to attempt full activity before he is physically able to do so.

The following case study illustrates how a businessman responded to a sudden heart attack with inappropriate and excessive denial.

Case Study   *Physical Illness*

Mr. Z, age 43, was chairing a board meeting of his large, successful manufacturing corporation when he developed shortness of breath; dizziness; and a crushing, viselike pain in his chest. The paramedics were called, and he was taken to the medical center. Subsequently, he was admitted to the coronary care unit with a diagnosis of impending myocardial infarction.

Mr. Z is married, with three children. He is president and the majority stockholder of a large manufacturing corporation. He has no previous history of cardiovascular problems, although his father died at age 38 of a massive coronary occlusion. His oldest brother died at the age of 42 from the same condition, and his other brother, still living, is a semi-invalid after suffering two heart attacks at the ages of 44 and 47.

Mr. Z was tall, slim, suntanned, and very athletic. He swam daily, jogged every morning for 30 minutes, played golf regularly, and was an avid sailor who participated in every yacht regatta, usually winning. He was very health conscious, had annual physical checkups, watched his diet, and quit smoking to avoid possible damage to his heart, determined to avoid dying young or becoming an invalid like his brothers.

When he was admitted to the coronary care unit, Mr. Z was conscious. Although in a great deal of pain, he seemed determined to control his own fate. While in the coronary care unit, he was an exceedingly difficult patient, a trial to the nursing staff and his physician. He constantly watched and listened to everything going on around him and demanded complete explanations about any procedure, equipment, or medication he received. He would sleep in brief naps and only when he was totally exhausted. Despite his obvious tension and anxiety, his condition stabilized. The damage to his heart was considered minimal, and his prognosis was good. As the pain diminished, he began asking when he could go home and when he could go back to work. He was impatient to be moved to a private room so that he could conduct some of his business by telephone.

Mr. Z denied having any anxiety or concerns about his condition, although his behavior in the unit contradicted his denial. Recognizing that Mr. Z was coping inappropriately with the stress of illness, his physician requested as consultant a therapist whose expertise was crisis intervention to work with Mr. Z to help him through the crisis period.

The therapist agreed to work with Mr. Z for 1 hour a week for 6 weeks. Their first session was scheduled the second day of his stay in the coronary care unit. The therapist reviewed Mr. Z's chart and talked with his physician before the first session to gain an accurate assessment of Mr. Z's physical condition and to gain some knowledge of factors (e.g., socioeconomic status, marital status, family history) to assist in assessing his biopsychosocial needs.

In the first session the therapist observed Mr. Z's overt and covert signs of anxiety and depression and determined, through discussion with him, his perception of what hospitalization meant to him, his usual patterns of coping with stress, and available situational supports. Through direct questions and reflective verbal feedback, she was able to elicit the reasons for his behavior and reactions to his illness and to his confinement in the coronary care unit.

Observing his suntanned, youthful appearance and the general physical condition of a very active and persistent athlete, the therapist questioned him about his lifestyle before his hospitalization. Mr. Z was quite adamant about his "minor" condition and the possibility of curtailed activity. He stated that he was very aware of his family's tendency toward cardiac conditions but added, "I have always taken excellent care of myself to avoid the possibility of becoming a cardiac cripple like my brother." Apparently he was not too concerned about the prospect of dying; in fact, he might prefer it to the overwhelming prospect of being a useless, dependent invalid.

He expressed concern about the length of time he might have to spend in the hospital. When questioned about his concern, he stated: "I *have* to be in good shape by the second of December (in approximately 3½ months). I've entered the big yacht race, and I plan to win again!"

When he was asked how his wife and children were reacting to his illness and hospitalization, Mr. Z's facial expression and general body tension relaxed noticeably. He smiled and said, "My wife, Sue, is simply unbelievable; she takes everything in stride. She is always cool, calm, and collected. She even met with the board of directors and told them to delay any major decisions until I return . . . but that she could handle any minor decisions!" The therapist asked if she could meet his wife. Mr. Z replied that his wife would be in to see him soon and suggested she stay and meet her.

After meeting with them briefly, the therapist asked Mrs. Z to stop by her office before leaving. Mrs. Z arrived at the office and sank gratefully into a chair, losing the bright, cheerful, and optimistic manner she had maintained while with her husband. Observing her concerned expression and slumped posture, the therapist inquired, "You are very concerned about your husband, aren't you?" Mrs. Z readily admitted that she was concerned but did not want her husband to know. When asked what specifically concerned her, she replied: "Jim's inability to accept any type of forced inactivity and his refusal to accept the possibility that he might have to change his hectic lifestyle. He can't *bear* the thought of being ill or being dependent on anyone or anything!"

The therapist explained that it is difficult for many patients to accept a passive, dependent role while ill and that it takes time for them to adjust to a changed lifestyle. She then explained to Mrs. Z that the physician had arranged for Mr. Z to have therapy sessions for the next 6 weeks to help him through his crisis. Mrs. Z seemed relieved that someone else recognized the problems confronting her husband and would help him as he worked through his feelings about his illness and unwanted but inevitable changes in lifestyle. The therapist suggested that Mrs. Z might also need some support, as she too had to adjust to Mr. Z's illness. They agreed to meet for an hour each week so they could work together toward a resolution of the crisis. A convenient time was arranged each week when Mrs. Z came to visit her husband.

Mr. Z's denial of the possibility that he might die like his father and oldest brother or that he might become an invalid, "useless and dependent," like his other brother was considered of prime importance. It was felt that the first goal of intervention was to assist Mr. Z to ventilate his feelings about his illness and hospitalization. A second goal was to assist him to perceive the event realistically. A third goal was to give support to Mrs. Z and assist her in coping with the stress induced by her husband's hospitalization.

It was believed that Mr. Z's high anxiety level would interfere with his ability to express his feelings about his illness and his hospitalization. In an attempt to reduce his anxiety, the therapist made two recommendations to his physician, which were accepted. The first recommendation was that Mr. Z be moved out of the coronary care unit to a private room as soon as possible. The environmental surroundings in the coronary care unit, with its overwhelming and complex equipment, strange sounds, and constant activities of the staff, apparently increased Mr. Z's anxiety. Because of the stressful situation, he was not getting sufficient rest. After his move to a private room later that afternoon, he began to relax noticeably, became much less demanding of the staff, and began sleeping and eating better.

The second recommendation was that he be permitted to use the telephone for 30 minutes three times a day. Thus he was able to conduct some of his business from his bed. This apparently made him feel less dependent, and the increased mental activity relieved some of his anxiety about becoming a "helpless" invalid.

In the next sessions Mr. Z began to discuss—hesitantly at first and then more freely—his feelings about his illness and his reaction to hospitalization. He discussed his father's sudden death when he was in his teens and how lost he would have felt if his older brother had not stepped in and taken over. All three brothers were very close, and the death of the oldest one, while Mr. Z was in college, reactivated the grief he felt for his father. He was just beginning to accept his oldest brother's death when, a year later, his other brother had a severe heart attack and was unable to continue in the family business. As Mr. Z saw it, his brother was a "helpless" invalid. Mr. Z, the youngest son, then became president of the corporation and controlled the majority of the stocks. He stated that although he certainly didn't *want* to die, he was less afraid of dying than he was of becoming useless, helpless, and a burden to his family.

Through discussion and verbal feedback, Mr. Z was able to view realistically his illness and the changes it would make in his life. No, he was *not* an invalid. Yes, he *would* be able to work and to live a normal life. No, he would not have to give up sailing; he would just have to have someone else do most of the crewing. Yes, he would be able to resume his activities but would continue them at a more leisurely pace. For example, instead of scheduling fifteen things to do in a day, schedule seven. Gradually he became more accepting as he began to realize that the mild myocardial infarction was a warning he should heed and that with proper care and some diminishing of his usual hectic pace, he could continue to live a productive and useful life.

The therapist continued to meet with Mrs. Z to give her support and began anticipatory planning for her husband's convalescence at home. They discussed Mr. Z's strong need to feel independent and in control of all situations, and the therapist encouraged her to continue to let her husband make decisions for the family. She assured Mrs. Z that he would be able to continue a relatively normal life and that she did not need to protect and "coddle" him, something he would greatly resent. When asked how their children were reacting to their father's hospitalization, Mrs. Z replied, "At first they were terribly concerned and silent; now they are beginning to ask, "When is he coming home, and what can we do?" It was obvious that Mr. Z had strong situational support in his family.

Mr. Z's recovery progressed fairly smoothly, and he began to ambulate and take care of his basic needs. Although more accepting of his need for some assistance, he still became upset and impatient if the staff attempted to assist him in routine care.

Mr. Z was discharged after his second week, with instructions for his convalescence at home. The therapist continued to meet with Mr. and Mrs. Z at their home during the rest of the sessions to assist the family toward stabilization as Mr. Z adjusted to his new regimen of reduced activity and to provide anticipatory planning for their future.

By the end of the fifth week, with the strong support of his family and the therapist, Mr. Z was able to view his illness and his feelings about curtailing some of his hectic activities in a more accepting and realistic manner. His family still consulted him for advice and opinions about family decisions. This made him feel that he was still an active, participating member of the family.

He was able to conduct a large part of his business from his home by having board meetings there and by having periodic telephone conversations with his office staff. His secretary came to his home 3 days a week to take dictation and to secure his signature when it was needed on documents. He also telefaxed materials and orders to his office employees. Thus he still remained in control of his business life, which contributed greatly to his self-esteem.

The children and Mrs. Z were encouraged to continue in their usual daily activities so that Mr. Z would not feel that his being at home was disrupting to their lives. It also helped Mrs. Z to cope with her feelings and her desire to protect her husband from stress. Gradually, she was able to realize that he was capable of coping with some stress and that he was not as fragile as she had believed him to be.

Before termination, the therapist and Mr. Z reviewed the adjustments he had made and the insights he had gained into his own behavior. He was intellectually able to understand the reasons for his denial and dependence-independence conflicts. He was very optimistic about his future and believed that he could adjust to a reduced-activity schedule. He still, rather wistfully, was hoping his physician would approve his entering the yacht race. He was realistic about his physical condition and the possibility that a coronary attack could occur again, stating, "At least now I've learned to relax and roll with the punches."

Mrs. Z and the children felt they would be able to cope with the occasional bouts of frustration and temper flare-ups of Mr. Z. They were now aware of how difficult it was for him to make the many adjustments necessary to his new way of life.

Mr. Z's fear of becoming a "cardiac cripple" like his brother distorted his perception of the event. He was unable to relax and be dependent in the coronary care unit; his anxiety and tension made him unable to accept the fact that he had a myocardial infarction. His family and his colleagues—his usual situational supports—were unable to be with him because of hospital rules and his restricted activity. He used denial excessively because he was unable to accept the fact that he might have to change his lifestyle. Because this was his first hospitalization and the first time he had to be in a dependent role, his anxiety increased considerably.

That dire disease, whose ruthless power
Withers the beauty's transient flower.

–Oliver Goldsmith

Complete the paradigm in Figure 8-3 for this case study, then compare it with the completed one in Appendix D. Refer to the paradigms in Chapter 3 as needed.

Alzheimer's Disease

Alzheimer's disease is a progressive, degenerative disease that attacks the brain and impairs judgment with mental functioning. Its victims generally experience confusion and personality and behavioral changes. They ultimately require full-time supervision or custodial care. The cause is still unknown. Although researchers have linked two different susceptibility genes to the disease, it is clear that unknown environmental factors also play a major role. Based on researchers' studies of brain cells grown in the laboratory, electromagnetic fields (EMFs) can disturb the normal concentrations of calcium ions within cells. The increased concentration of calcium within the cells produced by EMFs, researchers speculate, triggers a well-known cascade of reactions that ultimately leads to the accumulation of damaging plaques and tangles (Maugh, 1996).

Alzheimer's disease afflicts as many as 4 million Americans; most are over the age of 65. It is characterized by memory loss, disorientation, depression, and deterioration of bodily functions. It is ultimately fatal, causing approximately 100,000 deaths each year (Maugh, 1996).

Unless a cure or means of prevention are found for Alzheimer's disease, 12 to 14 million Americans will be affected by the year 2000. Approximately 10% of the population over 65 years of age are afflicted with Alzheimer's disease. The percentage rises to 47.2% in those over the age of 85, which is the *fastest-growing* segment of the U.S. population. This is significant because the nation's entire elderly population is increasing rapidly, and it is estimated that by the year 2050, the United States will have 67.5 million people over the age 65, compared with 25.5 million at present. It is truly the "graying of America!" More than 50% of all nursing home patients are victims of Alzheimer's disease or a related disorder. The annual cost of nursing home care ranges between $24,000 and $36,000.

Financing for care for Alzheimer's disease, including costs of diagnosis, treatment, nursing home care, informal care, and lost wages, is estimated to be more than $580 billion each year. The federal government covers $4.4 billion and the states another $54.1 billion. Much of the remaining costs are borne by patients and their families.

The initial symptoms of Alzheimer's disease are insidious and often imperceptible as organic changes start to occur in the brain and a decline in many areas of intellectual and physical abilities begins. Initially, no objective or subjective

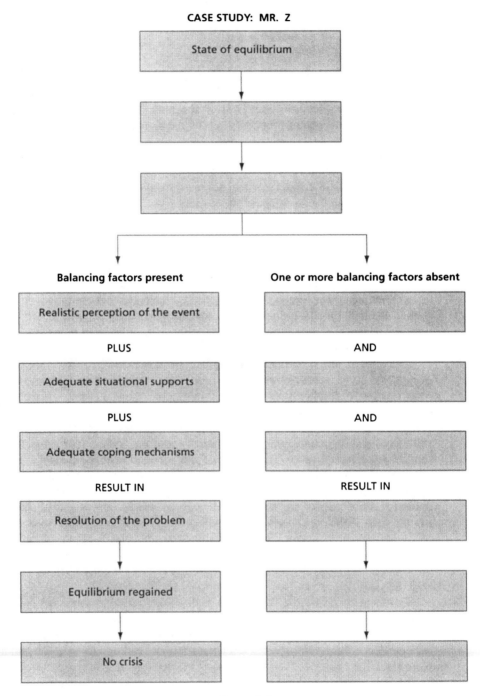

Figure 8-3

symptoms are reported. As the disease progresses, the earliest noticeable symptoms are generally related to memory impairment. Although motor activities are not affected at this time, subjective awareness of memory loss begins to interfere more and more with the person's daily living activities. It is a rare person among us who has not occasionally misplaced needed items, forgotten familiar addresses and telephone numbers, and even forgotten the names of close friends. If these lapses do not happen too often, the usual response can be momentary embarrassment or irritation. We blame it on being tired or under stress or on just having too much on our minds to remember, but there is always a sense of self-confidence that the memory will return.

For the Alzheimer's disease patient, however, such forgetfulness begins to become chronic, something that cannot be shrugged off so easily as only temporary. As subjective awareness and concerns over memory loss increase, self-confidence in an ability to recall lost memories diminishes. For many, written checklists and notes of things to do become a way of life. Eventually, however, these no longer suffice as memory supports as they, too, become lost and forgotten.

As memory loss increases, signs of early confusional behavior begin. A person easily becomes lost in unfamiliar places and needs to depend increasingly on others for help in finding his way when away from home or other familiar locations. Changes to new environments create much anxiety, particularly when combined with stressful events such as an illness requiring hospitalization. The person's forgetfulness begins to be noticed by others and can no longer be seen simply as temporary or "normal" behavior. At the same time, recent memory loss becomes much more subjectively noted. Ability to concentrate decreases, and the use of denial as a defense mechanism increases.

From this stage in intellectual decline, identifiable overt symptoms of Alzheimer's disease begin, and regression progresses into a late confusional stage. The person can still handle his own immediate physical needs, yet motor skills gradually decrease. Language becomes affected, and it becomes increasingly difficult for the person to find the right words. The ability to concentrate diminishes greatly, and the ability to handle finances, cooking, and other daily decision-making activities suffers accordingly. The individual becomes more withdrawn and anxious. Frustration and anger increase as the use of denial becomes less effective. No longer can he deny to himself or to others that something is wrong with him.

Inevitably, whether slowly or rapidly, regression progresses into a period of early dementia. At this stage such persons can survive no longer without assistance from others. Now there is time disorientation and frequently forgetfulness of familiar family names. Although the person is still capable of handling the basic functions of daily living (such as feeding himself, bowel and bladder control, and bathing), caretaking needs increase greatly as intellectual and motor skills continue to decline. For many this is a period of rapid decline as the disease progresses toward the stage of middle dementia.

By this time there are symptoms of hallucinatory types of perceptions, which are responded to with fear, agitation, and even violence. Familiar faces may be recognized, but name recall is nearly nil. Variable awareness of recent events and past memories may be sketchy and incomplete.

As motor skills decrease, bowel and bladder incontinence begins. Constant attendance becomes necessary for all activities of daily living. Caretaking activities may exceed the abilities of family and friends; institutionalization may be the only family recourse. In the final, late dementia stage of Alzheimer's disease, the person becomes increasingly vegetative and requires total care. Speech decreases to one or two words, all intellectual skills disappear, and motor skills decline until full assistance is needed to eat, drink, and even turn in bed. Eventually, there is coma and finally death.

A diagnosis of Alzheimer's disease for a family member means that the whole family, as well as the patient, must learn to live with the condition. Alzheimer's is insidious in its onset; a misdiagnosis of early symptoms can create added stress for everyone concerned. Too often the early symptoms of memory loss, depression, passive dependency, and emotional lability are misunderstood or passed off as transient reactions to situational stress.

As the disease progresses, a person with Alzheimer's becomes impaired in his ability to control the appropriate expression of his own emotions and to comprehend the effect of his behavior on others. He is emotionally labile, overreacts, and often appears insensitive to others' feelings. Emotional changes often appear as exaggerations of previously established behavioral characteristics. For example, the passive and withdrawn person may become even more dependent, suspicious, and depressed; the characteristically independent, aggressive person may appear demanding, hysterical, and even manic in behavior.

As organic changes in the brain occur, dependency on others increases. This may not be too disturbing for one whose past personality characteristics were those of passive dependency. However, for one whose personality characteristics emphasized independent, aggressive behaviors, feelings of frustration and anger increase as dependency needs increase. This can lead to what has been termed *catastrophic reaction,* which is best described as an emotional overreaction, one that is obviously out of proportion to an anxiety-provoking situation. It occurs as intellectual impairment increases and emotional control decreases. This is a fairly common response as the affected individual is increasingly confronted with failure in achieving what formerly were, to that person, simple tasks. Often believing that the individuals concerned have full control over their behavioral changes, family and friends may, in turn, respond inappropriately. Such a reaction may only serve to increase stress and, consequently, the severity of the symptoms exhibited. Family members almost invariably need to cope at some time with feelings of fear, anger, guilt, shame, and isolation, as well as persistent feelings of grief and mourning. These feelings may arise intermittently and in varying degrees, dependent on each member's past experiences, values, personal resources, and current life situation.

Any unusual problems arising with the patient may, in fact, be a symptom of family dysfunction. It would not be unusual for family members, no longer able to relate to each other openly and directly, to relate through problems as they arise in the patient. It is as though there is a need for the patient to have problems in order for family members to continue to relate. This only serves to reinforce the patient's problematic behaviors.

Once the diagnosis of Alzheimer's disease has been confirmed and denial of the illness diminishes, each family member begins to face the reality of its consequences for himself, as well as for the patient. Each member strongly feels a need to find a satisfactory reason or meaning for the occurrence of the illness. Until one is found—real or imagined—feelings of helplessness, powerlessness, and insecurity exist. It is realistic for family members to be anxious, confused, and fearful and to feel alone with the situation. It is not at all unusual for them to be completely uninformed when a diagnostic label like this is attached to one of their members. Their only source of knowledge could be one of hearsay misinformation. There may also be misperception of correct information provided them at the time of the diagnosis.

Natural outcomes are feelings of anger and aggression, which can mobilize members toward constructive actions, thereby reducing feelings of helplessness and powerlessness. Another outcome may be outwardly destructive behavior, which leads to increased feelings of helplessness and anger that are compounded by feelings of guilt. Depression and discouragement are the most common feelings for close relatives or friends of those with chronic, irreversible diseases. Anger and frustration leading to rage reactions or internalized toward feelings of suicide are not uncommon during the progressive course of the illness.

Family members are faced with the need to identify the meaning of the functional loss of one of their members and what it will mean to each member as family roles are redefined and functions are redistributed. Until these are dealt with, conflict and chaos are inevitable. The family system becomes less cohesive and could eventually break up or disintegrate. Any one role change, subtle or otherwise, almost invariably leads to change in those of other members. Welcome or unwelcome, planned or unplanned, a role change can affect each member's usual ways of thinking, feeling, and behaving. Feelings in particular strongly affect perceptions and the thinking processes.

If a parent is affected and children are involved in the caretaking process, role reversal becomes an inevitable problem with which they must deal. This occurs as responsibilities and control—from the more abstract, intellectual, decision-making responsibilities to, eventually, basic physical functions—gradually must be taken from the affected person. This is particularly difficult for many to accept because of the relatively early age at which Alzheimer's occurs and the insidious nature of its onset and progress. It would not be unusual to find strong feelings of ambivalence, anger, and reluctance to accept the loss of the child role and the reversal of dependency roles with the parent. These feelings are compounded by the fact that the parent may physically appear quite well and capable of self-care until the later stages of the illness. To accept the reversal in roles is also to acknowledge anticipation of an ultimate desertion by death.

Family members experience many conflicting and unique feelings as the disease progresses. Emotions may run the gamut from hopeful optimism to hopeless despair. All of these emotions are as highly complex and variable as is each member's perception of the situation and its effect on his own life. There may be feelings of frustration and anger as the caregiver's patience wears thin and the caregiving chores continue to increase.

Denial is not an uncommon initial response when a person is overwhelmed with a stressful situation. However, for those who do not cope through the use of denial, the grief process may begin in anticipation of the loss. The more a person is emotionally invested in the loved one, the more threatened that person may feel in anticipation of the loss.

The extraordinary demands of caregiving to a family member with Alzheimer's or a related disorder are known to be a source of strain to caregivers. Caregivers are resentful of behavioral symptoms that they often perceive as demanding or manipulative, and they often respond with anger or avoidance. Examples of these patient behaviors include intermittent incontinence, the exaggeration of physical illness to gain sympathy or to stop the caregiver's activities, or "putting on a sweet image in front of other people" while being unpleasant to the caregiver. These behavioral symptoms were perceived as related to the poor quality of the previous relationship or the manifestation of the caregiver's unpleasant temperament (Jivanjee, 1994).

Caregivers' perceptions strongly influence their responses to patient behavioral symptoms, indicating the importance of looking at the meaning of behaviors for individual caregivers. Education about the behavior causes and consequences of dementia may help caregivers to modify their negative responses. Mintzer and others (1993) suggest that the agitated behaviors of dementia patients may be triggered, sustained, or extinguished by elements in the environment. Attitude change may be difficult for those who have been in long unhappy relationships, but with training these caregivers may increase their understanding of the effects of environmental stimuli on patient behavioral symptoms. They may also be able to modify the home environment and their own reactions. Caregivers may also increase their assertiveness in dealing with demanding behaviors and benefit from increased support from family members.

Social work intervention needs to be available at the beginning of the caring process to support, educate, reduce abrasive situations, and enhance well-being. Extensive community education about Alzheimer's and related disorders and the effects of caregiving will help to create awareness and a higher level of community support. At the policy level, caregivers' varied needs and preferences can be met by a coordinated array of supportive services including individual, family, and group support and low-cost home care, respite, and institutional care. Caregivers need financial support to minimize their overall stress level and to permit them to obtain the services they need.

The four phases of grief and mourning are responses to any situation involving loss, not just the death of a loved one. Families of patients with Alzheimer's disease are faced with prolonged periods of grief and mourning. This greatly differs from an overwhelming feeling of grief that gradually lessens as time passes after a loved one's death. Grief and mourning for death is sanctioned by our society, but overt, prolonged grief and mourning for a chronically ill person, particularly one who looks physically well, are rarely accepted as connected with death. More often, such mourning may be perceived as self-pity or weakness.

When the stresses of caring for the affected person become so great that a family or personal crisis is precipitated, professional counseling may be required to avert maladaptive problem-solving behavior. The case study that follows depicts a crisis that was precipitated by a daughter who could not cope with caring for her mother, who had Alzheimer's disease.

Case Study   *Alzheimer's Disease*

Frank was referred to a community crisis clinic by his family physician because of his increasing symptoms of tension, anxiety, and depression. When he arrived, he appeared quite tense, with visible hand tremors. The receptionist contacted a therapist, and Frank was directed to the therapist's office.

When the therapist asked why he had come to the clinic that day, Frank replied in a very depressed tone of voice, "My whole world is collapsing around me. My wife, Molly, is sick, but I've been able to handle it—until now. My daughter has always been such a help, but now she is walking out on us. I just can't handle much more; I can't do it alone." He became increasingly agitated as he spoke, his voice rising in anger. After a long pause, he seemed to regain his composure. In response to direct questioning by the therapist, he slowly described the problem that led up to this visit to the clinic for help.

Frank said that he and Molly, who were both 56 years of age, had been married for 20 years. They had one daughter, Kim, who was 17 years old and had just graduated from high school. He described his family life as "good, no more problems than most people," until about a year ago when Molly had to quit her job. She had worked for the same person all of their married life. When that person retired a year ago, Molly was reassigned to a new office in the same company. Within a few days, she began to complain that her new boss was very disorganized and seemed to go out of his way to find fault with her work. She said that she was even accused of such ridiculous things as misplacing records and forgetting to tell him of his appointments. She started going to work earlier and staying later in an effort to "get the boss organized," but he continued to criticize and complain about her work. Frank said that Molly became increasingly irritable, preoccupied, and forgetful at home during that time. It seemed as though she were scapegoating him and Kim for all of her problems at work.

Finally, she came home one day and told him that she was given the option of resigning or being demoted. With Frank's encouragement, she decided to resign and take a few weeks' vacation before looking for another job. Frank hoped that, with time and some rest, she would "pull herself together and eventually become her cheerful, organized self again." This, however, was not to be the case.

As the weeks passed, Molly seemed to become even more disorganized and forgetful. She never again spoke of looking for a new job. She argued increasingly, accusing him and Kim of misplacing her personal items, losing telephone messages, and so on. Bills were left forgotten and unpaid in her desk until Frank learned to watch for them in the mail.

Neither he nor Kim seemed able to reason with her any longer about these incidents. Any references to her forgetfulness were met with denial and angry responses. Finally, they learned to cope as best they could with her erratic, irresponsible behaviors. Over time, they gradually took over many of her household responsibilities.

Molly first displayed overt signs of confusion, disorientation, and memory loss when she was hospitalized for elective surgery, about 6 months before Frank came to the clinic. Nurses had found her late at night wandering down the halls in her bare feet, "looking for *her* bedroom." When the nurses suggested that she had lost her way, she became verbally abusive to them for saying that to her. Before dawn, she was found fully dressed and sitting on a chair in the hallway. When questioned, she replied that she was "waiting for Frank to drive *her* to work." Further questioning revealed that she was disoriented as to place, could not recall the day of the week or her physician's name, and had forgotten why she had come to the hospital.

Following this episode, further tests and examinations were completed, and a diagnosis of Alzheimer's disease was made. Findings suggested that Molly had progressed into the early confusional stage.

When asked how he and Kim responded to this news, Frank said that their initial feelings were quite mixed. "We were glad to finally find a physical reason for her behavior changes but were shocked and really couldn't believe that there was no known cure for it. It made me really angry that this could happen to any of us."

When it was strongly suggested that Frank contact a local Alzheimer's support group for ongoing support and information about Molly's care at home, Frank saw no immediate need to do so. To him, Molly appeared quite healthy. As he perceived it, all that he and Kim would need was "a little more patience with Molly when she forgot things or lost her temper." Over time, they had learned to help her avoid stressful situations, even though it sometimes made life more stressful for them. Gradually, however, the relationship between him and Kim became distant as he spent increasing amounts of time away from home at his job.

At first, Kim never complained about having to spend more time at home with her mother. Neighbors and friends visited often, and she could still leave Molly alone for brief periods. As Molly's memory loss increased, however, Molly's frustration tolerance decreased. Her unprovoked irritability became much more frequent; soon, visitors rarely came to see them. At the same time, Kim found herself having to assume an increasing number of the household roles and responsibilities formerly held by her mother. Any attempts to bring in a housekeeper or a companion for her mother were met with overt antagonism from Molly.

Two evenings ago, Frank came home late and was confronted by a tearful, angry Kim. She told him that she "couldn't take it anymore" and was going to move out if he didn't find someone else to take care of her mother. He said that her outburst really took him by surprise. When he asked her the cause of this sudden change in attitude, she angrily responded, "Sudden? There is nothing sudden about this! For weeks I've been telling you how I feel, but you never listen to me anymore. You're always too busy at work, and when you come home, you seem to ignore just how much mother has changed. She's become like a spoiled, demanding little child. I feel more like a live-in babysitter than like her daughter. I have no life of my own anymore—and you don't seem to care what happens to me!" The conversation was abruptly ended by Kim leaving the house and slamming the door behind her. She called her father about an hour later to say that she was going to spend the night at a friend's house. She added that she still had a lot to think over but would be home the next morning.

Frank said that he never slept that night and that his mind was in a turmoil, thinking about what Kim had said. He felt shocked and overwhelmed with strongly ambivalent feelings toward Molly, who slept quietly upstairs in their bedroom. He said that he "suddenly faced reality—and hated it." He felt completely alone and trapped, with no way out of the whole situation. As he described it, "By morning I had the shakes, couldn't concentrate on anything, and felt like hell."

When Kim came back the next morning, neither mentioned what had been said the night before. He left for his office as quickly as he could. For the next several hours, he drove his car randomly about the city, thinking about what had been happening to his life for the past year. It was only then, he said, that he finally faced the reality that he had lost forever the Molly whom he had loved and married. Now he was in danger of losing Kim, too. He suddenly felt so overwhelmed with grief that he pulled the car to the side of the street and parked. He felt so sick and trembled so severely that he was afraid to drive. As soon as he felt able, he drove directly to his physician's office, where he was seen immediately. It was from there that he had been referred to the clinic.

The therapist's assessment was that, until his confrontation with Kim, Frank had successfully used denial to cope with Molly's illness. This evaluation was supported by his avoidance of opportunities to obtain more information about Alzheimer's disease from one of the local support groups.

As Molly's symptoms became more overt, he avoided having to "do something about it" by extending his time at work. When Kim tried to communicate her need for help and understanding, he effectively managed to tune her out. As a result, he was not consciously lying when he said that he was shocked at the "sudden change in Kim's attitude."

Frank's crisis was precipitated by the threatened loss of his daughter and compounded by unresolved feelings of grief and mourning for the anticipated loss of his wife. The goals of intervention were to assist Frank to identify and ventilate his unrecognized feelings about his wife, to help him obtain appropriate situational supports for himself and Kim as he dealt with plans for Molly's future care, and to help him obtain an intellectual understanding of role reversal because it was affecting Kim's relationship with her mother.

During the first session, the therapist determined that Frank was not suicidal. When asked to describe himself as he "usually was," he said that he was a person who prided himself on being able to maintain control over his life. He believed that, to be successful, a person should be able to set goals and, with good planning, achieve them. Reflecting further on his feelings about Molly, he admitted to the therapist that, deep down, he had always believed that Molly could have controlled her behavior if she had really wanted to do so. He felt that her failure to do so was, in some way, a personal rejection of him. No longer able to communicate with her about his feelings, he had used denial and avoidance to cope. As Molly's condition deteriorated, he felt more angry and frustrated with her and used his work to justify the increasing amount of time spent away from home.

With further discussion and reflection about Molly's behavioral changes, it became very apparent that Frank had little factual information about Alzheimer's disease. When he was first informed by the doctors, his anxiety was so high that he remembered hearing little other than that her memory loss would continue to get worse and that there was no cure.

As Molly's increasing episodes of unprovoked anger increased, their few remaining friends gradually began to avoid contact with her. Recalling this now with the therapist, he acknowledged that, in fact, this had been a relief for him. He no longer had to worry about what she might do or say to their friends if she became upset.

What he had failed to realize, though, was the added stress that this had placed on Kim. After further questioning and reflection, he said, "Could it be that I didn't listen to Kim because I didn't want to know? I didn't want to hear how bad things had really become?" He paused, and then said softly, "The Molly that I loved so much left me long ago. I miss her so much and wish that she could come back, even for a little while. There's so much I want to say to her. While I stay away from home, I can make believe that she's still there waiting for me. Going home hurts so very much."

It was suggested that he contact the local Alzheimer's support group to learn about alternative ways available to him for Molly's care at home. He was made to realize that, unless he began to face the reality of Molly's illness and the situation at his home, he might well lose Kim, too.

When questioned further about his confrontation with Kim the evening before, he seemed unable to understand why Kim felt so angry about her mother. Further discussion focused on the way Kim's roles and responsibilities in the family had changed during the past few months. As he slowly identified these changes for the therapist, he began to obtain an intellectual understanding of parent-child role reversal and its effect on the child, particularly on one as young as Kim.

Gradually he began to recognize Kim's confrontation for what it was: a cry for his understanding of what was happening to her. She was overwhelmed by her inability to meet the ever-increasing dependency needs of her mother without some help from him. Unable to communicate her own dependency needs to either him or her mother, she saw escape from the entire situation as her only solution.

It was suggested to Frank that one of his first priorities was to find someone else to assume major responsibility for Molly's care and supervision. Until this happened, he could expect further confrontations with Kim and should not be surprised if Kim carried out her threat to leave home.

As an interim measure, Frank decided to take a few weeks of long overdue vacation time and stay home to help out until he could find someone to provide full-time help with Molly's care.

During the second session, Frank appeared much more optimistic as he described his past week at home. He said that he and Kim had talked together "for hours" the evening after his first session at the clinic. He reflected that it had been difficult at first for both of them to face the other with their feelings. "But," he added, "it was such a relief when we did. Until then, neither of us had realized just how far apart we had become and how much we needed to stick together to work things out."

During the past week, Frank also contacted the local Alzheimer's support group. By prearrangement, two members visited his home to meet with him, Kim, and Molly. He recalled his surprise at how easily Molly appeared to accept the "stranger's" visit and the apparent ease with which they included her in the conversation. As a result of the visit, appropriate resources were identified for assistance in Molly's care. After several interviews with applicants for a housekeeper's position and with Molly's agreement, they finally hired a woman who seemed best able to cope with Molly's needs. The woman moved in 2 days before this session and, he reported, "Molly hasn't scared her off yet." However, he would continue to remain at home for another week to help Molly adjust to any new changes in her daily activities.

Frank and Kim also attended a meeting of the local Alzheimer's group. It surprised them both to find several other young people of Kim's age present. When asked to describe his feelings about the meeting, he said that both he and Kim went to the meeting "not expecting much, maybe coffee, cake, and sympathy, but that's all." Instead, they found a group of people who, he said, seemed to know exactly what his family had been going through. He learned that many of his experiences were not unique but common to all of them. "For the first time," he said, "I was able to get some answers that were useful to us. Maybe no one could tell us why she got this disease, but this group of people could give me some good suggestions on how to help all of us deal with it." Most important for both him and Kim, as they left the meeting, was their feeling that they were no longer alone with their problems and that now a support group was available to them as problems arose.

Before the end of the session the therapist and Frank reviewed and assessed the adjustment that he had made and his insights into his own feelings about Molly and the effects of her illness on his future. They also discussed his understanding of the effect that the process of role reversal with her mother was having on Kim. It was strongly suggested that he encourage Kim's continued attendance at the Alzheimer's group meetings. The purpose was to provide her with ongoing peer support as she dealt with her changing relationship with her mother.

He was commended for taking direct action during the past week and for obtaining appropriate resources to help him with his ongoing situation at home. Such action strongly suggested that he no longer was coping solely through denial and avoidance but was making a conscious effort to perceive the situation realistically. Frank was encouraged to continue to be more direct in his communications with Kim and to let her know that he was recognizing that she had needs, too. Before termination he was reassured that he could return for help with any future crises should the need arise.

Frank had used denial and avoidance as methods for coping with his feelings about Molly's illness and eventual death. Kim saw his behavior as a rejection of her efforts to communicate to him the realities of her mother's deteriorating condition and its effect on her own unmet dependency needs. Failing to recognize the extent to which the process of role reversal with her mother had affected Kim's life, Frank perceived her threat to leave home as yet another rejection and threatened loss of someone close to him. Lacking any previous coping experience with his new role demands, his anxiety and depression increased to an intolerable level; Frank was in a state of crisis.

Intervention focused on helping him to identify and understand his unrecognized feelings toward Molly, to obtain an intellectual understanding of the effects of role reversal on Kim, and to obtain appropriate situational supports for the family because they, individually and as a unit, would undoubtedly be confronted with more stress-provoking situations as Molly's illness progressed.

Old age and the wear of time teach many things.

–Sophocles

Complete the paradigm in Figure 8-4 based on this case study, then compare it with the completed one in Appendix D. Refer to the paradigms in Chapter 3 as needed.

Suicide

SUICIDE IN ADOLESCENCE

Suicide is the eighth leading cause of death in the United States; it is the third leading cause of death for young individuals 20 to 24 years of age and the third leading cause for adolescents 15 to 19 years of age (National Institute of Mental Health, 1996). Youth suicide is clearly a significant public health problem in the United States worthy of the concern and attention of parents, educators, and mental health professionals. The suicide rate for people 15 to 24 years of age has more than tripled over the last 30 years. Suicide rates for individuals 15 to 19 years of age increased from 8.7 : 100,000 to 14.96 : 100,000 in 1994. It is suspected that the actual suicide rate among young people is even higher than reported. In a review of coroners' reports for all suicides, undetermined cause of death, and questionable accidents over a period of 24 years, it was concluded that suicides were underreported by approximately 24% (Ladely and Puskar, 1994). The Statistical Abstract of the United States (1995) lists suicide as 33.6 : 100,000 deaths in the population.

Now approaching epidemic proportions, suicide is currently the third leading cause of death among teenagers in the United States. It is estimated that 300 to 400 teen suicides occur per year in Los Angeles County; this is equivalent to one teenager lost every day. Evidence indicates that for every suicide, there are 50 to 100 attempts at suicide (Student Health and Human Services Divisions, 1996). Due to the stigma associated with suicide, these statistics may well be understating the problem. Nevertheless, these figures do underscore the urgent need to seek a solution to the suicide epidemic among our young people.

The majority of adolescent suicide completers exhibit symptoms of some psychiatric disorder before their deaths, although only a small percentage ever received mental health treatment. The focus for suicide prevention programs clearly must be on the ability of parents and teachers to recognize symptoms that indicate that the adolescent may be at risk for suicidal behaviors. Adults should look for sudden changes in the adolescent's behavior that are significant, last for a long time, and are apparent in all or most areas of his life (pervasive). Parents, teachers, and mental health professionals should be alert to the danger signs of suicide listed as follows:

- Previous suicide attempts
- The verbalization of suicide threats

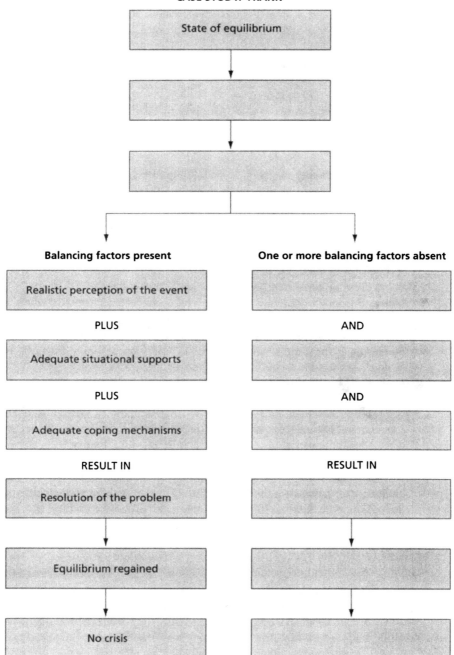

CASE STUDY: FRANK

State of equilibrium

Balancing factors present

One or more balancing factors absent

Realistic perception of the event

PLUS

Adequate situational supports

PLUS

Adequate coping mechanisms

RESULT IN

Resolution of the problem

Equilibrium regained

No crisis

AND

AND

RESULT IN

Figure 8-4

- The giving away of prized personal possessions
- The collection and discussion of information on suicide methods
- The expression of hopelessness, helplessness, and anger at oneself or the world
- Themes of death or depression evident in conversation, written expressions, reading selections, or artwork
- Statements or suggestions that the speaker would not be missed if he were gone
- The scratching or marking of the body or other self-destructive acts
- Recent loss of a friend or a family member (or even a pet) through death or suicide; other losses, for example, the loss of a parent resulting from divorce
- Acute personality changes, unusual withdrawal, aggressiveness, or moodiness; new involvement in high-risk activities
- Sudden dramatic decline or improvement in academic performance, chronic truancy or tardiness, or running away
- Physical symptoms such as eating disturbances, sleeplessness or excessive sleeping, chronic headaches or stomach aches, or apathetic appearance
- Use or increased use of substances

When a child or adolescent talks of suicide you should:

- *Listen.* Encourage the child to talk to you or some other trusted person. Listen to the child's feelings. Don't give advice or feel obligated to find simple solutions. Try to imagine how you would feel in the child's place.
- *Be honest.* If the child's words or actions scare you, tell him. If you're worried or don't know what to do, say so. Don't be a cheerful phony.
- *Share feelings.* At times everyone feels sad, hurt, or hopeless. You know what that is like; share your feelings. Let the child know he is not alone.
- *Get help.* Professional help is crucial when something as serious as suicide is considered. Help may be found at a suicide prevention or crisis center, local mental health association, or through clergy. Become familiar with the suicide prevention program at the child's school. Contact the appropriate person or persons at the school. Knowledge that help is available to him means that he is unlikely ever to reach a time in life during which he perceives suicide to be the only option. Remind him that suicide is a permanent solution to a temporary problem.

SUICIDE IN MIDLIFE

Midlife is usually a time when power peaks. By age 40 most of us are pretty much what we are ever going to be, with a few notable exceptions. Most developmental social psychologists have focused on early childhood not on midlife development. At roughly ages 40 to 45 we need to make changes in our life dreams that will modify existing early adult life structure, to appraise the past and rid ourselves of our illusions, accommodate other given life changes (such as divorce, job plateauing, children leaving home, diminished life energies, and job shifts), turn more inward and be less concerned with mastery of the external environment, and resolve four basic polarities (i.e., young-old, creation-destruction, masculine-feminine, and attachment-separation). At midlife we need to modify our dream and realize that success does not necessarily entail happiness.

Middle age people are not as observable as the dependent young or the elderly nor are they usually in schools or institutions. Those of us in midlife tend to be society's guardians and accordingly are routinely not ourselves guarded. When middle age people get into trouble, often no one is even watching or expecting it.

Some subtypes of midlifers that require special assessment for their suicidal potential follow (Maris, 1995).

- *Executive suicides,* especially males who tend to be "control freaks," authoritarian, and rigid thinkers, including police officers
- *Menopausal females,* who may perceive themselves as having outlived or grown weary of their reproductive and nurturing usefulness or responsibilities
- *Younger midlife urban inner city African-Americans,* who are often angry (rageful), drug and alcohol abusers, are estranged from their families, and are inclined to violence
- *AIDS patients* (and others with physical impasses and little future or hope, e.g., cancer and heart disease patients) (Note that most of the physically ill do not resolve their life problems by suiciding.)
- *The pseudodeveloped,* who tend to be stagnated and have accumulated excessive developmental debits, are chronically depressed, and are chronologically older than their achievements or emotional maturity
- *Midlife males in crisis or burnout,* who have estranged adult children and spouses, are often substance abusers, and have work and economic problems concomitant with interpersonal and sexual problems

Of course, some of these midlife suicidal types overlap, and one has to consider the 15 or so generic predictors of suicide, as well as the more ad hoc characteristics of a particular midlife suicidal type. Many of these types of midlife suicide are poorly understood and are underresearched. One consequence is that some important types of midlife suicide may have been overlooked. Shneidman (1992) likes to say that the "four letter word" in suicidology is "only," as in, "It was the only thing I could do."

RELATED FACTORS

Age and gender.   Statistics indicate that women *attempt* suicide more often than men but that men *commit* suicide more often than women. Currently, this trend is changing because women are beginning to feel the same stresses in their changing social roles that men feel. They are also beginning to use more lethal methods in their suicide attempts. It is also known that the rate for completed suicide rises with increasing age. Consequently, an older man presents the greatest threat of actual suicide and a young woman the least. Within this framework, age and sex offer a general, although by no means clear-cut, basis for evaluating suicidal potential. One must remember that young women and young men do kill themselves, even when their original aim is to manipulate other people. Each case requires individual appraisal.

Suicidal plan. How an individual plans to take his life is one of the most significant criteria in assessing suicidal potential. The therapist must consider the following three elements.

1. Is it a relatively lethal method? An individual who intends to commit suicide with a gun, by jumping from a tall building or bridge, or by hanging is a far greater risk than someone who plans to take pills or cut his wrists. Because the person who plans either of the latter two methods is amenable to treatment or resuscitation, these methods are less lethal than the irrevocable consequences of putting a gun to one's head.

2. Does the individual have the means available? It must be determined if the method of suicide the individual has considered is in fact available to him. A threat to use a gun, if the person has one, is obviously more serious than the same threat without a gun.

3. Is the suicide plan specific? Can the individual say exactly when he plans to do it (e.g., after the children are asleep)? If he has spent time thinking out details and specific preparations for his death, his suicidal risk is greatly increased. Changing a will, writing notes, collecting pills, buying a gun, and setting a time and place for suicide suggest a high risk. When a patient's plan is obviously confused or unrealistic, the therapist should consider the possibility of an underlying psychiatric problem. A psychotic person with the idea of suicide is a particularly high risk because he may make a bizarre attempt based on his distorted thoughts. The therapist should always find out if the patient has a history of any emotional disorder and whether he has ever been hospitalized or received other mental health care.

Stress. The therapist needs to find out about any stressful event that may have precipitated the suicidal behavior. The most common precipitating stresses are losses: the death of a loved one; divorce or separation; loss of a job, money, prestige, or status; loss of health through illness, surgery, or accident; and loss of esteem or prestige because of possible prosecution or criminal involvement. Not all stresses are the result of bereavement. Sometimes increased anxiety and tension are a result of success, such as a promotion with increased responsibilities. Always investigate any sudden change in the individual's life situation. Learning to evaluate stress from the individual's point of view rather than from society's point of view is necessary. What may be minimal stress for the therapist could be perceived by the patient as severe stress. The relationship between stress and symptoms is useful in evaluating prognosis.

Symptoms. The most common and most important suicidal symptoms relate to depression. Typical symptoms of severe depression include loss of appetite, weight loss, inability to sleep, loss of interest, social withdrawal, apathy and despondency, severe feelings of hopelessness and helplessness, and a general attitude of physical and emotional exhaustion. Other persons may exhibit agitation through such symptoms as tension; anxiety; guilt; shame; poor impulse control; or feelings of rage, anger, hostility, or revenge. Alcoholics and all other substance abusers tend to be high suicidal risks. The patient who is both agitated and depressed is particularly at high risk. Unable to tolerate the pressure of his feelings, the individual in a state of agitated depression shows marked tension, fearfulness, restlessness, and pressure of speech.

He eventually reaches a point where he must act in some direction to relieve his feelings. Often he chooses suicide.

Suicidal symptoms may also occur with psychotic states. The patient may have delusions, hallucinations, distorted sensory impressions, loss of contact with reality, disorientation, or highly unusual ideas and experiences. As a baseline for assessing psychotic behavior, the therapist should use his own sense of what is real and appropriate.

Resources.   The patient's environmental resources are often crucial in helping the therapist decide how to manage the immediate problem. Who are his situational supports? The therapist must find out who can be used to support him through this traumatic time: family, relatives, close friends, employers, physicians, or clergy. To whom does he feel close? If the patient is already under the care of a therapist, the new therapist should try to contact him.

The choice of various resources is sometimes affected by the fact that the patient and the family may try to keep the suicidal situation a secret, even to the point of denying its existence. As a general rule, this attempt at secrecy and denial must be counteracted by dealing with the suicidal situation openly and frankly. It is usually better, for both the therapist and the patient, if the responsibility for a suicidal patient is shared by as many people as possible. This combined effort provides the patient with a feeling that he lacks: that others are interested in him, care for him, and are ready to help him.

When there are no apparent sources of help or support, the therapist may be the person's only situational support, his one link to survival. This is also true if available resources have been exhausted or family and friends have turned away from the individual. In most cases, however, people will respond to the situation and provide help and support if given the opportunity.

Lifestyle.   How has the person functioned in the past under stress? First, has his style of life been stable or unstable? Second, is the suicidal behavior acute or chronic? The stable individual describes a consistent work record, sound marital and family relationship, and no history of previous suicidal behavior. The unstable individual may have had severe character disorders, borderline psychotic behavior, and repeated difficulties with major situations, such as interpersonal relationships or employment.

A suicidal person responding to acute stress, such as the death or loss of someone he loves, bad news, or loss of a job, presents a special concern. The risk of early suicide among this group is high; however, the opportunity for successful therapeutic intervention is greater. If the suicidal danger can be averted for a relatively short period, individuals tend to emerge without great danger of recurrence.

By contrast, individuals with a history of repeated attempts at self-destruction may be helped through one emergency, but the suicidal danger can be expected to return at a later date. In general, if an individual has made serious attempts in the past, his current suicidal situation should be considered more dangerous. Although individuals with chronic suicidal behavior benefit temporarily from intervention, the emphasis should fall more on continuity of care and the maintenance of relationships.

Acute suicidal behavior may be found in either a stable or an unstable personality; however, chronic suicidal behavior occurs only in an unstable person. In dealing with a stable person in a suicidal situation, the therapist should be highly responsive and active. With an unstable person, the therapist needs to be slower and more thoughtful, reminding the patient that he has withstood similar stresses in the past. The main goals are to help him through this period and assist him in reconstituting an interpersonal relationship with a stable person or resource.

Communication.   The communication aspects of suicidal behavior have great importance in the evaluation and assessment process. The most important question is whether communication still exists between the suicidal individual and his significant others. When communication with the suicidal patient is completely severed, it indicates that he has lost hope of any possibility of rescue.

The form of communication may be either verbal or nonverbal, and its content may be direct or indirect. The suicidal person who communicates nonverbally and indirectly makes it difficult for the recipient of the communication to recognize or understand the suicidal intent of these communications. Also, this type of communication in itself implies a lack of clarity in the interchange between the suicidal person and others. At the same time, it raises a danger that the individual may act out suicidal impulses. The primary goal is to open up and clarify communication among everyone involved in the situation.

The patient's communications may be directed toward one or more significant persons within his environment. He may express hostility, accuse or blame others, or demand openly or subtly that others change their behavior and feelings. His communication may express feelings of guilt, inadequacy, and worthlessness or indicate strong anxiety and tension.

Significant other.   When the communication is directed to a specific person, the reaction of the recipient becomes an important factor in evaluating suicidal danger. One must decide if the significant other can be an important resource for rescue, if he is best regarded as unhelpful, or if he might even be injurious to the patient.

The unhelpful significant other either rejects the patient or denies the suicidal behavior itself by withdrawing, both psychologically and physically, from continued communication. Sometimes this other person resents the patient's increased demands, insistence on gratification of dependency needs, or the demands to change his own behavior. In other situations the significant other may act helpless, indecisive, or ambivalent, indicating that he does not know what the next step is and has given up. A reaction of hopelessness gives the suicidal individual a feeling that aid is not available from a previously dependable source. This can increase the patient's own hopelessness.

By contrast, a helpful reaction from the significant other is one in which the other person recognizes the communication, is aware of the problem, and seeks help for the individual. This indicates to the patient that his communications are being heard and that someone is doing something to provide help (Yu-Chin and Arcuni, 1990).

In the following case study, Carol attempted suicide because of lack of communication with a significant other. She anticipated a rejection because of a similar past experience.

Case Study   *Suicide*

Carol was referred to a crisis center for help by a physician in the emergency room of a nearby small suburban hospital. The night before, she had attempted suicide by severely slashing her left wrist repeatedly with a large kitchen knife, and she had severed a tendon as a result.

When she was first seen by the therapist at the center, her left wrist and arm were heavily bandaged. She appeared tense, disheveled, very pale, and tremulous. She described her symptoms as insomnia, poor appetite, recent inability to concentrate, and overwhelming feelings of hopelessness and helplessness. Carol, a 30-year-old single woman, lived alone. She had come to a large midwestern city about 4 years ago, immediately after graduating from an eastern university with a master's degree in business administration. Within a few weeks she had obtained a management trainee position with a large manufacturing distribution company. During the next 3 years, she advanced rapidly to her current position as manager of the main branch office. She stated that her co-workers considered her highly qualified for the position. She denied any on-the-job problems other than "the usual things that anyone in my position has to expect to deal with on a day-to-day basis." As a result of her rapid rise in the company, however, she had not allowed herself much leisure time to develop any close social relationships with either sex.

About a year ago, Carol met John, a 40-year-old widower who had a position similar to hers with another company. His office was on the same floor as hers. Within a few weeks, they were spending almost all of their leisure time together, although still maintaining separate apartments.

Carol's symptoms began about 2 weeks ago, when John was offered a promotion to a new job in his company, which he accepted before mentioning it to her. It meant that he would be transferred to another office about 30 miles away in the suburbs. She stated that she did feel upset "for just a few minutes" after he told her of his decision; "I guess that was just because he hadn't even mentioned anything about it to me first."

They went out that evening for dinner and dancing to celebrate the occasion. Before dinner was over, John had to bring her home because she "suddenly became dizzy, nauseated, and chilled" with what she described as "all of the worst symptoms of stomach flu."

Carol remained at home in bed for the next 3 days, not allowing John to visit her because she felt she was contagious. After she returned to work, she continued to feel very lethargic, had difficulty concentrating, could not regain her appetite, "and felt quite depressed and tearful for no reason at all." Convincing herself that she had not yet fully recovered from the "flu," she canceled several dates with John so that she could get more rest. She described him as being very understanding about this, even encouraging her to try to get some time off from work to take a short trip by herself and really rest and relax.

During this same time, John had begun to spend increasing amounts of time at his new office. Their coffee break meetings at work became very infrequent. Within the next week, he expected to be moved completely. The night before Carol came to the Crisis Center, she had come home from work expecting to meet John for dinner; instead, she found a note under her door written by her neighbor. It said that John had telephoned him earlier and left word for her that he had "suddenly been called out of town—wasn't sure when he would be back but would get in touch with her later."

She told the therapist, "Suddenly I felt empty . . . that everything was over between us. It was just too much for me to handle. He was never going to see me again and was too damned chicken to tell me to my face! I went numb all over—I just wanted to die." She paused a few minutes, head down and sobbing, then took a deep breath and went on, "I really don't remember doing it, but the next thing I was aware of was the telephone ringing. When I reached out to answer it, I realized I had a butcher knife in my right hand and my left wrist was cut and bleeding terribly! I dropped the knife on the floor and grabbed the phone. It was John calling me from the airport to tell me why he had to go out of town so suddenly—his father was critically ill."

Through the sobs she told him what she had done to herself. He told her to take a kitchen towel and wrap it tightly around her wrist. After she had done that, he told her to unlock the front door and wait there, that he would get help to her.

He immediately called the neighbors, who went to her apartment and found her with blood soaked towels around her wrist and sitting on the floor beside the door. They took her to the hospital, and John continued on his trip. After being treated in the emergency room, Carol went home to spend the night with her neighbors. They drove her to the Crisis Center the next morning.

During her initial session, Carol told the therapist that she had no close relatives. Her father and mother had died within a few months of each other during her last year in college. Soon after, she had fallen in love with another graduate student, and at his suggestion they had moved into an apartment together. She had believed that they would marry as soon as they had both graduated and had jobs.

Just before graduation, however, her boyfriend had come home and informed her that he had accepted a postdoctoral fellowship in France and would be leaving within the month. They went out for dinner "to celebrate" that night because, she said, "I couldn't help but be happy for him—it was quite an honor—I just couldn't tell him how hurt I felt."

The next morning after he had left for classes, she stated that she "suddenly realized I would never see him again after graduation—that he had never intended to marry me—and I was helpless to do anything about it." She took some masking tape and sealed the kitchen window shut, closed the door and put towels along the bottom, and turned on all of the stove gas jets.

About an hour later, a neighbor smelled the gas fumes and called the fire department. The firemen broke into the apartment, found her lying unconscious on the floor, and rushed her to the hospital. She was in a coma for 2 days and remained in the hospital for a week. Her boyfriend came only once to see her. When she returned to the apartment, she found that he had moved out, leaving her a note saying that he had gone home to see his family before leaving for France. He never contacted her again. A month later Carol moved to the Midwest.

For the first few months after meeting John, Carol was very ambivalent about her feelings toward him. She frequently felt very anxious and fearful that she was "setting myself up for another rejection." Even when John proposed marriage, she found herself unable to consider it seriously and told him that they should wait a while longer "to be sure that they both wanted it." Continuing, she stated, "Until about 2 days ago I had never felt so secure in my life. I'd begun to seriously consider proposing to him! Then, suddenly, the bottom began to fall out of everything."

When John accepted the new job without telling her first, Carol saw this as the beginning of another rejection by someone highly significant in her life. As her anxiety increased, she withdrew from communication with John "because of her flu." John's well-intentioned agreement to cancel several dates so that she could get more rest further cut off her opportunities to communicate her feelings to him. His suggestion that she take a trip alone compounded her already strong fear of imminent rejection by him.

Finding the neighbor's note under the door was, for her, "the last straw," final proof that he was leaving her, "just like *her* boyfriend did in college." Unable to cope with overwhelming feelings of loss and anger toward herself for "letting it happen to *her* again," she impulsively attempted suicide.

Carol's two suicide attempts, except for the method used, were quite similar. Both were precipitated by the threat of the loss of someone highly significant in her life; both were impulsive, maladaptive attempts to cope with intense feelings of depression, hopelessness, and helplessness; and both demonstrated an inability to communicate her feelings in stressful situations. When asked by the therapist how she coped with anxiety in the past, Carol said that she would keep herself so busy at work that she did not have much time to worry about personal problems. This had been her method of coping with anxiety at school, too, until her first suicide attempt. Because she had been too ill to work full time the past 2 weeks, her previous successful coping mechanisms could not be effectively used.

The goal of intervention was to help Carol gain an intellectual understanding of the relationship between her crisis and her inability to communicate her intense feelings of depression and anxiety caused by the threat of losing John.

Before the end of the first session, the therapist's assessment was that Carol was no longer acutely suicidal. However, because of her continuing feelings of depression, a medical consultation was arranged and an antidepressant prescribed. A verbal contract was agreed on; Carol was to call the therapist if she felt suicidal again. Carol agreed to the suggestion that she have a friend move into her apartment to help her out until her arm was less painful. Before leaving, she assured the therapist that she would call him immediately if she again began to feel overwhelmed by anxiety before her next appointment.

When Carol returned for her next session, she was markedly less depressed. She told the therapist that John had called her soon after she came home from the center the week before. Although he had expressed great concern for her, she had been unable to tell him exactly why she had attempted suicide. "I just couldn't tell him that I thought he had left me for good. He'd think that I was trying to blame him. After all, I've been telling him for months that we both should keep our independence!" However, she said she felt much more reassured of his love for her. John expected to be back in about 2 more weeks.

During this and the next few sessions, the therapist explored with Carol why she found it difficult to communicate her feelings to someone so significant in her life.

Carol was reluctant at first to admit that this was a problem that could have contributed to her recent crisis. She saw herself as someone who was completely self-sufficient and denied any dependency needs on John. As a child, she had been expected to control her emotions, to appear "ladylike" and composed at all times. Efforts on her part to communicate her feelings as she passed through the normal maturational crises of childhood and adolescence were met with rejecting behavior from those most significant in her life—her parents. Slowly, she began to gain insight into the ways in which she had learned maladaptive methods to cope with stress, such as withdrawing from contact with others whenever she felt threatened by a stressful situation, by somatizing her anxiety rather than admitting it was more than she could handle. By the end of the third session, she reported that she had been able to communicate her feelings to John more openly and honestly than she had ever done in the past. She appeared to be surprised and pleased that John had responded so positively to her. When asked what she would have done if he had not responded this way, she paused thoughtfully, then answered, "It was a risk I had to take. I just had to find out for sure if I could handle it this time." She added that, although she had been very anxious while talking to him, she at no time felt as though she could not go on living if things had turned out differently.

By the end of the fourth session, John had returned to the city, and Carol had returned to her job full time. She no longer felt depressed, and her wrist was slowly regaining its functioning. They were seeing each other frequently despite the distance between their offices, and Carol now said that she felt much more comfortable talking things out with him.

Because Carol had attempted suicide once before under much the same crisis-precipitating stressful situation, she continued in therapy for the full 6 weeks. The purpose was to ensure that she could depend on situational support from the therapist while adjusting to the fact that she would no longer be seeing John every day. She was encouraged to telephone the therapist at any time she began to feel a recurrence of her earlier symptoms and felt unable to communicate these feelings to John.

Because she now seemed to have a better understanding of the relationship between her suicide attempts and the precipitating events, she said that she felt more secure in being able to cope with stressful situations in a more positive manner.

Carol's distorted perception of rejection by John was compounded by her previous experience in losing someone highly significant in her life. Unable to directly communicate her feelings to John, her anxiety and depression increased. Lacking adequate coping mechanisms and situational supports, she became overwhelmed with feelings of hopelessness and helplessness. Anticipating another rejection, Carol, entering a state of crisis, impulsively attempted suicide. Intervention was focused on getting her to understand why she was unable to communicate and cope with her intense feelings of inadequacy in interpersonal relations.

O death, where is thy sting?
O death, where is thy victory?

–*Holy Bible*

Complete the paradigm in Figure 8-5 for this case study, then compare it with the completed one in Appendix D. Refer to the paradigms in Chapter 3 as needed.

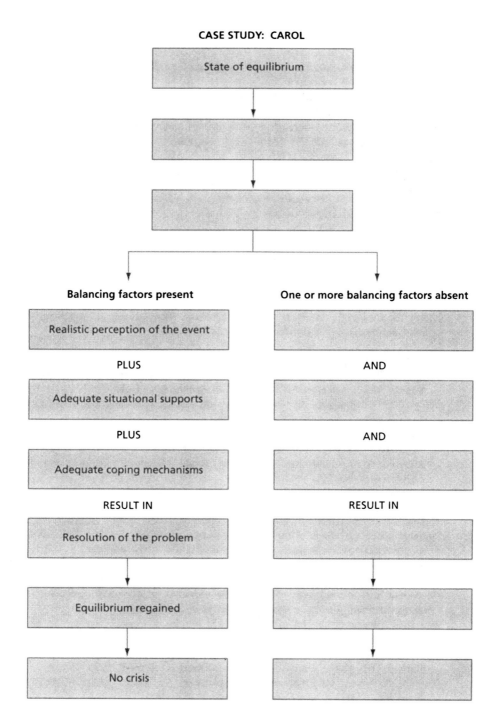

Figure 8-5

REFERENCES

Becker V, Kaplan M: Rape victims: issues, theories, and treatment, *Annu Rev Sex Res* 2:267, 1991.

Calhoun KS, Atkeson BM: *Treatment of rape victims: facilitating psychological adjustment,* New York, x, 1991, Pergnon.

Hellerstein H, Goldstone E: Rehabilitation of patients with heart disease, *Postgrad Med* 15:265, 1954.

Hollender MH: *The psychology of medical practice,* Philadelphia, 1958, WB Saunders.

Jivanjee P: Enhancing the well-being of family caregivers to patients with Alzheimer's disease, *J Gerontol Soc Work* 23:31, 1994.

King SH: *Perceptions of illness and medical practice,* New York, 1962, Russell Sage Foundation.

Koss MP, Harvey MR: *The rape victim: clinical and community interventions,* ed 2, Newbury Park, Calif, 1991, Sage.

Koss MP, Woodruff WJ, Koss PG: Criminal victimization among primary care medical patients: prevalence, incidents, and physician usage, *Behav Sci Law* 9:85, 1991.

Kotchick BA and others: Coping with illness: interrelationships across family members and predictors of psychological adjustment, *J Fam Psychol* 10(3):358, 1996.

Kubie LS, Cited by Kaufman JG, Becker MD: Rehabilitation of the patient with myocardial infarction, *Geriatrics* 10:355, 1955.

Ladely SJ, Puskar K: Adolescent suicide: behaviors, risk factors, and psychiatric nursing interventions, *Issues Ment Health Nurs* 15:497, 1994.

Lee P, Bryner S: Introduction to a symposium on rehabilitation in cardiovascular disease, *Am J Cardiol* 7:315, 1961.

Maugh TH II, Times medical writer: Worldwide study finds big shift in causes of death, *Los Angeles Times,* September 16, 1996, World Health Organization.

Maugh TH II, Times medical writer: Study says EMF may be linked to Alzheimer's, *Los Angeles Times,* December 18, 1996.

McIver J: Psychiatric aspects of cardiovascular diseases in industry. In Warshaw LJ, editor: *The heart in industry,* New York, 1960, Harper & Row.

Munton AG, West A: Innovations and personal change: patterns of adjustment to reolocation, *J Organiza Behav* 16(1):363, 1995.

Munton AG and others: *Job relocation: managing people on the move,* Chichester, United Kingdom, 1993, John Wiley & Sons.

National Center for Health Statistics, Hyattesville, Md, 1994, Public Health Service.

National Institute of Mental Health, Student Health and Human Services Division, Personal communication: *Suicide facts: unpublished data,* 1996, The Institute.

Parson F: *The social system,* New York, 1951, Free Press.

Reiser MF: Emotional aspects of cardiac disease, *Am J Psychiatry* 107:781, 1951.

Shneidman ES: *A conspectus of the suicidal scenario.* In Mans RW and others, editors: *Assessment and prediction of suicide,* New York, 1992, Guilford Press.

Statistical Abstract of the United States, ed 115, Bureau of Census, Washington, DC, 1995, US Government Printing Office.

Stermac CE, Segal ZV, Gillis R: Cultural factors in sexual assault. In Marshall WR, Laws DR, Barbaree HE, editors: *Handbook of sexual assault,* New York, 1990, Plenum.

Yu-Chin R, Arcuni OJ: Short term hospitalization for suicidal patients within a crisis intervention service, *Gen Hosp Psychiatry* 12:153, 1990.

ADDITIONAL READING

Alzheimer's Disease and Related Disorders Associated, Inc. (ADRDA). Scheibel A, Chair: Statistics, Los Angeles, 1996, The Association.

Ambuel B, Lewis C: Social policy of adolescent abortion, *Child Youth Fam Serv Q* 115:2, 1992.

Ambuel B, Rappaport J: Developmental trends in adolescents' psychological and legal competence to consent to abortion, *Law Human Behav* 16:129, 1992.

Archer J, Rhodes V: The grief process and job loss: a cross-sectional study, *Br J Psychol* 84:395, 1993.

Archer J, Rhodes V: A longitudinal study of job loss in relation to the grief process, *J Community Applied Soc Psychol* 5:183, 1995.

Baker JE and others: Psychological tasks for bereaved children, *J Orthopsychiatry* 62:105, 1992.

Carroll JL, Loughlin GM: Sudden infant death syndrome, *Pediatr Rev* 14:88, 1993.

Chaplin JP: *Dictionary of psychology,* ed 2, New York, 1985, Dell.

Cummings EM, Davies PT: Maternal depression and child development, *J Child Psychol Psychiatry* 35:3, 1994.

Eisenberg L: The social construction of the human brain, *Am J Psychiatry* 152:1563, 1995.

Farran CJ and others: Finding meaning: an alternative paradigm for Alzheimer's disease family caregivers, *Gerontologist* 31(4):483, 1991.

Frazier A, Burnett W: Immediate coping strategies among rape victims, *J Counsel Dev* 72:633, 1994.

Horowitz MJ: A model of mourning: change in schemas of self and other, *J Amer Psychoanal Assoc* 38:297, 1993.

Mace NL, Rabins PV: *The 36 hour day,* Baltimore, 1981, Johns Hopkins University Press.

Maris RW: Suicide Prevention in Adults (Age 30-65), *Suicide Life Threat Behav* 25(1):171, 1995.

Miles MS, Funk SG, Carlson J: Parental stressor scale: neonatal intensive care unit, *Nurs Res* 42:148, 1993.

Mintzer JR and others: Behavioral Intensive Care Unit (BICU): A new concept in the management of acute agitated behavior in elderly demented patients, *Gerontologist* 33(6):801, 1993.

Sadowski C, Kelley ML: Social problem solving in suicidal adolescents, *J Consult Clin Psychol* 61:121, 1993.

Scott ES: Judgment and reasoning in adolescent decision making, *Villanova Law Rev,* 37:1607, 1992.

Seiffge-Krenke I: Coping behavior in normal and clinical samples: more similarities than differences? *J Adolesc* 16:285, 1993.

Stroebe W, Stroebe M: *Bereavement and health: processes of adjusting to the loss of a partner.* In Montada L, Filipp SH, Lerner MJ, editors: *Life crises and experiences of loss in adulthood,* Hillsdale, NJ, 1994, Erlbaum.

Tracey N: The psychic space in trauma, *J Child Psychother* 17(2):29, 1991.

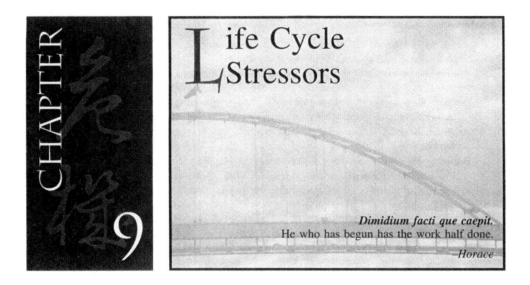

CHAPTER 9

Life Cycle Stressors

Dimidium facti que caepit.
He who has begun has the work half done.

—Horace

An overview of the literature relating to life-cycle stressors and coping requires a brief restatement of some definitions of the more pertinent concepts. *Life cycles* refer to the various phases of human life from the perinatal period through approaching death. *Stress stimuli (stressors)* are threat or loss conditions—circumstances or situations that produce various degrees of bodily reactions that indicate that an individual is experiencing *stress* or a *state of stress*. Stress, then, is a set of nonspecific physiological and psychological responses of the body to any demands made on it, whether these responses are pleasant or unpleasant experiences. As people proceed through Selye's general adaptation syndrome, they experience (1) an alarm reaction that involves marshaling the body resources, (2) a stage of resistance during which the bodily resistance to the stress response rises above normal, and (3) a stage of exhaustion during which the adaptation response energy is used up or dissipated. Persons have *adapted* positively to the stressor situation when their bodily alterations have ensured their safety or survival and have increased their functioning and enjoyment within their environment. They have *maladapted* when the bodily responses or alterations have resulted in internal disharmony (illness) or disharmony between them and their environment.

All people are exposed to a variety of stressors virtually all the time throughout the course of their life spans. Both pleasant and unpleasant stimuli may produce stress responses, and individual perceptions of and psychophysiological reactions to these stimuli may vary quite widely. The problem seems to lie not so much in the fact that people are exposed continually to life stressors; more accurately, the problem is in the degree and duration of these stressor situations and in the variable range of personal responses and capacities to withstand and cope with such stimuli. Although most people have the capacity to sustain relatively high degrees of stress for short periods of time, a prolonged stress response or an overly strong stimulus can be maladaptive or destructive. The literature cited in the following sections focuses on the adaptive capacities of people in several phases of the life cycle beginning with prepuberty.

Prepuberty

Prepuberty years are characterized as the learning stage; that is, "I am what I learn" (Erikson, 1959, 1992). The child wants to be shown how to do things both alone and with others; he develops a sense of industry in which he becomes dissatisfied if he does not have a feeling of being useful or a sense of his ability to make things and make them well, even perfectly. He now learns to win recognition by producing *things*. He feels pleasure when his attention and diligence produce a completed work.

Slow but steady growth occurs as maturation of the central nervous system continues. In terms of psychosexual development, pressure is reduced in the exploration of sensuality and the gender role while other skills are developed and exploited.

The cognitive phase of development includes the mastery of skills in manipulating objects and the concepts of his culture. Thinking enters the period of *concrete operations* (Piaget, 1963, 1989), and the ability to solve concrete problems with this ability increases, so that toward the end of this period the child is able to solve abstract problems. The solution of real problems is accomplished with mental operations that the child was previously unable to perform. By puberty, the child exhibits simple deductive reasoning ability and has learned the rules and basic technology of his culture, thus reinforcing his sense of belonging in his environment.

Self-esteem is derived from the sense of adequacy and the beginning of "best" friendships and sharing with peers. This also marks the beginning of friendships and loves outside the family, as he begins to learn the complexities, pleasures, and difficulties of adjusting himself and his drives, aggressive and erotic, to those of his peers. By learning and adjusting, he begins to take his place as a member of their group and social life. In making this adjustment, he seeks the company of his own sex and forms groups and secret societies. The gangs and groups, especially with boys, fight each other in games, baseball, and cops and robbers, working off much hostility and aggression in a socially approved manner (Homonoff, 1991).

Feelings of inadequacy and inferiority may begin if the child does not develop a sense of adequacy. Family life may not have prepared him for school, or the school itself may fail to help him develop the necessary skills for competency. As a result, he may feel that he will never be good at anything he attempts.

In general, children are better able to cope with stress when normal familial supports are available. Any real or imagined threat of separation from a nuclear family member could drastically reduce a child's abilities to cope with new or changing psychosocial demands. Children are particularly vulnerable to crisis-precipitating situations such as the loss of a parent through death. Equally as stressful are recurring partial losses of a parent from the child's usual environment. Examples of the latter are repeated episodes of parental hospitalization or frequent, extended absences from home by one or both parents (Cassell, 1991).

An increasingly common source of emotional distress for children of this age group is the entry or reentry of the "homemaker" parent into the work field. This major change in the parenting role demands reciprocal changes in the child's role. For some children, externally imposed demands to assume increased independence and responsibility for self may be more than the child is maturationally able to cope with. Not yet able to assume the level of expected independence, the child may actually perceive this action as a form of rejection by the parent.

A common symbol of this role change is the home "latchkey" that is bestowed upon the child, much like a rite of passage and with the accompaniment of new social rules and regulations. In general, such rules and regulations focus on protection of the child and the home, with the child given implicit or explicit responsibility for ensuring that neither is violated in the parent's absence.

The following case study is about an 8-year-old boy for whom the latchkey symbolizes only rejection.

Case Study   *Prepuberty*

Billy B, 8 years old, was referred with his mother to the school counseling psychologist by his homeroom teacher. For the past few weeks, she reported, Billy had changed from his usual cheerful, outgoing, alert behavior to moodiness and apparent preoccupation. He was falling behind in his schoolwork, and twice during the past week he had failed to return to his classes after the lunch hour. The first time that he had done this, the school had contacted his mother at her place of work. She told them that Billy had already telephoned her from home. He told her that his stomach was upset, so he had decided to go home and call her from there. She was planning to go directly home when the call came from the school.

Yesterday, the counselor was told, Billy again failed to return to his classes after the lunch hour. This time he did not call his mother, and he did not go home. After being notified by the school, his mother had telephoned home. She thought that Billy would be there, as before. Failing to get any answer, she went directly home from work to begin looking for him around the neighborhood. About an hour later, while making his routine security rounds, the apartment house custodian heard muffled sounds coming from a basement stairway and went to investigate. He found Billy crouched on the top steps, his head on his knees and sobbing. He was taken immediately to his mother. When questioned, he denied having been threatened by anyone or being injured, and he showed no signs of physical abuse. He refused to say why he had left school early again, or why he had not gone directly home.

Mrs. B immediately called the school and told them that Billy had been located and was safe. She was asked, and agreed, to come to school the next day with Billy to meet with his homeroom teacher. At the teacher's request, during the meeting the following day a referral was made for Billy and his mother to meet with a counseling psychologist.

Billy was seen initially without his mother present. He was average in height and weight, appeared physically healthy, although pale, and spoke hesitantly. He sat slouched in his chair, his eyes downcast, and appeared rather depressed. When asked why he had left school without permission twice that week, he muttered, "I don't know what everyone is so excited about. I can take care of myself—ask my mother—I can go home alone because I have the house key and can get in when my mother isn't home."

He stated that he had always liked school, got A's and B's, particularly enjoyed gym and outdoor sports, such as soccer and football. Until a week ago, he had attended an afterschool boys' sport group with many of his friends. This, however, had been suddenly canceled when the group director had resigned and moved to another city. He also said that his parents had been divorced when he was "a little kid" (4 years old) and that he now lived with his mother. He had frequently visited with his father, who lived nearby, until about 4 months ago. At that time his father had remarried and, a month later, his father's company had transferred him out of state.

After seeing Billy alone, the counselor talked to Mrs. B to verify and clarify this information and to assess her feelings about his problems and her ability to cope with them. Mrs. B was a tall, attractive, well-dressed woman who gave the impression that she was deeply concerned about the recent changes in Billy's behavior. She stated that Billy, an only child, had always been considered "well-adjusted," got along well with his friends, and, until recently, could always be depended on to keep up with his schoolwork. She went on to say that she and the boy's father had been particularly concerned about what effect their divorce might have on him. They had met regularly with a family therapist during that period to help Billy through their separation and eventual divorce.

Mrs. B had met her husband in college, and they had married right after graduation. He was an electronics engineer and she had majored in business administration. During the 3 years before Billy was born, she had advanced to a well-paying position as administrative assistant to the director of a large advertising company. When she learned that she was pregnant, she arranged to take a 6-month leave of absence after his birth. However, as she described it to the counselor, Billy was not a healthy baby and seemed to have one medical problem after another for more than 2 years. She described Billy's father as very possessive and domineering whenever they had decisions to make about Billy's care. "In fact," she said, "when the time came that I felt that I could safely leave Billy with a sitter and go back to work, it became clear to me that our marriage was in for a lot of rocky days."

After many days of arguing and eventual compromise, they agreed that she would return to work on a part-time basis and only if they were both satisfied that the babysitter was giving Billy the best of care.

Furthermore, the father completely refused the idea of a day nursery, insisting that they get a sitter to come to their home, stating, "It's his home as much as it is ours, and he is entitled to be here—not in some stranger's house where I can't check up on things whenever I want."

By the time Billy was 3 years old, his mother reported, both parents realized that he was being emotionally "Ping-Ponged" between them and that her returning to work, even for a day, would always be a point of conflict. Her husband had grown up in a very patriarchal family, with his mother never daring even to dream of any other role than that of "Kinder, Kirche, und Kuche." Considering any other role for his wife, now that they had a family, was difficult for him.

By contrast, Billy's mother had grown up in a family that encouraged equal rights for women. Her mother was a practicing attorney while rearing four children, and her father had managed a produce company. She just could not understand why she and her husband were having so many conflicts with only one child. By the time Billy was 4 years old, they had separated, and they were eventually divorced when he was 5. The final decree provided Mr. B with ample visitation rights, and they shared equally the responsibility for child support funds.

Until 4 months ago, Billy's mother had been able to manage on part-time work and was able to be home each day when he returned from school. However, earlier this year Mr. B had remarried and, when he transferred out of the state 4 months ago, he was more than 6 months delinquent in payments for his share of child support. Being, as she put it, "a very realistic person," Mrs. B decided that she could no longer depend on Billy's father for regular payments in the future. Three months ago she went to her boss and asked if she could be reassigned to full-time work on an ongoing basis as soon as possible. She stated that Billy had never expressed any particularly negative feelings about his father remarrying and moving away, only that he would miss seeing him as often as he had in the past. She had taken particular care in planning with Billy for her return to full-time work. She knew, for example, that she would not be able to be home before he got back from school at the end of the day, so they planned for him to join an afterschool supervised sport group. This was one that would pick him up at the school and return him to his home by suppertime each day. "By that time," she said, "I would be home and he wouldn't come home to an empty apartment." This, she felt, also took care of her worry about his playing unsupervised in the neighborhood without her there to "keep an eye on things."

Three weeks ago Mrs. B had started her full-time work. She had always managed to get home before Billy returned from the sports group. She thought that they would have no major changes for either of them to adjust to. One week ago, however, the director of the sports group suddenly resigned without notice. A replacement had not yet been found, and the group had been temporarily canceled. As the only interim choice that she could think of, Mrs. B decided to give Billy his own key to the apartment.

Worried about all of the real and imagined things that might happen to him before she got home, she accompanied the key with many admonishments about coming directly home from school, checking in with the apartment manager, and being sure to keep the door locked until she got home. She said that Billy did not seem to object to this at all. In fact, he had purchased a key chain to hook on his belt just like the one the building manager wore.

When the school called her the first time Billy cut classes and went home, she had counseled him to remain at school the next time he felt ill, and she would pick him up there. She had told him that he must "never go home alone again without first telling her or someone at the school. I don't like the idea of your being alone and sick. You know I would worry about you." She had also reminded him that they had planned this together and that they both had certain responsibilities to each other in working out this new living schedule. "Neither of us had much choice in this, you know," she told the counselor. "I'm making the best of things that I know how, and Billy is just going to have to cooperate. I just don't know why he is acting this way now."

The sudden, rapid changes in Billy's life during the past few months had forced him into assuming a degree of independence and self-responsibility beyond his maturational level of skills. Not yet accepting the loss of his father and perceiving it as a rejection of himself, he was forced into full dependence on his mother for any sense of security and all decision making. The timely entrance into the after-school sports group had provided him with opportunities to express his feelings of anger and hostility about the situation through the competitive, aggressive sports activities with his peers. Unfortunately, the group was canceled about the same time his mother started her new job, and he lost his normal outlet for expressing such feelings. Not only did he lose the situational support of his peers when he most needed it, but also he had the further situational loss of his mother from her familiar roles. He could no longer depend on her being at home when he might need her during the day. His anxiety increased, as he perceived this to be another sign of rejection from a parent figure. Billy had no coping mechanisms in his repertoire with which to handle these feelings of added anxiety and depression. At the particular time when he needed to use his usually successful coping behaviors, the opportunity was not available because of the demand by his mother that he "come home directly after school. You can't play in the neighborhood after school with your friends."

The therapist thought that Mrs. B needed assistance in gaining a realistic, intellectual understanding of the situation as it related to Billy's current behaviors. Increasingly anxious about the added responsibility that had been placed on her during the past few months, she was possibly projecting her own feelings of insecurity into overprotective behaviors toward Billy; that is, "It is Billy, not I, who should not be out alone and unprotected. Something terrible might happen to *him* when there is no longer a strong, dependable person nearby to help keep an eye on things."

Billy would need to explore his perceptions and feelings about the psychosocial losses of both parents from the usual family roles that they had occupied in his life. He needed to be helped to express his feelings constructively and to make a positive adaptation to the new role demands made of him. During the first session, the counselor focused on identifying with Mrs. B the many critical changes that had occurred in Billy's life during the past few months and their impact on his level of maturational skill development. The goal was to provide her with insight into how Billy might be perceiving such events at his level of comprehension and concrete thinking. Although he was old enough to be fully aware of the events happening, he was still too young to deal with them abstractly. For example, when his father had remarried and then moved away soon after, Billy most likely had perceived these actions as signs of complete rejection by his father and blamed himself in some way. In his mind, he may have wondered, "Why else would my father marry someone else and then move away, abandoning both me and my mother?"

It was also suggested to Mrs. B that her comments at the time (e.g., "If I don't go back to full-time work, we won't have a roof over our heads or food to eat") were probably taken quite literally by Billy. So, also, was her later admonishment to him always to come straight home from school, implying that he was one more source of problems for her.

In the next two sessions, through the use of direct questioning and reflection of verbal and nonverbal clues with Mrs. B, she became able to express her own feelings about the recent chain of events in her life and to begin to relate them to Billy's behavioral changes. Her counselor suggested that she try to find some alternative supervised peer group activities for Billy after school. The purpose was to reinstate, for him, the opportunity for some normal, acceptable outlets for the angry, hostile feelings that he must still be having from the recent losses in his life.

The counselor met with Billy at the beginning of each session to discuss with him how he was doing in school classes and what things he was doing to occupy his time after school before his mother got home from work. Billy's feelings of rejection and insecurity were dealt with during this time.

The remaining time was spent with Mrs. B. She was encouraged to continue to provide Billy with as much independence as feasible, yet not expect him to assume any more than he could comfortably cope with at this time. The importance of providing Billy with every opportunity to learn new social skills and to develop strong feelings of competency and self-adequacy was emphasized. The fact that closing off his access to usual afterschool activities with his peers would greatly limit his chances for new learning experiences was discussed. It might also precipitate his return to the same maladaptive coping behaviors that he had been demonstrating during the past few weeks.

Mrs. B was not able to locate another supervised activity group for her son to attend after school. However, she did make arrangements with a retired gentleman who lived in the same apartment house to keep an eye on Billy and to be a contact for him when he came home and played in the neighborhood with his friends after school.

An important focus of anticipatory planning was to review with Mrs. B the maturational changes that she could expect to see developing in Billy over the next few years. The need for her to continue to allow him normal opportunities for growth and development was stressed. The fact that Billy was now a member of a single-parent family should not create any particular peer-group problems, because this situation was increasingly common among children his age. However, potential stressful situations were identified and discussed in terms of how she might approach coping with them as they arose, both for herself and in her dealings with Billy.

Billy was encouraged to be more direct in questions to his mother and in letting her know when he felt confused or angry about things that were happening to him. He understood that he could stop in and talk to the counselor whenever the need arose, but that he should also be expected to keep in close touch with his mother about his feelings in the future.

Billy had perceived his father's remarriage and move out of state as a rejection of himself. Unable to express his feelings to his mother, he coped by acting out his anger and hostility in competitive, aggressive sports activities with his peers. Despite Mrs. B's assumptions to the contrary, planning with Billy for her return to full-time work had served to reactivate his fears of another rejection. No longer having his sports activities available to him as before, his anxiety increased. Lacking any other available coping skills, he became overwhelmed.

Boys are nature's rare material.

–Saki

Complete the paradigm in Figure 9-1 for this case study, then compare it with the completed one in Appendix D. Refer to the paradigms in Chapter 3 as needed.

Adolescence

The individual is probably more aware of change during adolescence than during any other period in life. Adolescence is a period that confronts both the individual and the family with numerous problems and challenges. Erikson (1963, 1992) describes the main task of adolescence as that of identity formation, and identifies four primary components:

1. The physical and emotional separation from parents
2. The acquisition of socially oriented attitudes and opinions
3. The preparation for a working role
4. The definition of the sexual role

Unfortunately, these major psychological adjustments are expected to take place during a time when everything else is changing—when a person is no longer a child but not yet an adult. Adolescents are confronted almost simultaneously with rapid physiological changes, increased cognitive development, increased peer group pressures and activities, and changes in family and societal attitudes and expectations, all of which serve as stressors during this phase of their development and may interfere severely with the task of identity formation.

Emancipation from the family tends to be desired and feared by both the adolescents and their parents. Adolescents frequently find themselves expected to continue in the child role or to assume both the adult and child roles simultaneously. This mixed role expectation often leads to aggressive behaviors and to conflicts within the family structure because the adolescent is constantly pulled between the need for adult support and the desire for independence (Peterson, 1972). Actual as well as feigned illness tends to increase parental controls and promote more positive relationships with siblings, even though the adolescents themselves continue to be socially active.

In the search for identity, adolescents frequently attempt to submerge themselves in a peer group identity, which provides them with a temporary feeling of importance and belonging. The peer group serves a dual purpose: both insulating the adolescent from the adult world and building its own norms for its members. Although the group standards, values, and opinions can provide a positive background for testing out adolescent roles and styles for future adult life, the group pressures for untoward experiences (e.g., use of drugs and sex) may also have the negative effect of promoting a sense of alienation from the rest of society (Starr and Goldstein, 1975).

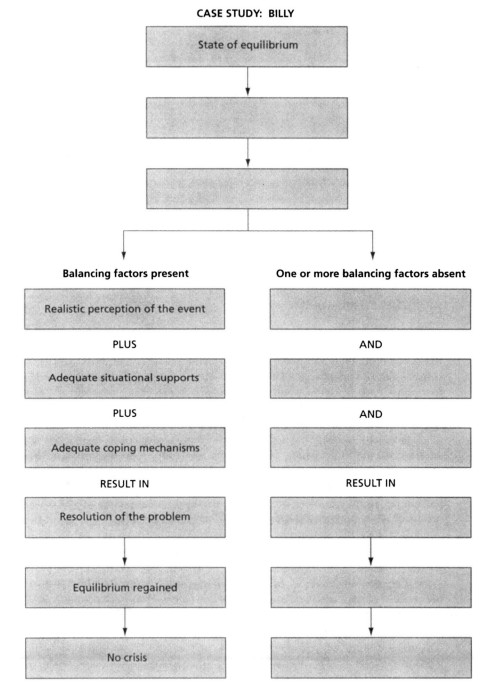

Figure 9-1

Tests of mental ability show that adolescence is also the period of greatest ability to acquire and make use of knowledge. The adolescent is capable of a high degree of imaginative thinking, which, although somewhat oversimplified and unoriginal, sets up the structure for adult thinking patterns and the work role (Piaget, 1963). Differences in cognitive skills development among male and female adolescents (e.g., verbal skills among females, quantitative and spatial skills in males) are seen as the result of interest, social expectations, and earlier training, rather than as variations in the innate mental abilities.

The adolescent has a strong need to find and confirm his identity. Rapid body growth equals that of early childhood, but it is compounded by the addition of physical-genital maturity. Faced with the physiological revolution within himself, the adolescent is also concerned with consolidating his social roles. He is preoccupied with the difference between what he appears to be in the eyes of others and what he believes himself to be. In searching for a new sense of continuity, some adolescents must refight crises left unresolved in previous years (Adler and Clark, 1991).

Changes that occur while secondary sex characteristics emerge make the adolescent self-conscious and uncomfortable with himself and with his friends. Body image changes, and the adolescent constantly seeks validation that these physiological changes are "normal" because he feels different and is dissatisfied with how he thinks he looks. If sudden spurts of growth occur, he concludes he will be too tall; conversely, if growth does not occur as expected, he thinks he will be too short, or too thin, or too fat. In this period of fluctuation, half-child and half-adult, the adolescent reacts with childish rebellion one day and with adult maturity the next (Lau, 1991).

The adolescent is as unpredictable to himself as he is to parents and other adults. On the one hand, he seeks freedom and rebels against authority; on the other, he does not trust his own sense of emerging maturity and covertly seeks guidelines from adults. In his struggle for an identity, he turns to his peers and adopts their mode of dress, mannerisms, vocabulary, and code of behavior, often to the distress of adult society. The adolescent desperately needs to belong, to feel accepted, loved, and wanted.

This is the age for cliques and gangs. The in-group can be extremely clannish and intolerant of those who do not belong. Banding together against the adult world, its members seek to internalize their identity, but because of different and often rebellious behavior they are frequently labeled incorrectly as delinquent.

Having achieved a sense of security and acceptance from peers, the adolescent begins to seek heterosexual involvement. This occurs first at group-oriented social events, such as dances, parties, and football games. As comfort and confidence increase, the adolescent progresses to more meaningful and deeper emotional involvements in one-to-one heterosexual relationships. Because of conflict between sexual drives, desires, and the establishment norms of society, this stage can be extremely stressful, and again the adolescent is faced with indecision and confusion (Rose-Gold, 1991).

Occupational identity also becomes a concern at this time. Continual queries by parents and school authorities arise about career plans for the future. Uncertainties are compounded when a definite choice cannot be made because of an inability to identify fully with the adult world of work. Having only observed or participated in fragments of work situations, the adolescent finds it difficult to commit himself to the reality of full-time employment and its inherent responsibilities. To state what is not wanted rather than what is wanted as a career is easier and more realistic (Baack, 1991).

Piaget (1963, 1989) refers to the cognitive development at this stage as *formal operations,* the period in which the capacity for abstract thinking and complex deductive reasoning becomes possible. At this time, the goal is "independence," and in midadolescence acceptance of the idea that to love someone and at the same time be angry with that person is possible. If this stage is successfully negotiated, the individual develops a capacity for self-responsibility; failure at this stage may lead to a sense of inadequacy in controlling and competing.

Because of the number and wide variety of stimuli and rapid changes to which he is exposed, the adolescent is in a hazardous situation. A crisis situation may be compounded by the normal amount of flux characteristic of adolescent development (Cameron, 1963; Erikson, 1950, 1959, 1963, 1989; Piaget, 1963, 1989; Zachry, 1940).

The following case study illustrates some of the conflicts that adolescents face while trying to find their identity, strive for independence, and win acceptance from their peer group. It also points out the need for understanding and patience on the part of parents as their adolescents grow up.

Case Study   *Adolescence*

Mary V, a 14-year-old high school sophomore, was referred to a crisis center with her parents by a school nurse. During the past few weeks, she had shown signs of increased anxiety, cried easily, and had lost interest in school activities. That morning, for no apparent reason, she had suddenly left the classroom in tears. The teacher followed and found her crouched in a nearby utility closet, crying uncontrollably. Mary seemed unable to give a reason for her loss of control and was very anxious. When her mother came in response to a call from the school nurse, they agreed to follow her advice and seek family therapy.

During the first session, the therapist saw Mary and her parents together to assess their interaction and communication patterns and to determine Mary's problems.

Mrs. V was quiet and left most of the conversation up to her husband and Mary. When she attempted to add anything to what was being said, she was quickly silenced by Mr. V's hard, cold stare or by Mary exclaiming in an exasperated tone, "Oh, Mother!" Mr. V spoke in a controlled, stilted manner, saying that he had no idea what was wrong with Mary, and Mrs. V responded hesitantly that it must be something at school.

Mary was particularly well developed for her age, a fact that was apparent despite the rather shapeless dress she was wearing. She might have been very attractive if she had paid more attention to her posture and general appearance.

When questioned, Mary said that she had not been sleeping well for weeks, had no appetite, and could not concentrate on her schoolwork. She did not know why she felt this way, and her uncontrolled outburst of tears frightened and embarrassed her. She was also afraid of what she might do next, adding that her crying that morning was probably because she had not slept well for the past two nights. At first, she tried to brush this off as final exam jitters.

She evaded answering repeated questions about sudden changes in her life in the past few days. When the therapist asked if she would be comfortable talking alone, without her parents, she gave her father a quick glance and replied that she would. Mr. and Mrs. V were asked if they objected to Mary talking to the therapist alone. Both agreed that it might be a good idea and went to the waiting room.

For a time, Mary continued to respond evasively. It was obvious that she had strongly mixed feelings about how to relate to the male therapist. Should it be "woman to man" or "child to adult"? Throughout this and the following sessions, she alternated between her child and adult roles. The therapist recognized the role ambivalence of adolescence and adjusted his role relationship, using whichever was most effective in focusing on the problem areas and making Mary more comfortable.

Mary eventually relaxed and began to talk freely about her relationship with her family, her activities at school, and some of the feelings that were troubling her. She said that she had two older brothers. The younger of the two, Kirk, was 16 years old and a senior in high school. She felt closer to him because "he understands and I can talk to him." Mary said that she had had "as good a childhood" as the rest of her friends. However, she did think that her father kept a closer eye on her activities than did the parents of most of her friends. He still called her his "baby" and "my little girl" and lately had begun to place more restrictions than usual on her friendships and activities.

She admitted that during the past year she had gone through a sudden spurt of body growth and development. She was keenly aware of these differences in her appearance and sensed the changing attitudes of her father and her friends. She felt her father was worried about her growing "up and out so fast." He was the one who insisted that she wear the almost shapeless dresses. She said she knew "it wasn't really because I outgrow things so fast right now—he thinks I look too sexy for my age!"

About 3 weeks ago, she had been invited to the junior-senior prom by a friend of her brother Kirk. She liked the boy and wanted to go but was not sure Kirk would approve because he would be at the prom too. Another problem was getting her parents' permission to buy the necessary formal. She had looked at dresses and knew exactly the one she wanted but knew her father would not let her have it.

Mary was asked if she felt able to tell her parents these things that were bothering her if the therapist were present to give her support. She thought that she could if he would "sort of prepare them first" and explain how important it was for her to go dressed like the rest of her girlfriends. He suggested that Mary discuss the situation with Kirk to see how he felt about her going to the prom with his friend, and she agreed to do this before the next session. The therapist assured her that he would spend the first part of the next session with her parents to discuss and explore their feelings about the prom.

It was thought that Mary needed support to assist her in convincing her parents that she be allowed to grow up. Mr. and Mrs. V needed to gain an intellectual understanding of some of the problems that adolescent girls face as they search for an identity, seek independence, and feel the need to be like their peers. Mrs. V would have to be encouraged to give support and guidance to Mary and help to resist Mr. V's attempts to keep Mary as the baby of the family.

At the next session the therapist went to the waiting room to get Mr. and Mrs. V and saw that Mary had brought her brother Kirk with her. She asked if he could come in with them at the last half of the session when the family would be together. The therapist agreed, realizing that Mary had brought additional support and that apparently Kirk had approved of her going to the prom.

The first part of the session was spent discussing with the parents the general problems of most adolescents, as well as the reasons behind their often erratic and unusual behavior. Both parents seemed willing to accept this new knowledge, although Mr. V said that he had not noticed any of this with the boys. Mrs. V said, "No, but you treated them differently. You were glad they were becoming men." The therapist supported Mrs. V and said that this was one of Mary's specific problems. He then repeated to the parents what Mary had said about the things that were bothering her. Both parents seemed slightly embarrassed, and Mr. V's voice and manner became quite angry as he tried to explain why he wanted to "protect" Mary. "She's so young, so innocent—someone may take advantage of her," and so on.

Discussion then focused on Mary's anxiety and the tension she was feeling because her father had made her feel different from her friends. Compromise between Mr. and Mrs. V and Mary was explored when Mary and Kirk joined their parents in the last half of the session. Mary was more verbal with Kirk present to support her, and Kirk told his father, "You are too old-fashioned. Mary's a good kid, you don't have to worry about her. You make her dress like a 10-year-old," and so on. Mr. V was silent for a while and then said, "You may be right, Kirk. I don't know." He then asked him, "Do you think I should let her go to the prom?" Kirk answered, "Yes, Dad. I'll be there. She can even double with me and my date." Her father agreed, adding that Mrs. V should go with her to pick out a "fairly decent dress." Mary began to cry, and Mr. V in great consternation asked, "What's wrong now?" She replied, "Daddy, I'm so happy. Don't you know women cry when they are happy too?"

The next few sessions were spent in supporting the family members in their changing attitudes toward each other. Anticipatory planning was directed toward establishing open communication between the parents and Mary to avoid another buildup of tensions and misunderstandings. Mary was encouraged to use Kirk as a situational support in the future, because he and his father were not in conflict. The family was told they could return for help with future crises if necessary and were assured that they had accomplished a great deal toward mutual understanding.

Mary suffered acute symptoms of anxiety because she had to ask her father for permission to go to a dance. She wanted to be a member of her peer group but felt uncomfortable because she was not allowed to dress as they did. She wanted independence but was inexperienced and afraid to make a decision that would oppose her father. Because the situation involved possible conflict with her brother, she did not feel comfortable talking with him about her problem.

Intervention was based on exploring areas of difficulty with the family and assisting them to recognize, understand, and support Mary's adolescent behavior, her bid for independence, and her need to become a member of her peer group.

Youth is wholly experimental.

–Robert Louis Stevenson

Complete the paradigm in Figure 9-2 for this case study, then compare it with the completed one in Appendix D. Refer to the paradigms in Chapter 3 as needed.

Adulthood

Because adulthood begins in the late teens and continues to the end of the life cycle, talking about stressors in relation to the usual age-group phases—early, middle, and late adulthood—may be considered more practical. What cannot be denied, however, is that major changes or shifts in life circumstances very often occur at different periods for different individuals. Moreover, a particular experience that is highly threatening for one person may just as often be relatively innocuous for another, depending on how each perceives and appraises the personal effect of the experience. A life change need not be particularly undesirable to induce stress (Dohrenwend and Dohrenwend, 1974). In addition, certain types of stressors or life strains can occur repeatedly throughout a person's total life period.

A number of investigators have focused on identifying which types of life situations seem to present the greatest threats to human psychophysiological stability and have developed lists of life events weighted according to the degree of experienced stress among their study populations. Perhaps the most widely known of these lists is the forty-third-item Social Readjustment Rating Scale (SRRS) developed by Holmes and Rahe (1967). The scale consists of a mix of pleasurable and undesirable life events identified by people as productive of bodily stress responses (e.g., marriage, new job, job loss, death of a loved one, etc.). Since its publication in 1967 the SRRS has generated considerable public and professional interest and criticism as well as an extensive body of research. For example, Dohrenwend and Dohrenwend (1974) found that both ethnicity and the degree of life experience affected the rating of life events as stressors. In analyzing a number of studies that focus on social class and ethnic group membership and their judgments of the magnitude of stressful life events, Anderson and others (1977) found that cultural judgments about this magnitude are even greater than the various reports have suggested. In pretests of a more extensive list of 102 life events actually experienced in a number of populations, group differences were found to vary more by ethnicity than by sex or social class.

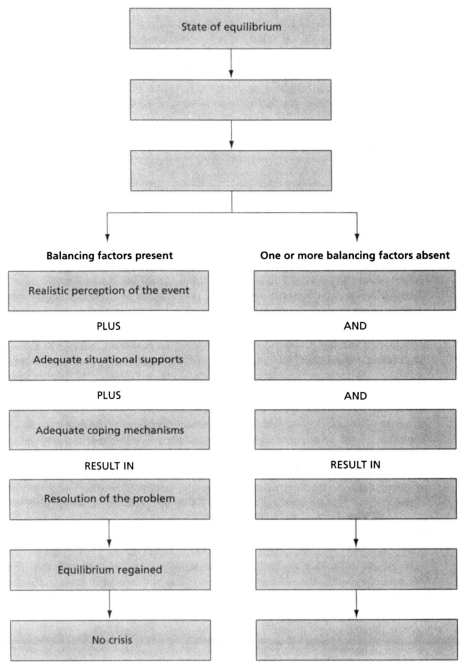

Figure 9-2

An important resource for preventing or moderating responses to stressful life events is that of social support. Cobb (1976) defines social support as "information leading the subject to believe that he is cared for and loved, esteemed, and a member of a network of mutual obligations." In his review of over 50 studies, Cobb cites findings identifying the mechanism of social support as a moderator of acute stress situations throughout the life cycle. The variable of social support too often has been neglected as a mitigating or even preventive factor in the relationships between stressful life events and illness, which suggests that considerable empirical research needs to be done in this area. In this context, two of the many possible hypotheses that could be tested concerning the reasons that social support may play a positive role in the prevention of illness are that (1) social norms may affect group member health behaviors and that (2) social interaction may provide preventive healthcare information.

Many problem situations such as nutritional deficits, rest and sleep problems, sexual difficulties, moral-religious conflicts, self-image problems, divorce, and bereavement can be experienced at any time during the life cycle, since these stressor events are neither predictable nor universally experienced. Moreover, other types of life circumstances including environmental settings, educational preparation, and economic resources can mitigate, submerge, or exacerbate life crises.

Discussions about the stages and stressors of life development are always somewhat arbitrary at best, but are even more so when discussing the age 30-to-65 phase, or middle adulthood. In general, it can be said that the decisions made in young adulthood tend to give shape and direction to life during the 30s. Certain expectations have been fulfilled, certain skills have been learned, and a number of achievements have been accomplished. Gratifications during the 30s and early 40s include success in a job, a marriage, a family, which constitute fulfillment of earlier hopes and expectations. Nevertheless, new decisions and lifestyle adjustments have to be made, disappointments and discontentments occur more frequently, and ambition for success may turn into desperation. The concomitant incidence of anxiety, depression, and other symptomatology (e.g., psychosomatic complaints, fear reactions, and other emotional reactions), which seemed high in the 30s, may reach maximum heights during the 40s when a person begins to sense that life is finite and that health and even interpersonal decrements are more permanent than temporary. However, certain types of stressors including career and work-related stressors, changes in the family unit structure (through death, divorce, departure of the last child, etc.), physical aging, and the like, do tend to occur more frequently in this period of middle adulthood.

Although a number of studies report that good work relationships can buffer some occupational stresses and their related psychological strains, research into specific occupations suggests that other factors such as personality and prior experience may be more important in the development of effective coping mechanisms.

Adulthood is the usual period in life when the responsibilities of life and/or of parenthood are assumed, involving the abilities of a man or woman to accept the strengths and weaknesses of one another and to combine their energies toward mutual goals. It is a crucial time for reconciliation with practical reality.

Maturity is always relative and is usually considered to develop in adulthood. Many adults who marry and have children never do achieve psychological maturity, whereas others who choose not to marry may show a greater degree of mature responsibility than many of their married peers.

Adult normality, like maturity, is also relative. Normality requires that a person achieve and maintain a reasonably effective balance, both psychodynamically and interpersonally. The normal adult must be able to control and channel his emotional drives without losing his initiative and vigor. He should be able to cope with ordinary personal upheavals and the frustrations and disappointments in life with only temporary disequilibrium. He should be able to participate enthusiastically in adult work and adult play, as well as have the capacity to give and to experience adequate sexual gratification in a stable relationship. He should be able to express a reasonable amount of aggression, anger, joy, and affection without undue effort or unnecessary guilt.

In actuality, expecting to find perfect normalcy in any adult is unreasonable. Absolute perfection of physique and physiology are rare rather than normal, and an adult with a perfect emotional equilibrium is equally as exceptional.

This case study concerns a young woman whose lack of psychosocial maturity created problems when she was faced with the responsibility of motherhood. Her husband's competence and pleasure in caring for their baby increased her feelings of inadequacy and rejection.

Case Study   *Adulthood (Motherhood)*

Myra and John, a young married couple, were referred by Myra's obstetrician to a crisis center because of her symptoms of depression. Myra said she was experiencing difficulty in sleeping, was constantly tired, and would begin to cry for no apparent reason.

Myra was an attractive but fragile blonde of 22 years whose looks and manners gave her the appearance of a 16 year old. John, 28 years old, had a calm and mature demeanor. They had been married 1½ years and were the parents of a 3-month-old son, John, Jr. John was an engineer with a large corporation. Myra had been a liberal arts major when they met and married. John was the oldest of four children and was from a stable family of modest circumstances; Myra was an only child who had been indulged by wealthy parents.

When questioned by the therapist specifically about the onset of her symptoms, Myra stated that they had really begun after their baby was born, with crying spells and repeated assertions that she "wasn't a good mother" and that taking care of the baby made her nervous. She said she felt inadequate and that even John was better with the baby than she. John attempted to reassure her by telling her she was an excellent mother and that he realized she was nervous about caring for the baby. He suggested that he get someone to help her. Myra said she did not want anyone because it was her baby, and she could not understand why she felt as she did. When questioned about her pregnancy and the birth of the child, she said there had been no complications and had added hesitantly that it had not been a planned pregnancy. When asked to explain further, she replied that she and John had decided to wait until they had been married about 3 years before starting a family. She went on to explain that she did not think she and John had had enough time to enjoy their life together before the baby was born.

After she recovered from the shock of knowing she was pregnant, she became thrilled at the thought of having a baby and enjoyed her pregnancy and shopping for the nursery. Toward the end of her pregnancy, she had difficulty sleeping and was troubled by nightmares. She began to feel uncertain of her ability to be a good mother and was frightened because she had not been around babies before.

When she and John brought the baby home, they engaged a nurse for 2 weeks to take care of the child and to teach Myra baby care. She thought that basically she knew how, but it upset her if the baby did not stop crying when she picked him up. When he was at home, John usually took care of the baby, and his competency made her feel more inadequate. The precipitating event was thought to have occurred the week before, when John had arrived home from work to find Myra walking the floor with the baby, who was crying loudly. Myra told him she had taken the baby to the pediatrician for an immunization shot that morning. After they returned home, he had become irritable, crying continuously and repeatedly refusing his bottle. When Myra said she did not know what to do, John told her the baby felt feverish. After they took the baby's temperature and discovered that it was 102° F, John called the pediatrician, who recommended a medication to reduce the temperature and discomfort. John got the medication and gave it to the baby; he also gave the baby his bottle. The baby went to sleep, but Myra went crying and upset to their bedroom.

Myra's mixed feelings toward the baby would be explored in addition to her feelings of inadequacy in caring for him. She apparently resented the responsibility of the parental role, which she was not ready to assume. Unable to express her hostility and feelings of rejection toward the baby, she turned them inward on herself, with the resulting overt symptoms of depression. Bringing these feelings into the open would be a necessary goal. Myra also needed reassurance that her feelings of inadequacy were normal because of her lack of contact and experience with infants and also because most new parents felt this same inadequacy in varying degrees. John obviously was comfortable and knowledgeable in the situation as a result of his experience with a younger brother and sisters; he would be used as a strong situational support.

The therapist, believing that a mild antidepressant should help to relieve Myra's symptoms, arranged a medical consultation. It was not thought that she was a threat to herself or to others, and intervention was instituted.

Myra's mention in the initial session that she and John had not had enough time to enjoy each other before the baby was born was considered to be an initial reference to Myra's negative feelings regarding her pregnancy and the baby. In subsequent sessions, through the therapist's use of direct questioning and the reflection of verbal and nonverbal clues, Myra was able to express some of her feelings about their life as a family with a baby in contrast to her feelings when she and John were alone.

Their previous life pattern revealed much social activity before the birth of the baby and almost none afterward. Myra said that although this had not really bothered her too much at first, recently she had felt as if the walls were closing in on her. John appeared surprised to hear this and asked why she had not mentioned it to him. Myra replied with some anger that it apparently did not seem to bother him because he obviously enjoyed playing with the baby after he came home from work. The possibility of reinstating some manner of social life for Myra and John was considered essential at this point. John told her that his mother would enjoy the chance to babysit with her new grandson and that he and Myra should plan some evenings out alone or with friends. Myra brightened considerably at this and seemed pleased at John's concern.

The therapist also explored their feelings about the responsibilities of parenthood and Myra's feelings of inadequacy in caring for the baby. Myra could communicate to John and the therapist her feelings that the baby received more of John's attention than she and that she resented "playing second fiddle." John explained that he had originally assumed care of the baby so that she could get some rest and that he enjoyed being with her more than with the baby. He told her that he loved her and that she would always come first with him.

Myra was eventually able to see that she was being childish in resenting the baby and that she was competing for John's attention; as her social life expanded, her negative feelings toward the baby lessened, and she said she was feeling more comfortable in caring for him. After the fourth session, the medication was discontinued, and Myra's symptoms continued to decrease.

Because of John's maturity, it was thought important that he should be aware of the possibility that Myra could occasionally have a recurrence of feelings of rejection. If the original symptoms returned, he would recognize them by the pattern they would take and would be able to intercede by exploring what was happening, discussing this openly with Myra. When the progress and adjustments they had made in learning to cope with the situation were reviewed with them, both expressed satisfaction with the changes that had occurred. They were told that they could return for further help if another crisis situation developed.

Myra was an only child who had rarely had to accept responsibility for others before her marriage. Because she had planned to wait 3 years before having a child, she had strong, mixed feelings about the responsibilities of motherhood before that time and felt unprepared. Her husband's adequacy in caring for the baby when she failed reinforced her mixed feelings. Loss of the social life shared with her husband, combined with the diversion of his attention from her to the baby, reinforced her strong feelings of rejection. Because she was unable to recognize and accept her feelings of ambivalence and was also unable to tell her husband of her anger and frustration, she turned them inward. Lack of previous experience in caring for infants made her unable to cope with the situation, increased her frustration and anger, and resulted in overt symptoms of depression and anxiety.

But I was one and twenty, No use to talk to me.

–Alfred Edward Housman

Complete the paradigm in Figure 9-3 for this case study, then compare it with the completed one in Appendix D. Refer to the paradigms in Chapter 3 as needed.

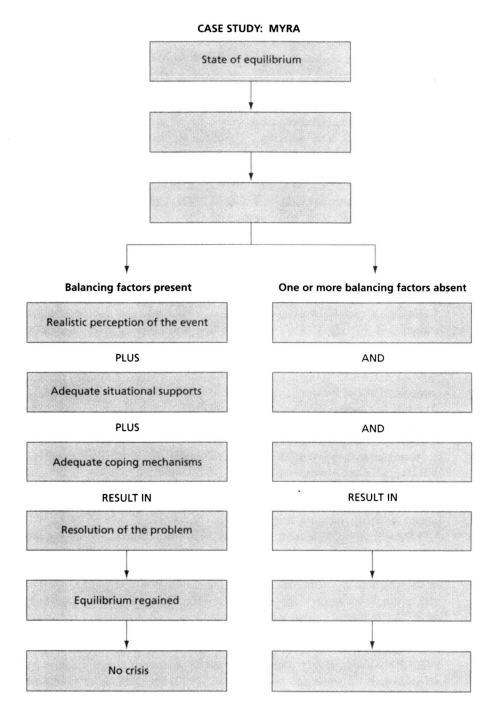

Figure 9-3

To the average person, reaching late adulthood implies that life patterns have been fairly well set and are no longer open to choices for change. Anxiety results if a man or woman has not demonstrated some capacity for success in either family or career roles. Symptoms of this are frequently noted in such forms as excessive use of alcohol, psychosomatic symptoms, feelings of persecution, and depression (English and Pearson, 1955).

Our culture seems unable to place any firm boundary lines on phases of the aging process. The general tendency is to view a life as uphill from infancy and over the hill and declining after reaching the peak of the middle years. With our cultural emphasis on youthfulness, it is not unusual for a person of 50 years to view his future with regret for things left unaccomplished. Hahn (1963) refers to this state as "heads against the ceiling," a time when "the realization strikes home that the probability for appreciable advancement is remote. . . . The ceiling is encountered relatively early by some and at an amazing late time by others, but for all of us the ladder eventually ends at a ceiling." He further describes this as a period when "younger men and women are beginning to crowd into the competitive economic, political and social arenas." With the rapid technological changes affecting business and professions, younger persons are often better prepared to supply the necessary knowledge and skills.

Family life changes as children grow up and become involved with school, careers, and marriage. For parents, it is a time when specific tasks of parenthood are over, and they must return to the family unit of two, making reciprocal changes in role status in relation to their children and to the community. New values and goals must be developed in the marriage to replace those values no longer realistic in the present; failure to recognize this need can open the way to frustration and despair. The wife and mother now has freedom from parental responsibility, but, if her entire lifestyle was centered around the parental role, she may lack interests, skills, and abilities with which to make the role change.

Menopause, or the cessation of the menstrual cycle, is often thought of as a dividing point between young adulthood and middle age. The actual termination of menstruation, however, occurs over a wide age range, usually between 45 and 55. Menopause marks the abrupt loss of fertility in women, while in men the climacteric occurs gradually and at a later age.

Menopause can represent a hazard for women because of its psychological repercussions. For some, the end of fertility may represent the end of sexuality and the loss of role identity. For women who have chosen not to have children the loss of fertility may represent the closing of the door to bearing children, perhaps giving rise to doubts about their choice. Women who have been raised to view menopause as the beginning of middle age and the end of youth may well experience it as a negative event and be thrown into a crisis (Pruett, 1980).

No definite evidence exists that sexual gland activity in the male undergoes similar rapid decline and cessation; however, men can experience symptoms similar to those of women at the same age period. Pruett (1980) considers these syndromes to be neuroses rather than a result of any changes in the sexual gland activity.

The unmarried person who has had thoughts of eventual marriage and family is now faced with the reality of advancing years. This is a particularly critical time for anyone who has relied strongly on physical attractiveness. He or she now faces the inevitability of physical decline. A person in this stage of life can continue to pursue career interests but may face limitations to further career advancements.

The following case study concerns a 40-year-old wife and mother whose planned changes in her family role after the marriage of her daughter seem to be threatened by the onset of early menopause.

Case Study   *Adulthood (Menopause)*

Mrs. C, a 40-year-old, youthful-appearing mother of three daughters (ages 17, 20, and 22 years) was referred to a crisis center by her physician because of severe anxiety and depression, as evidenced by recent anorexia, weight loss, insomnia, crying spells, and preoccupation, which had begun after a visit to her physician 3 weeks earlier. At that time, she had been told that she was entering early menopause. Her youngest daughter was to be married in a month; the two older ones were already married and living out of state.

She described herself to the therapist as having always been socially active both in community affairs and in her husband's business and social life. Mr. C was employed as a senior salesman for a nationwide firm selling women's clothing. His work required frequent trips out of town and much business entertaining while at home. She seldom traveled with him (because of the children) but was deeply involved with planning and hostessing his in-town social engagements. She said that she enjoyed this and had always been confident of her ability to do it well. Part of her wife role was to wear the clothes of her husband's company as an unofficial model, and her husband had always expressed his pride in her attractiveness.

In recent weeks, she had begun to feel inadequate in this role, and strong feelings of doubt regarding her ability had begun to plague her. At the same time, she sensed that her husband was becoming indifferent to her efforts to keep herself and their home attractive to him. Her symptoms had overtly increased in the 2 days just past, until now she feared a complete loss of emotional control.

Mr. C was 2 years older than Mrs. C. He was socially adept, and her women friends frequently told her they thought he was "such a youthful, good-looking, and considerate person." She herself felt fortunate to have him for a husband. He was aggressive in business and could be sure of advancement. She said they had always been sexually compatible and shared interests and mutual esteem.

When asked about what had occurred in the past 2 days to increase her symptoms, she said that her husband had come home 2 nights ago and found her disheveled and crying and not ready to go to a scheduled business dinner for the second time in a week. He angrily told her that he did not know what to do and to "pull yourself together and find someone to help you because I've tried and I can't!" Then he left for the dinner alone. The next day he left town on a business trip after securing her promise to see a physician.

Mrs. C said that she had seen several physicians during the past few months because of various physical complaints. None had found any organic cause, but all had advised her to get more rest, and one even told her to find a hobby. The last physician, whom she saw 3 weeks ago, told her she was entering early menopause.

Mrs. C had not told her husband of this because she feared his reaction in view of her own negative feelings; her initial reaction had been disbelief. This was followed by fear of "change of life," as she had heard of so many unfortunate things that could happen to a woman during this time. In common with other women, she did not want to become old and unattractive and was angry that it could be happening to her so soon. She thought that she would no longer be an asset to her husband in his work because his clothes were not designed for middle-age women.

Mrs. C had looked forward to traveling with her husband after their youngest daughter's marriage. They had planned such a future together enthusiastically, and she felt proud to have contributed to his success but was now afraid that he would not need her anymore and that all her plans were ruined.

Her expressed feelings of guilt and a fear of the loss of her feminine role were thought to be the crisis-precipitating events. She was not seen as a suicidal risk or as a threat to others, although she was depressed and expressed feelings of worthlessness. She was highly anxious but could maintain control over her actions.

Mrs. C had withdrawn from her previous pattern of social and family activities. Her husband was frequently out of town, and the last of the daughters living at home had transferred many of her dependency needs to her fiance. Mrs. C in the past 3 months had felt physically ill and had narrowed her social activities to infrequent luncheons "when I felt up to it." Her peer group was in the 35- to 40-year age level and were all actively involved in community affairs, family activities, and so on. Conversation with women friends still centered around problems of raising children, and she believed that because her children were grown she no longer had much to offer to the conversation.

Her goals for a role change from busy parenthood to active participation with her husband in his business-social world were threatened, and she had no coping experiences in this particular situation. Previous methods of coping with stress were discussed. She related that she had always kept busy with their children and either forgot the problems or talked them out with close friends or her husband. She could not recall a close woman friend who had reached the menopausal stage and with whom she could discuss her feelings, and she was too fearful of the reaction she imagined her husband would have to discuss it with him. Her inability to communicate her feelings and the loss of busy work with her children eliminated any situational supports in her home environment, obviating the use of previously successful coping mechanisms. The goal of intervention established by the therapist was to assist Mrs. C to an intellectual understanding of her crisis.

Obvious to the therapist was that Mrs. C had little knowledge of the physiological and psychological changes that occur in menopause. She had no insight into her feelings of guilt and fear of the threatening loss of her feminine role. Unrecognized feelings about her relationship with her husband would be explored. During the next 5 weeks, through the use of direct questioning and reflection of verbal and nonverbal clues with Mrs. C, it became possible for her to relate the present crisis and its effect to past separations from her husband (business trips) and her previous successful coping mechanisms.

Mrs. C had married when she was 17 years old. She described herself as having been attractive and popular in school, busy at all sorts of school activities. Mr. C had been what everyone considered quite a catch. He came from a prosperous family, had been a high school football captain and class president, and was sought after by many of her girlfriends. At the time of their marriage he was a freshman in college.

She always had a high regard for her physical attractiveness and her ability to fulfill the social role Mr. C expected of her. Throughout the years when he traveled alone, she felt left out of a part of his life and had looked forward with great expectations to being able to be with him all of the time. Knowing that his business brought him in frequent contact with attractive women buyers and models, she regarded her own physical attractiveness as a prime requirement to "meet the competition." With Mr. C's frequent trips away from home, she had magnified her role in the husband-wife relationship to be more on the physical-social level than in the shared role of parental responsibilities.

Mrs. C never questioned her physician after he informed her of his diagnosis of early onset of menopause, and obviously her knowledge was inadequate and based almost entirely on hearsay and myth rather than on fact. The physiological basis of the process of aging was discussed, and much of her fear was allayed. This was an important phase of anticipatory planning.

She was given situational support in which to talk out her feelings of insecurity in her marriage and to view it in much more realistic terms. Relationships between the precipitating events and the crisis symptoms were explored.

By the third week, Mrs. C had made significant progress toward reestablishing her coping skills. She no longer feared "getting old overnight" and was able to tell her husband that she was entering early menopause. His response was, "What the hell! Is that why you have been acting so peculiar lately? You might have told me; the way you've been carrying on anyone would have thought you had just been told you had 6 months to live!" Although her first impulse was to interpret this as evidence of his indifference to her as a woman, she later saw it as positive proof of her own unrealistic fears. She returned to her medical doctor as advised for continuing care and planning for physical problems that might arise in the future.

By the fifth week, she expressed confidence in her ability to meet the goals that she and her husband had set for their future. Their daughter was married, and Mrs. C was ready to leave town with her husband on a business trip. Before termination, the adjustments she had made in coping with the crisis were reviewed and discussed with her.

Mrs. C had been unable to cope with the combined stresses of early menopausal symptoms and the need to change her family role. She avoided communicating her fears to anyone who might have given her situational support for fear they would confirm her own negative reactions. Increasing feelings of inadequacy, resulting in anxiety and depression, led to a crisis level of disequilibrium.

Initial intervention focused on the exploration of Mrs. C's knowledge of the physical and psychological changes that could occur in menopause. As she was

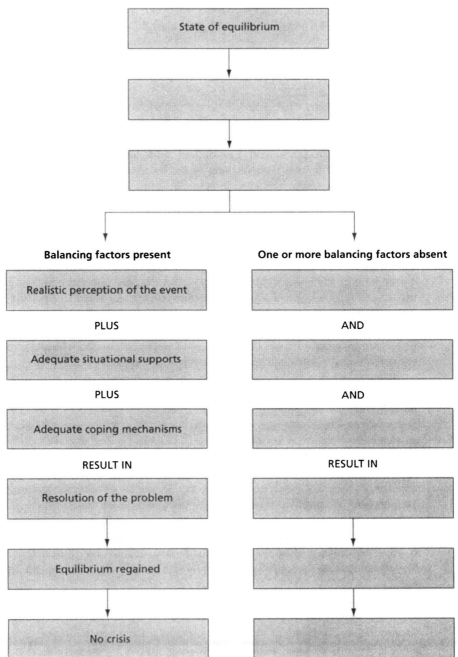

Figure 9-4

encouraged to explore and ventilate her feelings about her relationship with her husband, her perception of the stressful situation became more realistic and her coping skills were reintroduced successfully.

A fool at forty is a fool indeed.

–Edward Young

Complete the paradigm in Figure 9-4 for this case study, then compare it with the completed one in Appendix D. Refer to the paradigms in Chapter 3 as needed.

Old Age

Despite the fact that no clear line of demarcation exists between any of the phases of adulthood in our society, the later phase of adulthood has been identified chronologically as beginning at age 65. Decisions relating to autonomous functions and activities; occupational changes; choice of marital partners; and concerns about health, housing, and leisure activities take place throughout the whole of adulthood, and many of the associated stressors have the same magnitude, frequency, and impact on an individual's lifestyle regardless of chronological age. Decrements in the functioning of human organs or organ systems or in the psychosocial capacities of people can and do occur at any age, since as yet no empirically predictable limits related specifically to time of occurrence have been defined. What can be documented, however, is that certain major events, such as enforced retirement and loss of friends and intimate loved ones, become more likely with increasing age, and that these negative life events are perceived as more stressful than events classified as pleasant or positive. Coping with the confluence of physical, emotional, and social factors, which might otherwise sufficiently exacerbate each other to produce functional impairment, requires the ability to reintegrate one's goals, self-image, and life role. This ability to make such adjustments varies on an individual basis.

Seventy-five percent of the American population now lives to age 65, and 95% of those 65 years and older reside in a noninstitutional setting. The proportion of older persons has consistently increased more rapidly than that of younger persons; the 4% of those 65 years and older in 1900 had increased to over 10% by 1975, and projections show a continuation of this differential to at least 12% of the population by the year 2000. A review of the gerontological literature suggests that persons living beyond age 65 generally pass through three life stages: (1) Between ages 65 and 75, most people continue with normal activities unless they have a specific illness, (2) most people also can carry out normal activities through age 85, although many begin to show the effects of age even without an overt disease/illness condition, and (3) after reaching the age of 85, however, only a relative few people are seen as having the ability to carry on normal activities without some major assistance, including institutionalization. Aside from the variable illness or disability factor, differences between and within these stage-of-life cohort groups are often perceived as being related to such other influences as previous lifestyle, adaptation to loss of the work role, adjustment to minor ailments and stresses, openness to both feelings and ideas, and maintenance of social activities and contacts.

The illnesses and disabilities of older persons are predominantly age- or time-related, and tend to be chronic rather than acute. For the most part, chronic diseases limit mobility and comfort and are the most frequent causes of institutionalization. In general, despite the problems and hazards associated with aging, the large majority of older persons remain well enough for many years to participate in a variety of activities, are reasonably secure financially, and maintain social ties with family and friends.

Nevertheless, and regardless of their life stage, older persons with multiple losses (e.g., work role, mobility, health, vision, spouse, mental acuity, and home) are at greater risk for requiring some form of institutional support than are those with single or few losses. Probably the most compelling reason for institutionalization is that these persons either outlive or overwhelm their support systems. What is not known, however, is what those at risk of institutionalization actually do to remain in the community. The functional status of older persons living in the community can be quite high, despite the number and severity of their chronic disabilities. This high level of functioning is based on the mechanisms the person has developed in the past to cope with stressors and is now using to deal with the stressors accompanying chronic illnesses and other losses of aging.

The author's article on stressors in old age lists some of the needs of older persons who continue to function in the community, for example, adequate income, suitable housing, proper and adequate nutrition, and access to transportation. These persons must also carry out certain responsibilities, such as establishing and continuing in a range of physical and social activities, remaining flexible and adaptable in the face of societal and community changes, seeking and accepting healthcare and other helping services to ensure self-maintenance. Access to and use of social support factors thus appear to be important determinants of whether older people are relatively happy and self-sustaining. Certainly a strong need for companionship exists, and most older people are interested in sex, have sexual feelings, and need sexual outlets (Aguilera, 1980).

As is the case with people of any age, the healthcare needs of older persons range from periodic evaluations to maintain wellness status, through the complexity of services needed for acute care, to the supportive care needed for longer term chronic health problems. Because persons may carry into their older years the health problems of youth and early maturity, as well as being subject to health stresses related to the aging process, the number of health problems afflicting any one person may vary greatly. Although much can be done to alleviate or control some of the effects of the aging process, the increased likelihood of multiple health problems, combined with the slower recovery time associated with aging, often leads to more frequent and prolonged hospitalizations. For older persons who continue to need at least some medical surveillance and skilled posthospitalization nursing care, a number of new problems arise. While theoretical alternatives to institutionalization are available for many of the elderly, some form of congregate living and continued healthcare may become a practical necessity. Where family resources are inadequate, or where no suitable family substitute is available, the person's need for continued care may require placement in a skilled nursing facility.

The predictors of morale, life satisfaction, satisfaction with treatment, and survival were the patient's subjective perceptions of the facility and their preference and options for living in the facility itself or elsewhere. Loss of control among the institutionalized aged was at least partially responsible for depression, physical decline, and early death. This suggests a need for increased attention to the patients' cognitive and emotional status at application and entry periods, as well as throughout their institutional stay.

Probably the most common problem in later adulthood is depression. Concomitant with depression may be feelings of fatigue, lack of energy, low self-esteem, and insomnia. Depression following bereavement is common. Loss of a spouse is usually perceived as the single greatest loss that a person can experience throughout the life cycle.

The dependency related to being ill, or to being ill and institutionalized, often gives rise to fear of dependence and may be expressed in irritability, an unwillingness to cooperate in treatment, and a general dissatisfaction with life. When an illness brings into focus the probability of diminished life expectancy or impending death, indirect or even direct self-destructive behavior may occur. This may take many forms: active or passive, lethal or relatively innocuous, easily identified or obscure. Behavioral examples include alcoholism and drug abuse, hyperobesity, disregard for one's health or safety, and withdrawal from the social environment. Behaviors that appear to staff as uncooperative or belligerent and destructive to the patient's health may also serve a dual psychological purpose: that of being able to express anger and frustration at circumstances related to medical condition and institutionalization and of reestablishing some feelings of control and self-esteem.

A continuation of maturational stages of development would be more difficult to define for the aged than for younger groups because the processes of decline and growth occur concomitantly but not in equal balance. The process is highly individualized in all cases, and the variability of physiological, psychological, and sociological factors makes definite chronological relationships highly improbable.

When an elderly person seeks help, his symptomatology requires particularly close scrutiny before an interpretation for intervention is undertaken. The therapist must first be aware of his own tendencies to stereotype the client's appearance and symptoms as a normal aging syndrome. Determining which of the crisis symptoms may be the result of organicity is particularly important because rapid onset of behavioral changes is not infrequently caused by cerebrovascular or other organic changes associated with longevity. A professional review of the current medical history of the person must be part of the initial assessment phase.

Too often the person, because of organic changes, cannot gain an intellectual understanding of the crisis or recognize his present feelings; or those who directed him to the therapist may themselves be in crisis. If this is true, the therapist first may have to resolve the feelings of the referrer that have been projected toward the elderly person who seems to be in need of help.

In the aging process, the ego organization needs to withstand increasing biopsychosocial threats to its integrity; unfortunately, the person's coping abilities may fail to adapt to meet the threats. The ability to accept new value systems and adapt to necessary changes in the achieved maturational development of earlier years without loss of achieved integrity may indeed be a developmental task for the elderly.

The following case study concerns a couple who could be considered members of the older age group.

Case Study   *Old Age*

Sarah was accompanied to the crisis center by her husband, John, a former client who had come there for help when in crisis following the death of their only son about 10 years ago. Sarah was 69 years of age, 3 years older than John. She was neatly dressed, appeared to be slightly apprehensive, and walked with obvious difficulty, supported by a Canadian crutch and her husband's arm. After being assisted into a chair in the therapist's office, she quickly asked that John be allowed to remain with her during the session. She stated that it "had really been John's idea that we both come here today. I'm sure that he can explain the problem better than I." After a slight pause and several hesitations John began to speak. Sarah sat tensely forward on her chair, never taking her eyes from his face as he spoke.

According to John, their problem "probably first began" about 3 months ago, when Sarah had fallen in the house and fractured her hip. After a month in the hospital, she had been sent home in his care. The plan was for her to continue physiotherapy as an outpatient. Despite all of the therapy and exercises at home, she was apparently not making the progress they had expected. "Look at her, she still can't walk alone! She still needs someone to help her about or she might fall again, and God knows what would happen to us then! It's been a worry for both of us."

As John continued to speak, it became quite obvious that he was avoiding any direct references to himself. He described Sarah as having recent symptoms of insomnia, anxiety, and depression and expressed the fear that she might be going into the same crisis symptoms that he had been treated for at the center 10 years ago. "It was sheer hell to feel the way I did then. She doesn't deserve to go through what I did then if she can be helped now."

As he spoke, he was becoming obviously more agitated. He avoided eye contact with Sarah, kept moving about restlessly in his chair, and was becoming increasingly tense and tremulous. His eyes frequently became tearful, and his voice broke on several occasions. In almost direct contrast to his behavior, Sarah had assumed a very supportive role, reaching out several times to pat his arm in a calming gesture and, finally, holding his hand tightly.

At the point when it seemed he might begin to cry openly, he abruptly stood up and said, "OK. Sarah, I've told her all about the problem. Now I'm going to go take a walk for a while and let you do some of the talking, too." With that, he said he would be back in about 20 minutes and left the office.

As soon as John had left, Sarah began to cry quietly. Then she gave several deep sighs and, for the first time, relaxed back into her chair. "Please," she asked the therapist, "can you help him again like you did the last time?" She stated that for the past week he had not slept more than an hour at a time during the night, paced constantly, cried easily and often for no apparent reason, and had reached the point where he now seemed too anxious and too preoccupied to make even the simplest of decisions.

According to Sarah, she and John had been married for 42 years. They had had only one son, who had died, unmarried, 10 years ago. Although Sarah had never held a salaried job, she had always been very actively involved in both civic and church organizations in their community. After John's retirement from federal service, she had withdrawn from several of these organizations in order to devote more time to activities that they could participate in together. They had developed many new social interests and maintained a fairly active social life. Sarah felt that the past 10 years had included some of the best times in their life together. They had always seemed to be planning something "for the future" and had acquired many new friends. Their home was completely paid for; they had planned wisely for financial security "in their old age," and, until her accident, they had had few health problems to worry about.

Even after her hip fracture, they had apparently been able to provide each other with the situational support needed to cope adequately with the many new changes arising in their daily lives. "After all," Sarah said, "it wasn't as though our world was going to come to an end because of this—only that it might have to slow down a bit until we could catch up again."

After a month in the hospital, Sarah went home and arranged to continue therapy as an outpatient. Despite regular visits to physiotherapy and John's rigidly imposed schedule of exercising at home, her recovery had been much slower than they had anticipated. Last week her physician, also not satisfied with the rate of her progress, recommended that she seriously consider admission as a full-time inpatient to a well-known rehabilitation center in a nearby city. He was unable to guarantee how long she might have to remain, estimating only that it would be a minimum of 1 month.

She stated that at the time John seemed to be as much in agreement as she with the idea, although, she recollected, he had seemed a bit preoccupied on the drive home. He took her out to dinner that night to celebrate her improved chances for a full recovery. That same night she was awakened several times by John getting out of bed and pacing about the house. When she mentioned it to him in the morning, he quickly apologized for disturbing her and blamed it on "too much coffee and food" the night before. She noticed, however, that he seemed very preoccupied that day, even to the point of having to be reminded when it was time for her exercises. Several times he asked if she felt confident that they were making the right decision, or if they should try to find another physician for her who might suggest "better treatments."

His tension and anxiety continued to increase over the next few days. He seemed unusually concerned with how she felt about the decision, and no amount of reassurance from her could convince him that she really wanted to go into the hospital for treatment. Several times yesterday, she found him looking at her sadly with tears running down his face. His only explanation was that he felt "so sorry for you, having to go to a strange place, and I might not be there when you need me!" Last night he had not gone to bed at all but had sat in the living room. She had not dared go to sleep for fear he would go outside and wander around.

Several times during the past few days, she had suggested he contact the crisis center to speak to his former therapist. At first, he ignored her, then finally yesterday he had countered with the proposal that they go together. "I'm sure," he told her, "that you must be feeling just as anxious as I am about all of this." She said that she agreed to this because she could think of no other way to convince him to come alone. "Of course, I'm upset about having to go back to a hospital," she told the therapist. "Anyone in my condition would like to have some sort of guarantee that they are going to improve, but my greatest concern is what this all has done to John." After discussing her feelings a bit longer with her, the therapist determined that Sarah appeared to be coping adequately with the recent events in her life and, although anxious and concerned about them, was indeed not in crisis.

Finding that John had returned from his walk, the therapist arranged to have Sarah wait outside and called him back into the office. He still appeared very tense, yet when confronted with his evident symptoms of depression and anxiety, he at first denied their severity. Then, after several evasive responses, he began to openly describe just how frightened and overwhelmed he had been feeling for the past week. "I just don't know what's going to happen to us next. I don't think I'll be able to handle much more. I was so sure she'd be back walking by this time. We did everything that the doctors told us to do—I worked so hard with her to keep up with the exercises and all of the appointments—and they haven't helped. Now she has to go back to the hospital. I feel that some of this is all my fault. Maybe I didn't work hard enough with her, or maybe I was doing the exercises the wrong way. She hates being crippled like this. Sometimes I think she must hate me because she has to be so dependent on me for doing everything."

After Sarah had come home from the hospital 2 months ago, John had been kept very busy and involved in driving her to appointments, arranging the household schedules, and helping her exercise at home. He found many rewards in this role, feeling that he was contributing greatly toward her eventual recovery. However, as the weeks and months passed without much apparent improvement in her condition, he was disturbed to find himself angry toward her, even at times blaming her for not trying harder. Lately, he had been finding it increasingly difficult to hide these feelings from her and found himself wishing that he could just get away from the situation for a while, to take a trip like they used to, even if it meant going off without her! Now, because of her decision to go into the rehabilitation center for treatment, he was being given the opportunity to "get away from it all" for a while, to turn the responsibility for her daily exercises and care completely over to others, and he felt very guilty. Perhaps he had not really tried hard enough to help her walk; maybe he should have found ways to encourage her more. The more he ruminated on these thoughts, the more he convinced himself that her lack of progress was entirely his fault. Therefore, it was his fault that she had to go back to a hospital, and it would be completely his fault if she were never able to return home again!

The goals of intervention were to help John obtain a realistic perception of the situation, to assist him to ventilate his feelings about the effects of Sarah's disability on his life, and to provide him with situational support to help him cope with the pending loss of Sarah, albeit temporary at this point. Before the next session and with his consent, his personal physician was contacted to determine if there were any organic bases for his behavioral changes. The physician's report was negative.

During the next two sessions, through questioning and reflection, John was helped to ventilate his feelings about his fears that Sarah might never recover beyond her present level of functioning. With situational support supplied by the therapist, he was able to begin to discuss openly the anger that he had felt toward Sarah for "threatening the security of their future" with her accident. All of the careful planning they had done for their "old age" seemed to be falling apart more each day. "It wasn't just the financial security," he said, "we have enough insurance to take care of our illnesses. Our plans were all made for the *two* of us, *together*—not for just one of us, *alone!*" His fears of losing her had been displaced into anger against her for being the cause of his very unpleasant feelings.

It became quite apparent during the first session that John really did not have any clear idea as to the nature of Sarah's injury. To him, a broken bone was just that, regardless of which one. It broke, therefore it should heal! He had never sat down with her orthopedic surgeon to ask questions, leaving it to her to keep him informed. He was advised to make an immediate appointment with this physician to get direct information about Sarah's expected progress rather than to continue to rely on his own uneducated conclusions.

By the next session, he reported that he had followed through, kept the appointment, and was relieved to learn that, although Sarah's progress was a bit slower than expected, the physician expected her to return to a fairly normal level of functioning. He was advised that it would take time, however, and he would be expected to help Sarah have patience. The recommendation that she enter the rehabilitation center in the next city was made in an effort to speed up her progress and was not to be construed by him as a sign that she might never recover. As John's anxiety and depression decreased, he began to view the events leading up to his crisis in a more realistic manner. He realized that his anger was a normal response to his situation with Sarah but that what he *did* with that anger was not normal. Rather than openly discussing his feelings with Sarah as he would have at any other time in their lives, he found himself "protecting" her from them, yet blaming her for all of his misery. Because he lacked any other available situational support, his anxiety and depression had increased, even further distorting his perceptions of the event.

When the suggestion was made that Sarah enter a rehabilitation center for further therapy, John's anxiety level interfered with his ability to perceive this as anything other than the beginning of a final loss of Sarah from his life. As he later described it to the therapist, "I guess this is always in the back of a person's mind once they get around my age. When you're young, you go to a hospital and the odds are good that you come home again, but when you get to be Sarah's and my age, the odds aren't so good that you come home again! And she was asking me to help her make the decision to go to that hospital—me, who was already mixed up in my feelings about having to take care of her like this the rest of my life!"

By the end of the third session, John's symptoms had lessened greatly, and he was now able to help Sarah pack and move into the rehabilitation center without any increase in anxiety. He realized now that, in overprotecting her from his true feelings, he had only created anxiety for her as well as a crisis for himself. He planned to visit her three times a week. They agreed that this would give her full time to concentrate on "being able to walk at home," and he would begin to reestablish contact with their old friends so that he would not feel so lonely while she was away.

Exploration with John about his feelings concerning the possibility that Sarah might not improve beyond her current level of functioning helped prepare him for this eventuality. He was able to begin to consider alternative modes of life for the two of them. For example, he decided that they should seriously consider selling their two-story home. "After all," he said, "if it isn't her broken hip, sure enough it's going to be my arthritis in the next few years that is going to make those stairs seem like Mount Whitney!" Furthermore, John found himself faced with the realities of what he would have to be able to do for himself if Sarah ever left him forever. While she was in the rehabilitation center, he knew that he would have to begin learning how to plan a life for himself. Although she might outlive him, he recognized that this time without her was a sample for him of what life "might be for him—and only a complete idiot would not recognize that I had better learn what to do and learn pretty damned fast!"

Unprepared to assume his new role in caring for Sarah, John's increased anxiety distorted his perceptions of their stressful situation. When Sarah failed to make the progress that he had expected, he became frustrated and angry and saw himself as a failure in his new role. Unable to communicate these feelings appropriately, he displaced his anger on Sarah. When asked to help her decide about reentering a hospital, he felt threatened by a permanent role reversal and the eventuality of her loss. He lacked adequate coping mechanisms to deal with the increasing stresses of the situation; he became immobile and unable to make any decisions for their future.

Intervention focused on helping John ventilate his feelings and obtain a realistic perception of the event. As his anxiety and depression decreased, he became able to anticipate and plan for their future. The major focus of the last session was to help him recognize and accept that with increasing age future threats to his biopsychosocial integrity could occur and that he should learn to seek help as problems arose and not try to assume all of the responsibility himself.

Two months later, the therapist received a telephone call from John. Sarah had come home from the rehabilitation center about 2 weeks before. Her progress, unfortunately, was not what they had expected. However, according to John, she was at least able to stand in the kitchen and make the "best damned dinner I have eaten in a month" and that was "good enough for me!" They had already put their home up for sale and were looking for a large mobile home into which they could move and then travel around the country to begin living the retirement they had planned.

Pew de gens savent etre vieux.
Few people know how to be old.

–Duc de La Rochefoucauld

Complete the paradigm in Figure 9-5 for this case study, then compare it with the completed one in Appendix D. Refer to the paradigms in Chapter 3 as needed.

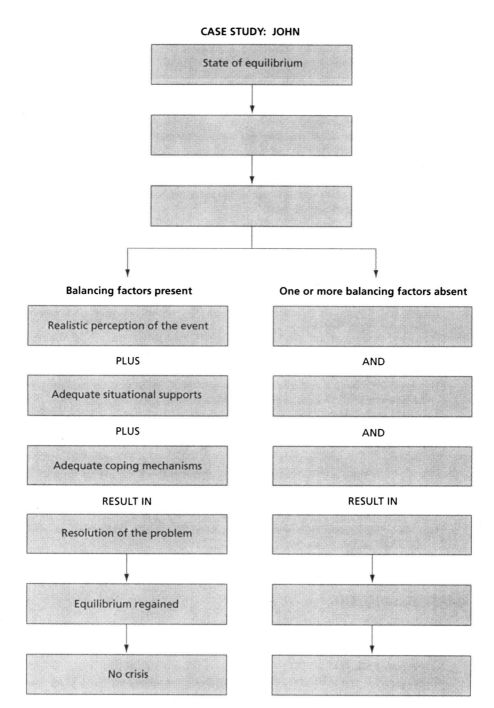

CASE STUDY: JOHN

State of equilibrium

Balancing factors present

Realistic perception of the event

PLUS

Adequate situational supports

PLUS

Adequate coping mechanisms

RESULT IN

Resolution of the problem

Equilibrium regained

No crisis

One or more balancing factors absent

AND

AND

RESULT IN

Figure 9-5

REFERENCES

Adler ES, Clark R: Adolescence: a literary passage, *Adolescence* 26:757, 1991.

Aguilera DC: Stressors in late adulthood. In Aguilera DC, editor: Coping with life stressors: a life cycle approach, *Fam Community Health* 2(4):61, 1980.

Anderson CR and others: Managerial response to environmentally induced stress, *Academy Management J* 20(2):260, 1977.

Baack D: The personal impact of company policies: a social penetration theory perspective, *J Managerial Issues* 3:196, 1991.

Cameron N: *Personality development and psychopathology,* Boston, 1963, Houghton Mifflin.

Cassell RN: The child "at risk" for drug abuse rating schedule (DARS), *Psychol A J Human Behav* 28:52, 1991.

Cobb S: Social support as a moderator of life stress, *Psychosom Med* 38(5):300, 1976.

Dohrenwend BS, Dohrenwend BP, editors: Stressful life events: their nature and effects, New York, 1974, John Wiley & Sons.

English O, Pearson: *Emotional problems of living,* New York, 1955, WW Norton.

Erikson EH: Growth and crises of the health personality. In Senn MJE, editor: *Symposium on the healthy personality,* New York, 1950, Josiah Macy Jr Foundation.

Erikson EH: Identity and the life cycle. In: *Psychological Issues,* vol 1, No. 1, mono 1, New York, 1959, International Universities Press.

Erikson EH: *Childhood and society,* ed 2, 1963, WW Norton.

Erikson EH: Maturational crisis. In Stantrock JW, editor: *Life span development,* ed 4, Dubuque, 1992, WC Brown.

Hahn ME: *Psychoevaluation: adaption, distribution, adjustment,* New York, 1963, McGraw-Hill.

Holmes TE, Rahe RH: Social readjustment rating scale, *J Psychosom Res,* vol 11, 1967.

Homonoff EE, Meltz P: Developing and maintaining a coordinated system of community based services to children, *Community Ment Health J* 27(5):347, 1991.

Lau S: Crisis and vulnerability in adolescent development: erratum, *J Youth Adoles* 20:561, 1991.

Peterson C and others: The attributional style questionnaire, *Cognitive Therapy Res* 6:287, 1972.

Piaget J: *The child's conception of the world,* Totowa, NJ, 1963, Littlefield, Adams.

Piaget J: The life cycle. In Carter B, McGoldrick M, editors: *The changing family life cycle,* ed 2, Boston, 1989, Allyn & Bacon.

Pruett H: Stressors in middle adulthood, *Fam Community Health* 2(47):53, 1980.

Rose-Gold MS: Intervention strategies for counseling at-risk adolescents in rural school districts, *Sch Counselor* 39:122, 1991.

Starr, Goldstein: Human development and behavior, *Psychol Nurs,* 1975.

Zachry CB: *Emotion and conduct in adolescence,* New York, 1940, Appleton-Century-Crofts.

ADDITIONAL READING

Barabander CS: Alcohol and drugs in the workplace. In Ashenberg Straussner SL, editor: *Clinical work with substance-abusing clients,* New York, 1993, Guilford.

Cowger CD: Assessing client strengths: clinical assessment for client empowerment, *Soc Work* 39:262, 1994.

Goldmeier J: Intervention with elderly substance abusers in the workplace, *J Contemp Human Ser* p 624, 1994.

Lewis JA and others: *Substance abuse counseling, an individualized approach,* ed 2, Belmont, Calif, 1994, Brooks/Cole.

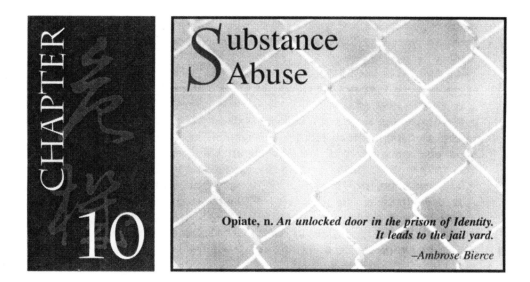

CHAPTER 10

Substance Abuse

*Opiate, n. An unlocked door in the prison of Identity.
It leads to the jail yard.*

–Ambrose Bierce

L ife is a never ending process in change. People change, fashions change—skirts are long and flowing one year, and the next year women and young girls are wearing microminiskirts. Men also change with "fashion," from wide lapels to small lapels, from cuffs on their trousers to no cuffs on their trousers. However, changes in fashions that we *wear* cause no harm. But they do make money for the fashion designers and retail stores.

A trend has occurred that is a *danger* to the youth and to those in the "Generation X." *Designer drugs* are now "in." Who has heard of "roofies" or "Scoop?" Of course, common to many are "pot," "crack," "sniffing," "uppers," and "downers," "H," and "smack." How much is known about these street drugs? Who takes them and why—*where* do they get them? What effect do some of them have? Is the effect a temporary or a *permanent* state? Can they cause the *death* of the person who takes them—or is given them?

California Attorney General Dan Lungren reported on the increased use of drugs by American teenagers less than a week after Senator Bob Dole released a similar finding in the Federal Report (1996). Much like the national statistics released, a disturbing trend of growing drug use is seen among *students.*

In the late 1980s, drug use among students decreased. In the early 90s, it mostly leveled off, with some warning signs of small increases. Over the past 4 years, a dramatic increase in drug use has occurred, back to levels that rival peaks of 10 years ago.

The federal study found drug use among 12 to 17 year olds escalated from 5.3% in 1992 to 10.9% in 1995. The state departments of alcohol and drug programs, education, and health services surveyed nearly 6000 students in schools scattered throughout California from November 1995 to March 1996. Among the findings:

- **Alcohol** use in the last 6 months: 67.2% of 9th graders, *down* from 68.6% reported in a 1993 to 1994 survey; 75.3% of 11th graders, *up* from 74.3% in 1993 to 1994.
- **Marijuana** use in the last 6 months: 34.2% of 9th graders, *up* from 30.4% in 1993 to 1994; 42.8% of 11th graders, *up* from 40% in 1993 to 1994.
- **Amphetamine** use in the last 6 months: 10.8% of 9th graders, *up* from 7.5% in 1993 to 1994; 10.4% of 11th graders, *up* from 10.1% in 1993 to 1994.
- **LSD** use in the last 6 months: 9.9% of 9th graders, *up* from 8.6% in 1993 to 1994; 10.8% of 11th graders, *down* from 12.2%, in the 1993 to 1994 survey.
- **Heroin** use in the last 6 months: 2.9% of 9th graders, *up* from 1993 to 1994; 2.2% of 11th graders, *up* from 1.4% in 1993 to 1994.
- **Cocaine** use in the last 6 months: 6.4% of 9th graders, *up* from 6.1% in 1993 to 1994; 7.2% of 11th graders, *up* from 4.9% in 1993 to 1994.

Marijuana

The danger has begun. Younger and younger students are drinking and getting "high," smoking cigarettes and pot to keep them high most of the time. Some students see their parents, older siblings, and peers drinking and smoking pot and apparently having a "good time." This is how it begins. It seldom stops without a great deal of help and strong self-discipline and self-motivation, or by accidental overdose and death.

Young pot smokers light up for laughs and the rush of a good high, not because of urban despair or lack of other pursuits (Ferrell, 1996). They tend to be articulate, self-assured, and free of any great worries about the future. For many of these teenagers, marijuana is nothing worse than a bit of spice—a secret ingredient in a lifestyle meant to be fun, daring, a bit on the edge.

Some are second-generation pot smokers, the children of baby boomers who first "blazed" in the 1960s. Others are influenced by friends, music, movies, and the shifting tide of popular opinion. They claim few misgivings over the double lives they lead, stashing "bud" in their closets and sock drawers, arranging deals over their own telephones, and slipping away to get high in garages, backyards, or in their own homes when their parents have stepped out for the night.

One 17-year-old senior, at a campus ranked among the top high schools in the nation said, "You've got every type doing it . . . the jocks, the brainiacs, the preppies, the surfers, the hippies . . . I know people who blow you away with their intelligence, and they're snapping bongheads every night." (Ferrell, 1996).

Some people manage to work marijuana into their lives without losing control. They pass their classes, hold down important jobs. This is part of what makes marijuana such an enigma—a reason why even many adults have trouble deciding how they feel about it.

Pot occupies a gray area in American thought. Scientific research has found evidence that pot is addictive and that it damages the lungs. But its status as a health threat is murky and subject to widely differing opinions, even among scientists. Tobacco and alcohol present some of the same problems, and these substances are legal. A significant number of marijuana users go on to harder drugs, but a large share do not. In January 1997, The American Medical Association announced their support for the use of marijuana for medical uses (Shuster, 1997). At the same time the federal government, represented by drug czar Barry McCaffrey, indicated its disagreement with the AMA's stance, saying that the change of a schedule status for marijuana was "premature" (p. A20).

Not only are more teenagers using pot, but they are also starting at a younger age. Ten years ago pot smokers seemed to begin at 17 or 18. Today they seem to start at 13 or 14. And 10 years ago the problem was limited to pot, alcohol, and some cocaine, or LSD. But nowadays kids get into everything. They are not as selective as they used to be and more are *risk-takers* (Ferrell, 1996).

While science is making progress toward understanding marijuana, science is also making marijuana more potent. Hybridizing and special growing techniques have enabled dealers such as *Hemp BC,* a cannabis *store* based in Vancouver, British Columbia, to offer 70 or more varieties of marijuana seeds. Customers can purchase them by catalog or over the Internet and grow pot that is far more potent than the marijuana of the 1960s.

Heroin

Federal drug czar Barry R. McCaffrey (Greenberg, 1996) has warned that heroin use is rising at an alarming rate nationwide and that dealers have found new and increasingly more successful ways to market the drug.

The average street price for heroin is so low and the quality is so high that new users can smoke or inhale it instead of injecting it, reported McCaffrey in releasing the latest *Pulse Check,* a quarterly report on drug use compiled by the White House Office of National Drug Control Policy.

The report also found that the increased availability and greater purity is aiding heroin's spread to blue-collar and suburban American. About three fourths of heroin users inject the drug rather than inhale it, and this may show that inhalation is a transition phase that switches to injection after a few years.

Some people who snorted cocaine during the mid-1980s are now using heroin. Heroin is the kind of drug that always appears after a stimulant epidemic like that we had with cocaine. Trends in illicit drug use in the United States are cyclical, with drugs going in and out of fashion. After the cocaine-related deaths of a number of athletes, actors, and musicians in the 1980s, cocaine use began to decline, and heroin replaced it as the drug of choice.

McCaffrey's survey also underscored the threat of methamphetamine (or "speed,"), which has almost replaced cocaine as the illegal drug of choice. "It's being called 'the poor man's cocaine.' It's an enormously lethal threat to people's health and mental stability and their ability to operate machinery." (Greenberg, 1996).

Most heroin in the United States came from Asia until about 1990, when the Colombians began producing it along with cocaine and shipping it through the southern U.S. border. Up to 70% of drug shipments now come through Mexico. The Colombians are getting into heroin to diversify their market, and now they're having their street-level people handle both cocaine *and* heroin. Selling the two different drugs through the same dealer, or "double-breasted," makes for a powerful marketing combination.

The death of a backup musician for *Smashing Pumpkins,* one of the country's most successful alternative rock bands, has spawned a macabre surge in sales of the very drug that killed him. Jonathan Melvoin, a 34-year-old keyboard player, died from an apparent overdose of heroin ("Red Rum" brand) in a plush New York hotel, and since, increasing numbers of users have been trying to buy the "Red Rum, that the Melvoin used." Melvoin's death has turned out to be a commercial for the drug, and is attracting buyers. Police called a news conference to warn of the potential consequences of the use of Red Rum, which they noted spelled "murder" backwards. They are trying to put out the word that it is very dangerous. It has a high potency, and people should not shoot it (Goldman, 1996).

Methamphetamine

Methamphetamine, also called crystal or crank, is an amphetamine derivative developed by a Japanese pharmacologist in 1919. Although it is prescribed to treat attention-deficit disorder and obesity, like other amphetamines, it has been abused since it came on the market in the 1930s.

An injectable, highly addictive form of "meth" used by "speed freaks" in the 1960s prompted the government to tighten controls on its manufacture in 1970. Abuse of meth fell off during the 1970s as cocaine became increasingly available.

But "meth" has become more popular in recent years, especially in California— now the nation's center for clandestine meth labs. The drug is easy to make, cheaper to buy than cocaine, and it produces a feeling of euphoria that lasts for hours—an effect strongly alluring to workers trying to keep up (Marsh, 1996).

Workers take the drug anywhere they do not expect to be caught—the restroom, a stairwell, a private office, in the car during break, and, for those who travel, the airplane bathroom. In one common pattern of abuse, an employee snorts speed before heading to work in the morning, takes it throughout the day as effects wear off, downs alcohol at night to counteract the buzz, wakes up hung over, and starts the cycle again.

When a speed user is in their midst, co-workers often sense that something is wrong but cannot put their finger on it. The paraphernalia are easily concealed: a small plastic bag or vial for carrying the stuff; a business card holder, mirror, or some other flat surface to hold a hit; a razor blade for pulverizing the powder and forming it into lines; and a short straw for sniffing it.

One clue is that a person disappears into the restroom stall but does not flush the toilet, and then returns to the office or assembly line sniffing or playing with the nose. Some users maintain their personal hygiene. But other heavy users, who stay awake for long hours, skip needed showers and appear at work with unkempt hair and wrinkled clothes. They often pick at their skin, leaving sores on the arms, legs, or face known as "speed bumps."

Normally, when people get very advanced into their use, you see them losing weight, looking pale and somewhat frail. They are very irritable, nervous, and anxious (Marsh, 1996). Normal situations, like going out to lunch with a group, are often avoided. Relations with co-workers often deteriorate as users get edgy, sometimes exploding at the slightest criticism and, in not-so-rare instances, lashing out physically. People taking crystalmeth can become emotionally and physically wrecked to the point where friends and neighbors cannot even recognize them anymore.

The increasing number of police raids on meth labs, chemical explosions, and emergency hospitalizations mark the rising epidemic of methamphetamine abuse; its impact is increasingly being felt in the workplace. Of 300,000 drug tests performed annually, about 15,000, or 5%, come up positive. Speed accounts for 35% of the positive results, up from 20% 2 years ago, and it has edged out cocaine, which has slipped about 5 percentage points to 30%. In virtually every industry, more people are abusing meth, as they are often deluded into believing it can help them work harder, better, faster, and longer.

Designer Drugs

ROHYPNOL

The drug Rohypnol, known among users as "roofies," has allegedly been used in a number of rape cases in which women reported their attackers slipped the small white pills into their drinks before the women lost partial memory of the hours that followed (Shuster, 1997). Los Angeles police say that they are seeing a great deal of it. They see people with it but are unable to do anything about it. The state Senate passed a bill by Senator Tom Hayden that makes the sale or possession of the hypnotic drug a crime. "We'd like to make the sale or possession of this dangerous drug—which has an insidious threat of violence with it—a crime," Hayden said. "There's a delusion out there that this is a cheap relaxant. But Rohypnol is really 10 times the power of Valium."

The drug is sold in 64 countries as a sleeping aid, but the manufacturer has not sought approval for sale in the United States. The pills gained notoriety when *Nirvana* singer Kurt Cobain overdosed on Rohypnol that he took with champagne, a month before killing himself. The pills, which can cause memory loss, are being sold for $1.00 apiece on the street. Because they can cause memory loss, some rape victims have trouble recalling the details of their attack, remembering just enough to be traumatized. No rape goes without serious pain and serious damage. No rape is forgotten.

Officials of Hoffman-LaRoche Inc., the firm that manufactures the 20-year-old drug, oppose Hayden's effort to place the drug in the same classification as substances such as LSD, saying it does little to address abuse of the pills. Company officials said they are working with authorities in Texas and Florida to develop a urine test for Rohypnol. The company is making a weaker version of the drug, about half the dosage, in Mexico and Colombia, where authorities believe traffickers are buying the drug to smuggle into the United States.

Roofies are being used by heroin addicts to expand the effects of low-grade heroin and by cocaine addicts to "cushion the crash" when the effects of that drug wears off. Young adults and teenagers also are taking the pills to boost the effects of alcohol and marijuana. This is not just a drug used for personal abuse. This is a drug used as a weapon in a violent crime (Shuster, 1997).

Law enforcement officials in Los Angeles County announced new procedures to collect evidence in sexual assault cases in which the use of disorienting and sometimes *lethal* "date-rape" drugs is suspected (Gold, 1996).

Beginning immediately, hospital caregivers are being asked to collect urine samples from rape victims, and police officers are being trained to look for evidence of these potent, invisible drugs when investigating sexual assaults.

GAMMA HYDROXYBUTYRIC ACID ("SCOOP" OR GHB)

Authorities are investigating whether four people who became ill in a bar—two of them critically—had downed drinks spiked with a designer drug. Urine tests on two of the victims showed the presence of an illegal drug known as Scoop. This liquid drug, which is odorless and tasteless, is known for its purported aphrodisiac and hallucinogenic properties (Tawa, 1996).

Drugs such as Rohypnol and GHB have drawn national attention as they circulate through party and nightclub circuits. Six people were rushed to a hospital after they consumed GHB at a club. The Los Angeles district attorney's office is prosecuting two rape cases involving these drugs, and the deaths of six people nationwide have been attributed to their use. After ingesting the tasteless and odorless drug, the victim feels dizzy and disoriented and may black out.

Beginning January 1, 1997, possession of Rohypnol (roofies), was illegal in California. However, GHB, known on the street as "cherry meth" or "liquid X," remains legal. Five to six sexual assaults a month involving the drugs have been reported. This is just the tip of the iceberg. Most victims do not report the rape because they feel shame and are uncertain about what happened.

Inhalants (The Silent Epidemic)

In the culture of drug use, sniffing (or huffing) has traditionally been regarded as kid's stuff—a stunt pulled by adolescents and preteens using felt tip pens and tubes of Elmer's glue. But drug counselors and treatment professionals say a different scenario is emerging nationwide—one of ignorant teenagers and parents, and a variety of readily available toxic substances (Brown, 1995).

Cutting across race and socioeconomic lines, huffing has evolved into what the National Inhalant Prevention Coalition has dubbed "the cocaine of the 90s." More than 1000 people nationwide die annually from sniffing substances found "right under the kitchen sink."

No longer a practice relegated to Third World slums, inhalants now rank as the third most used "drug" after alcohol and marijuana among students in the United States, grades 8 through 12. National surveys have found that 20% of all 8th graders have huffed toxic substances, with inhalants figuring prominently in the drug use of older teens.

More than 1000 household, office, and school products can be sniffed to get high, with gasoline, glue, aerosol, butane, and solvents such as toluene being the most popular. The most knowledgeable huffers seek out containers labeled with a skull and crossbones, which promises a bigger and *better* high.

Drug-treatment professionals tell of third graders sniffing "white-out" dabbed under their fingernails. Canisters of air fresheners, bottles of nail polish remover, and bags of moth balls all carry the potential for a cheap kick, without the stigma of being illegal or the threat of being physically addictive.

Yet, these substances can be far more dangerous and damaging than heroin, cocaine, or marijuana. Long-term and permanent neurological damage, akin to the type that produces multiple sclerosis, can result from huffing. A 1986 study of 20 chronic toluene sniffers found that nearly two thirds suffered damage to their nervous system. Toluene is generally found in lacquers and spray paints (Brown, 1995). Because the fumes of sniffed substances pass directly to the brain, death can result from just a single, overwhelming huff. Users can suffocate when they inhale chemicals that coat their lungs, thereby preventing oxygen from entering the bloodstream.

Huffing also has a high death rate among first-time users of 30%, according to a British study. Some users suffered heart failure triggered by adrenaline surges while under the influence of inhalants. Huffing gives pause for disbelief, just considering the effectiveness of delivery ("faster than an IV") and the type of chemicals being huffed.

This material is what people use to commit suicide. One will not know when a dose will kill. Ignorance of inhalants exists on all fronts, from users to physicians to law enforcement, and contributes to a wide-scale underreporting of usage. Few physicians or police are attuned to looking for the effects of inhalant abuse, even when faced with teen deaths resulting from automobile accidents or involving other drugs. If one dies from butane, no one will know. No one will detect it unless someone reports the deceased as a butane user.

Kids end up dead, and the death is labeled a suicide rather than an accident. A real lack of awareness exists on the part of law enforcement and the medical profession. Parents, too, are often in the dark and may not give a second thought to children with paint stains on their mouths and hands, or red or runny eyes and noses. Other symptoms of inhalant use include behaving dazed or drunk.

Because standard drug tests do not detect the presence of many inhalants, users can appear to be clean. Given the gamut of available, sniffable products, inhalant abuse experts are preferring to concentrate their efforts on education. Inhalants are like *Russian roulette*. One puts the bullet in and asks, "Do I feel lucky today?"

Substance Abuse in the Elderly

Behind the walls of sun-drenched retirement communities, the names of the latest life-numbing wonder pills—and the physicians who dole them out—are quietly swapped like favored formulas for hot toddies. This pill equals a pain-free afternoon. Another, a sure night's sleep (Weber, 1996).

If it is prescribed by the physician, how can it be wrong? Some senior citizens, unwilling to bother far-off and busy children or grandchildren, stumble into trouble self-medicating, and wind up hooked. The tablets they take for sleeplessness or pain diminish the dread of losing control, of being poor or ill, of seeing friends pass away.

Pill-taking becomes part of a comforting, physician-sanctioned ritual, part of a daily routine with dwindling options. Addiction specialists and some geropsychiatrists say physicians frequently do not have the time or the knowledge to diagnose underlying emotional problems such as depression. Pressed for time, they too often use pills as "bandages" for complaints of the elderly.

No one knows how many senior citizens might be abusing drugs. Usually retired, often widowed and without friends, elderly addicts are easily invisible: no co-workers to notice erratic behavior or absences; no brushes with the law over drugs procured legally; no telltale smell on their breath. They are the "closet junkies." They are at home. They are alone. They are afraid. They are hiding. Their drug pusher is their physician.

Shame and the fear of losing independence cause the many elderly abusers to deny or hide their problem—dirty laundry *no one* should see. Most never make it into treatment programs that cater to today's "let-it-all-hang out" therapy generation.

Family members in far-away cities, confident their aging parent is safely tucked into a retirement community or living contentedly in the family home, often mistake the fumblings, slurred speech, and memory loss of drug abuse for old age or senility. Or they may aggravate the problem because they prefer a sedated grandparent, rather than a cranky, complaining one. Drugs can cause or exacerbate depression in those least able to cope, perhaps bringing death much sooner. There is something wrong with the system for elderly. This is one of the great secrets of the geriatric community. Certainly it is one of the taboo subjects of physicians.

Geriatric specialists and some physicians say the push toward HMOs is forcing physicians to see more and more patients to make the same money. While such managed-care plans can preclude "doctor-shopping" by members, they also allow physicians less time to talk to patients and get to the real cause of aches and pains—especially if the patient is cranky and demanding.

It is extremely time-consuming and emotionally upsetting to find out what is really wrong. It takes 2 minutes to write a prescription, but it can take 2 years to convince people to stop taking drugs (Weber, 1960). Table 10-1 presents drugs that are considered inappropriate for patients older than 65 because safer and equally effective drugs exist.

Cocaine

Cocaine is physically and psychologically addictive. It can damage the liver, cause malnutrition, and increase the risk of heart attacks. Coming down from a high may cause such deep gloom that the only remedy is more cocaine. Bigger doses often follow, and soon the urge may become a total obsession. This pattern can lead to a psychological dependence, the effects of which are not all that different from physical addiction. Growing clinical evidence shows that when cocaine is taken in the most potent and dangerous forms—injected in solution or chemically converted and smoked in a process called free-basing—it becomes addictive.

Table 10-1 A Caution on Drugs for the Elderly

A panel of experts in geriatrics and pharmacology has identified drugs considered generally inappropriate for patients older than 65 because safer and equally effective drugs exist. They include 15 drugs the experts believe should be entirely avoided by the elderly. Doctors stress that patients should always consult their doctors before making changes in prescription medication. The 15 drugs to be avoided:

Drug	Brand name	Use	Reason to not use
Amitriptyline	Elavil	Treats depression	Other antidepressants cause fewer side effects.
Carisoprodol	Soma, Rela	Relieves severe pain caused by sprains and back injury	Minimally effective while causing toxicity; possible toxic reaction is greater than potential benefit.
Chlordiazepoxide	Librium	Tranquilizer or antianxiety	Shorter-acting benzodiazepines are safer alternatives.
Cyclobenzaprine	Flexeril	Relieves severe pain caused by sprains and back injury	Minimally effective while causing toxicity; possible toxic reaction is greater than potential benefit.
Diazepam	Valium	Tranquilizer or antianxiety medication	Shorter-acting benzodiazepines are safer alternatives.
Flurazepam	Dalmane	Sleeping pill	Shorter-acting benzodiazepines are safer alternatives.
Indomethacin	Indocin	Relieves rheumatoid arthritis pain and inflammation	Other nonsteroidal antiinflammatories cause fewer toxic reactions.
Meprobamate	Miltown, Equinal	Tranquilizer	Shorter-acting benzodiazepines are safer alternatives.
Methocarbamol	Robaxin	Relieves severe pain caused by sprains and back injury	Minimally effective while causing toxicity; potential for toxic reaction is greater than potential benefit.
Orphenadrine	Norflex	Relieves severe pain caused by sprains and back injury	Minimally effective while causing toxicity; potential for toxic reaction is greater than potential benefit.
Pentazocine	Talwin	Relieves mild-to-moderate pain	Other narcotic medications are safer and more effective.
Pentobarbital	Nembutal	Sleeping pill; reduces anxiety	Safer sedative-hypnotics available.
Phenylbutazone	Butazolidin	Relieves rheumatoid arthritis pain and inflammation	Other nonsteroidal antiinflammatories cause fewer toxic reactions.
Propoxyphene	Darvon	Relieves mild-to-moderate pain	Other analgesic medications are safer and more effective.
Secobarbital	Seconal	Sleeping pill; reduces anxiety	Safer sedative-hypnotics available.

From U.S. General Accounting Office, Washington, DC

Crack is not a new drug, but it does represent a new strategy in the sale and marketing of street cocaine. Crack is ready-made, free-base cocaine sold in the form of tiny pellets or "rocks," which can be smoked with no further chemical processing. The significance of this shift in cocaine vending patterns stems from the fact that it makes the practice of smoking cocaine free-base more readily accessible to potential users (Washton and Gold, 1987).

A cocaine high is an intensely vivid, sensation-enhancing experience; no evidence exists, as claimed, that it is an aphrodisiac. Indeed, evidence does suggest that the sustained use of cocaine can cause sexual dysfunction and impotence. Even casual sniffing can lead to more potent and potentially damaging ways of using cocaine and other drugs. Many cocaine users take sedative pills such as quaaludes to calm them down after the high and to take the edge off their yearning for more cocaine. A few smoke marijuana for the same purpose or mix their cocaine with heroin in a process called speedballing or boy-girl, which produces a tug-of-war wherein the exhilaration of cocaine is undercut by the heroin.

A few middle-class users who dabble with heroin in conjunction with cocaine smoke it rather than inject it; they believe this prevents addiction. This belief is false; heroin, however it is used, is a fiercely addictive drug. Treatment centers are receiving an influx of well-dressed, well-to-do men and women who have gravely underestimated heroin's effects. One of cocaine's biggest dangers is that it diverts people from normal pursuits; it can entrap and redirect a person's activities into an almost exclusive preoccupation with the drug.

New drugs and ways to get high appear at various times. Some remain for a length of time because of being "new" and their effect on the person using them. Two "soft" drugs have been introduced in the 1990s. One is "blond hash," which produces a "giddy high"; the second is "dark hash," which is used for a serious "zonking."

A newer illegal drug is "ice." Ice originated in the Philippines; from there it traveled to Hawaii, and from Hawaii to the mainland. It has at least three times the potency of speed, and has caused many deaths.

A second new drug is "cat," a powder that is easily produced from household chemicals such as battery acids and aerosols. Snorted like coke, it is relatively inexpensive to make ($25), and the "high" from cat can last 3 days. This, too, has resulted in many deaths.

A recent method being used to get high is called "autoerection ejaculation." This is done in a shower. The shower massage tubing is placed around the person's neck. He then hangs himself until he is almost unconscious, and he has a tremendous ejaculation. Unfortunately, he may be too unconscious to release the tubing and dies of hanging.

In Somalia, six or seven men gather every afternoon to gossip and to chew "qut" (sometimes spelled *khat* or *kat*) until they are in a narcotic euphoria. Qut is a pale green plant that when chewed provides the user brief moments of a feeling of well-being.

Qut is a way of life. The drug is cultivated in neighboring Kenya. Qut is a boon to dealers. It costs pennies to produce and abundant amounts of qut are flown into Somalia on charter planes costing $8000 a flight. No evidence exists that U.S. troops are bringing home any of Somalia's qut. One American civilian official said it might happen in the future because the drug now is finding a market in the United States (Freed, 1992).

Despite the influx of new uppers and downers, little likelihood exists that the cocaine blizzard will soon abate. A drug habit born of a desire to escape the bad news in life is not likely to be discouraged by bad news about the drug itself. Americans will continue to succumb to the powder's crystalline dazzle. Few are yet aware or willing to concede that, at the very least, taking cocaine is dangerous to their psychological health (Demarest, 1996).

Today's drug was yesterday's drug as well; we are now experiencing the third or fourth cocaine epidemic. Historically, it dates back 5000 years. Its real claims to fame occurred in the nineteenth century. Angelo Mariani, a Corsican chemist, may have come the closest to "turning the world on" by inventing an elixir with coca and alcohol. Numerous medical giants including Freud, Koller, Corning, Halsted, Crile, and Cushing praised the merits of the "discovery of the age"; cocaine's benefit to mankind would be incalculable. Its opponents labeled it the third scourge of mankind (after alcohol and morphine). The *New York Times* stated that it wrecks its victim more swiftly and surely than opium. CocaCola went "clean," replacing coca with caffeine. In the Harrison Tax Act (1914), cocaine was classified as a narcotic, and since then debate has continued about its abuse and addictive potential.

In the United States between 1982 and 1992, the number of people seeking treatment for cocaine abuse increased fivefold, the number of emergency room admissions fourfold, and the number of deaths fourfold. At least 1.5 million Americans are now profoundly dependent on cocaine, a new corps more numerous than heroin addicts. About 15% of high school seniors are regular users. Cocaine has become a $50 billion business, ranking it in sales among the top 10 U.S. companies. No longer is it the recreational drug of the affluent; 25% of blue-collar workers engage in frequent cocaine misuse. Men users outnumber women by a 3:1 ratio, with current profile remaining that of a white, college-educated man in his 30s with an annual income of $45,000.

A survey conducted by the National Institute on Drug Abuse (1992) revealed that 31 million Americans had used cocaine at least once. A 1996 survey revealed that 19% of American high school seniors had tried cocaine. The rising population of cocaine users has been accompanied by a similar increase in the number of heavy abusers who have had to seek medical treatment because of cocaine-related difficulties. The number of medical emergencies resulting from cocaine use increased by 900% between 1990 and 1995, while cocaine-related deaths increased by over 1100%. Cocaine has become a widely prevalent drug that is being used by all levels of our society, by men and women, adolescents, and adults, rich and poor (Statistical Abstract of the United States, 1995).

Cocaine is readily absorbed from all mucous membranes, although concomitant local vasoconstriction limits its rate of absorption. Despite this fact, absorption may easily exceed the rate of detoxification and excretion, leading to high toxicity. Cocaine undergoes rapid biotransformation in the body. Its two main metabolites, ecgonine and benzoylecgonine, are excreted in the urine in amounts equivalent to one fourth to one half the original dose within 24 to 36 hours. Depending on urine acidity, 10% to 20% of cocaine is excreted unchanged. To avoid detection, addicts attempt to enhance excretion by consuming large volumes of cranberry juice or ingesting megadoses of vitamin C. Physicians attempt to increase excretion by giving the patient intravenous ammonium chloride. After 100 mg of intravenous cocaine has been taken, a plasma peak occurs at 5 minutes; the distributional half-life is 20 to 40 minutes. The most popular routes for abuse purposes are intranasal (snorting), intravenous (running), and free-basing inhalation (smoking) (Hankes, 1984).

Cocaine is a beguiling drug that does not result in hangovers, lung cancer, or holes in the arm. Instead, a user takes a snort, and for the next 20 to 30 minutes has an increase in drive, sparkle, and energy without a feeling of being drugged. Reported subjective effects include mood elevation to the point of euphoria, decrease in hunger, increases in energy and sociability, indifference to pain, and significant decrease in fatigue. Users experience a feeling of great muscular strength and increased mental capacity, leading to an overestimation of their capabilities. The powerful experience of the cocaine high can lead the user into a pattern of regular and escalating use. The most commonly reported side effects of regular use include anxiety, dysphoria, suspiciousness, disruption in eating and sleeping habits, weight loss, fatigue, irritability, concentration difficulties, and perceptual problems. Increasing use may lead to hyperexcitability, marked agitation, paranoia, hypertension, and tachycardia. As the person becomes more and more "strung out," alcohol, sedatives, or other narcotics are often taken to combat the overstimulation.

Paranoid psychoses are manifested by a variety of symptoms such as visual distortion and hallucinations (geometric patterns such as "snow lights"), tactile hallucinations (sensation of insects on, in, or under the skin, called cocaine "bugs"), delusions (being chased by the police, or "bull horrors"), and violent behavior. Cocaine interacts with the catecholamine neurotransmitters, norepinephrine and dopamine, and alters normal interneuronal communication. It augments the effects of these catecholamines, probably by blocking (or prolonging) reuptake at the synaptic junction, leaving an excess of these neurotransmitters to restimulate receptors. Dopamine is a precursor of norepinephrine and is found in the corpus striatum, which is part of the network governing motor functions, and in that portion of the hypothalamus regulating thirst and hunger. Norepinephrine is the prime neurotransmitter of the ascending reticular activating system (RAS), regulating mechanisms of external attention and arousal. It acts as a vital transmitter as well in the hypothalamus, which regulates body temperature, sleep, and sexual arousal and, in general, mediates emotional depression. It also mediates neural activation in the median forebrain bundle of the hypothalamus, which is believed to serve as a person's "pleasure center."

When looking at a drug taken, but not prescribed, for a mood or behavioral change, one should consider the following: first, the potential for overdose; second, the potential for acute toxicity; third, physical derangements; fourth, its effects on mental status; and fifth, behavioral modification. That is, how much does it incapacitate a person or hinder his ability to function in an environment that was not a preexisting problem? Acute consequences include hyperpyrexia; hypertension with possible cerebrovascular accident, arrhythmia, or myocardial infarct; accidents because of impaired judgment and timing; and the dangers that lurk around some less than desirable purchase zones. Seizures are common and often progress to status epilepticus. Chronic complications depend on purity, route of administration, frequency of use, and sterility. All too often, users confuse cleanliness with sterility.

One of the frequent chronic medical complications is not strictly medical but dental. Cocaine is a powerful local anesthetic, and users often neglect their teeth because they are not aware of any discomfort or pain. They are often found to have missing fillings, cavities, loose teeth, impaction with inflammation, and even periodontal abscesses. A detailed oral examination is mandatory (Woods and Downs, 1973).

Malnutrition is common because food intake is ignored. Most patients are thin (rarely are they obese), and some are emaciated; 73% have at least one major vitamin deficiency, usually pyridoxine followed by thiamine and ascorbic acid. Intranasal users develop rhinorrhea, nasal septal necrosis, and perforation; hoarseness; aspiration pneumonia; and frontal sinusitis. Routine chest and frontal sinus x-ray examinations are suggested. Free-basing often results in burns from explosion of the volatile ether used in preparation of the base. Chronic users who prefer to smoke cocaine should be evaluated for pulmonary function. Intravenous users are subject to infections of the skin, lung, heart valves, brain, and eye by multiple unusual bacteria and fungi. Some 86% of intravenous coke users have antibody evidence of prior exposure to hepatitis B and human immunodeficiency virus (HIV). Talc and silicone adulterants produce granuloma formation in the lungs, liver, brain, and eye. Cocaine is metabolized by the liver and excreted by the kidney; any preexisting dysfunction exacerbates most conditions previously discussed.

Patients often "tank up" just before admission, that is, use very large doses in anticipation of "cold turkey" withdrawal. This increases the toxicity potential, and some centers are reluctant to admit patients on weekends and nights unless medical supervision is available. The lethal dose of cocaine is about 1.2 gm, but severe toxicity has occurred with an average dose of 20 mg. Tolerance and route of administration play an important role in the lethal dose. Sudden death from cocaine is so sudden that the only medical person to see the patient is often the coroner. Death occurs from status epilepticus, respiratory paralysis, myocardial infarction or irritability, and rarely, anaphylaxis. Antiepileptic medications do not appear to reduce or block cocaine-related seizures. The combined chronic lack of sleep and throat anesthesia may interact to cause a deep "crash" (sleep), which is accompanied by airway obstruction (suffocation) induced by a flaccid jaw or failure to remove secretions (drowning). The number of deaths resulting from the combined use of cocaine with other drugs has also rapidly increased but not as rapidly as the number of cocaine-related homicide victims. Death can and does occur in people who drink and use cocaine. The cocaine keeps the person awake enough to continue drinking and try to drive home; the cocaine wears off before the alcohol, and the high blood alcohol level oversedates, causing a fatal accident. Often only the blood alcohol level is analyzed, which falsely attributes the death to alcohol alone. Concomitant use of narcotics in an attempt to boost the cocaine high or to self-medicate its side effects often results in disaster. Another factor involved in cocaine-related deaths is cocaine-related suicides. These dependent people feel hopeless and helpless. Suicide may be seen as the only solution to deteriorating health and personal, domestic, or financial situations. However, fear of disability or disease from various sources does not deter use because most users discount these medical reports or doubt that any disability or disease will happen to them (Hankes, 1984).

The lifestyle generally accepted as normal involves major efforts to obtain and enjoy food, water, shelter, friendship, and a sexual partner. Researchers assume that a major function of the brain's reinforcement centers is to make it possible for the person to strive to achieve these goals despite the fact that their availability is limited. Cocaine's main danger is its bypassing of the normal reinforcement process. It reprograms or reprioritizes the person so that getting cocaine is supreme and all normal drives are subverted. People and their cocaine problems can be classified on the basis of access. People who have a lot of disposable income have the different problem of unlimited access; they can easily end up addicted. Cocaine is a drug of disposable income: What you have, the drug will soon dispose of (Zinberg and Robertson, 1972).

Many physicians and users debate whether cocaine is addicting, the underlying premise being that if it is not addicting, it is not dangerous. The definition of *addiction* encompasses three concepts: compulsive use, loss of control when using the drug, and continued use despite adverse consequences. Using this definition, cocaine is obviously very, very addicting. It lends itself to reinforcement. Toxic manifestations do not curtail use; taking cocaine leads to taking more cocaine. Drug-craving and drug-seeking behaviors are notable with cocaine, clearly indicating a high level of psychological dependence. This effect, coupled with cocaine's property to reinforce its own abuse, leads to disaster. Regular users, especially high-dose snorters, free-basers, and injectors, generally want to maintain the elation. Cocaine's price and pharmacology do not lend themselves to a self-regulated maintenance program. Users may "base" continuously for days or inject intravenously every 10 minutes. For some, the anxiety, suspiciousness, and hypervigilance become overwhelming. Even as the user comes down and recalls the paranoid experience, he generally starts up again with the notion that this time he will stop short of insanity. Success-oriented people who rarely use drugs may discover cocaine and in less than 2 or 3 years find themselves hopelessly involved in illicit activities or facing incarceration. Consistent use can result in a severe depressive reaction, which may be the result of depleted norepinephrine stores. This may lead to another temporary "cure," or another dose, perpetuating the habit. Others with mild depression self-medicate with cocaine. They quickly learn that they are nothing and that the drug is everything. Any subsequent success is misattributed to the drug, and these abusers come to believe that normal functioning without the drug is nearly impossible (Garwin and Kepler, 1984).

Physicians who abuse drugs are a problem and are as dangerous as physicians who are severely neglectful or incompetent. Drug abuse experts say that the culture of the medical profession can lead physicians, more so than the rest of the population, not only to abuse drugs themselves, but also to overprescribe to others. Fully 18% of physicians, or 14,000 of the 77,000 practicing in California, will develop dependency problems at some point in their lives. And the percentage is much higher among specialists whose work involves treating patients with narcotics (Bernstein, 1995).

The problems of physicians' drug abuse and overprescription of mood-altering drugs like tranquilizers and amphetamines for their patients have their roots in the way physicians are trained. Medical students are taught that pharmaceuticals often can be the answer to patients' problems, but remarkably little instruction is given on the nature of addiction. Many who develop dependency problems started in medical school or during grueling training periods as resident physicians in hospitals.

In 1994, 41 physicians were disciplined in California for overprescribing drugs to patients, and 23 for abusing drugs themselves. But those numbers are deceptively low. Most physicians who abuse drugs are "poly-drug abusers," people who abuse a variety of drugs. About half used alcohol, either in combination with drugs or alone. Of 202 drug- and alcohol-abusing doctors, 134 used prescription narcotics, including Demerol and Vicodin. Forty-three used cocaine, and 18 used marijuana.

Patients' lives can be ruined, and physicians who are drug-addled while practicing medicine can cause serious harm. Some physicians have admitted that they have performed surgery and had blackouts (Bernstein, 1995).

The case study that follows depicts the tragic circumstances that occurred when a young physician abused cocaine.

Case Study   *Substance Abuse*

Late one Thursday afternoon, Steve D, an open-heart surgeon, called his friend, a psychotherapist. He was quite concerned that no one hear their conversation; he wanted to talk to his friend but not at the hospital where other staff members might see him. They made arrangements for him to meet with the therapist at her home early that evening. The therapist recalled that Steve had a very distinguished background: his father, grandfather, and great-grandfather had been highly respected physicians; and Steve was a Phi Beta Kappa from a well-known and distinguished eastern school, had graduated magna cum laude, had married an intelligent and attractive woman, had three lovely children, had finished at the top of his class, and had done his residency with a famous cardiologist-surgeon. Everyone, including peers, nursing staff, and patients, respected and liked him. In other words, he had everything going for him.

When Steve arrived at his friend's home, she immediately noticed that he was tense and trembling. Then he lit a cigarette, which she had never seen him do before; he had always disapproved of smoking. He seemed hesitant about telling the therapist what was wrong. She reminded him that she could not help him if she did not know what the problem was, and he obviously had a problem.

Steve began by telling her that he had been indefinitely suspended from the hospital staff. His explanation started with his internship, when the hours were long and the physical and emotional demands were constant. He had started using cocaine then, "not every day or night, just when I was so tired I didn't think I could keep my eyes open from fatigue and complete exhaustion."

The therapist was shocked and saddened by his confession, but she made no outward sign of her feelings and told him to continue his story. His subsequent residency had been difficult; Steve had felt that nothing he did pleased the surgeon. However, when the residency was completed, the surgeon wrote a "glowing report," which stated that Steve had a "brilliant career" ahead of him and that he had been the surgeon's most outstanding resident. Steve told the therapist he had used cocaine while he was a resident, maybe a little more than when he was an intern, but not every day.

The therapist asked how he was using it and he replied, "I was just snorting it—then." She asked about the present, and he said, "Now I'm smoking it—free-basing—and injecting it." He also said that he was not combining heroin with it when he injected it because he was "not that crazy." He had been free-basing for about 2½ years and injecting for a little over a year.

She asked Steve who found out about his cocaine use and when. He started pacing up and down and asked for a drink. Since he had admitted to smoking some coke right before coming to see her, the therapist refused his request. She became very firm with him and offered him a choice of answering her questions right then or leaving. After only a moment's hesitation, Steve started talking. He had scheduled a triple bypass on a patient for the previous Monday morning. He explained that he never injected himself for 3 days before surgery, but he did free-base. He made it a point to be scrubbed early, before anyone else was around, and gowned so no one could see his arms (with tracks from injecting the cocaine). He said everything was going well in surgery on this particular morning until he accidentally cut his finger with a scalpel. He added that he had been a little shaky that morning for some reason (probably because of his heavy use of cocaine). One of his partners took his place to continue the surgery, and he went out to rescrub. Unfortunately, Dr. A, the chief of staff, was in the scrub room when Steve entered. Steve stripped his gloves and gown off and started to rescrub at a basin as far from Dr. A as possible. Dr. A asked him why he was rescrubbing, and Steve explained that he had cut his finger. Dr. A asked to see his finger. Steve quickly held up his hand and said it was nothing. However, the other physician apparently saw the tracks on Steve's arm and quietly but firmly asked him to hold out both his arms. Steve did as he was asked, and Dr. A looked at his arms and told him to stay where he was. Dr. A then called for a resident to replace Steve in surgery and told Steve to cancel all his appointments for the rest of the week and wait for Dr. A in his office. Dr. A arrived at his office and asked Steve what he had been shooting up on, how long, and why. After Steve related his story, Dr. A told him he had no excuse; they were all dealing with human lives and could not afford to make even one mistake. Dr. A called an emergency staff meeting of the ethics committee for an hour later. He made it clear that he was doing nothing to help Steve, who was to "try to explain" his behavior to the committee members.

Steve stopped talking at this point and had to be prodded into continuing. He said the committee meeting was "horrible," that the persons attending "stared at me as if they had never seen me before." All they had asked him was how much he was using and where he got his supply (by writing prescriptions for nonexistent patients). They informed him that he would have to enter a substance abuse facility and stay there until he was determined "clean" by the discharge clinic staff. He was automatically suspended from hospital privileges immediately. If he did not report to a facility by the end of the week, they would notify the Board of Medical Quality Assurance, and his license to practice medicine would be revoked.

The therapist asked him if he was going to do as the committee had told him by the next day. He replied, "I don't know. That's why I had to talk to you. Can't you work with me and get me over the need to use coke?" She answered firmly, "Absolutely not, it can't be done!" She explained that the amount he used, the methods, and the length of time all made outpatient psychotherapy inappropriate and dangerous. She told him he could die trying to get "clean" himself.

At that point, Steve said, "It would be better if I were dead." His friend pointed out to him that he would be leaving his wife and children a terrible legacy. She told him that he could continue to be a surgeon, but that it would not be easy. She then asked if he had discussed the matter with his wife, Jennifer, and he said "no." The therapist sent Steve home to talk to his wife and told him to bring her back with him that night. While he was gone, she would make some plans for him. He agreed to do as she said.

The first step would be to talk with Steve and Jennifer together to determine if his wife would stand by the decision that he enter a substance abuse facility. The next step would be to contact the best facility the therapist knew to see if a private room was available for Steve. She also needed to know if he could be admitted that night. The facility under consideration was approximately 125 miles away. The therapist did not think Steve would willingly accept a facility in the city.

The psychotherapist called the substance abuse facility and related her story to the director, Mr. B, a friend of hers. Mr. B informed her that he had a room and suggested that Steve might want to use an assumed name while there. He agreed that Steve and Jennifer should come that night; he would make the train reservations and meet them at the station.

Steve returned to the therapist's home with his wife. Jennifer was shaken by what her husband had told her, but she said they were very willing to do anything that the therapist suggested to help her husband. The therapist told them to make arrangements immediately to go to the facility that night. She told Steve that she would talk to the chief of staff and inform him of Steve's decision. Before leaving, Jennifer requested therapy after she returned from the facility; she did not understand how her husband could have become involved in using cocaine.

After they left, the therapist called Dr. A and told him what had happened that evening. He asked her what she felt the chances were for Steve to come out of his addiction really clean, with no desire to go back on cocaine. She responded that if he could get through the first week, he might make it. The length of time he had been using it and the methods he used made a more optimistic response impossible. However, the therapist felt they had done all they could for him.

During the night, the therapist received a call from the director of the facility. He informed her that Steve had died on the train; he had apparently "tanked up" and died in his sleep. Jennifer had been admitted to the hospital in a state of shock.

Because nothing could be done for Steve, anticipatory planning would involve helping his wife and children through the grief and mourning process. They would have to rebuild their lives without him.

My salad days when I was green in judgment.

−William Shakespeare

Complete the paradigm in Figure 10-1 for this case study, then compare it with the completed one in Appendix D. Refer to the paradigms in Chapter 3 as needed.

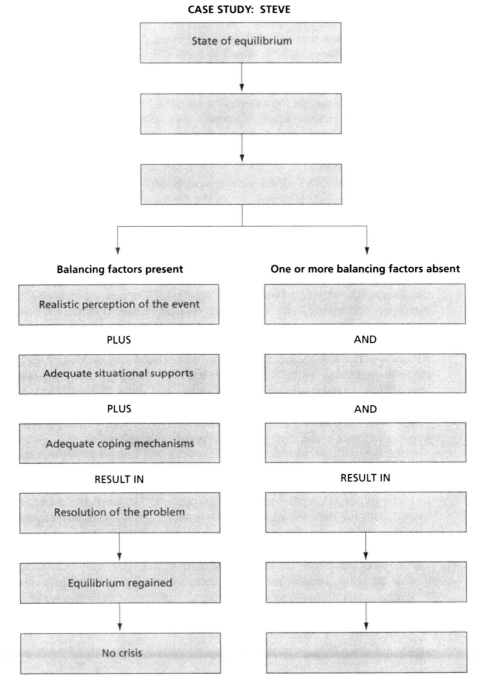

Figure 10-1

REFERENCES

Bernstein S, Times staff writer: Drug abuse by doctors a malady of the system, *Los Angeles Times,* September 18, 1995.

Brown SS, Times staff writer: In a fight against a silent epidemic, *Los Angeles Times,* April 2, 1995.

Demarest M: Cocaine: middle class high, *Time,* May 12, 1996.

Ferrell D, Times staff writer: Pot's deep roots in unlikely soil, *Los Angeles Times,* December 15, 1996.

Freed K: Chewing the fat, with a side of qut, *Los Angeles Times,* December 26, 1992.

Garwin F, Kepler H: Cocaine abuse treatment, *Arch Gen Psychiatry* 41:903, 1984.

Gold M: Special to the Times, New rules revealed in date rape drug checks, *Los Angeles Times,* December 12, 1996.

Goldman JJ, Times staff writer: Musician's death spurs heroin demand, *Los Angeles Times,* July 16, 1996.

Greenberg J, Times staff writer: Federal authorities see alarming trends in heroin use, *Los Angeles Times,* June 15, 1996.

Hankes L: Cocaine: today's drug, *J Fla Med Assoc* 71:235, 1984.

Marsh B, Times staff writer: Meth at work, *Los Angeles Times,* July 7, 1996.

National Institute on Drug Abuse: *National survey on drug abuse,* Rockville, Md, 1992, National Clearing House for Drug Abuse Information.

Shuster B, Times staff writer: Penalty sought for possession of date rape drug, *Los Angeles Times,* January 30, 1997.

Tawa R, Times staff writer: Police investigate illnesses at bar, *Los Angeles Times,* November 4, 1996.

U.S. Department of Commerce, Bureau of the Census: *Statistical abstract of the United States, 1995,* ed 115, Washington, DC, 1995, U.S. Government Printing Office.

Washton AM, Gold MS, editors: *Cocaine: a clinician's handbook,* New York, 1987, Guilford.

Weber T, Times staff writer: Addiction mars the golden years, *Los Angeles Times,* December 20, 1996.

Woods JH, Downs DA: The psychopharmacology of cocaine. In *Drug use in America: problem in perspective,* vol 1, Washington, DC, 1973, National Commission on Marijuana & Drug Abuse.

Zinberg NE, Robertson JA: *Drugs and the public,* New York, 1972, Simon & Schuster.

ADDITIONAL READING

Associated Press: Drug use among students up state poll finds, *Los Angeles Times,* August 27, 1996.

Jones E, Ackatz L: *Availability of substance abuse treatment programs for pregnant women: results from three national surveys,* Chicago, 1992, NCPCA.

Jones E and others: *Substance abuse treatment programs for pregnant and parenting women: a program guide,* Chicago, 1992, NCPCA.

Newcomb MD, Bentler PM: Impact of adolescent drug use and social support on problems of young adults: a longitudinal study, *J Abnorm Psychol* 97:64, 1988.

Sheehan M, Oppenheimer E, Taylor C: Why drug users sought help from one London drug clinic, *Br J Addict* 81:765, 1986.

Shelowitz PA: Drug use, misuse, and abuse among the elderly, *Med Law* 6:235, 1987.

Snyder CA and others: "Crack smoke" is a respirable aerosol of cocaine base, *Pharmacol Biochem Behav* 29:93, 1988.

Ventrua WP: Cocaine use: your choice now—no choice later, *Imprint* 35:28, 1988.

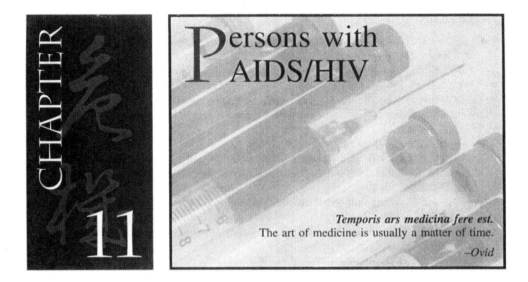

CHAPTER 11

Persons with AIDS/HIV

Temporis ars medicina fere est.
The art of medicine is usually a matter of time.

–Ovid

On December 22, 1996, the Associated Press announced in the *Los Angeles Times* that *Time Magazine's* 1996 Man of the Year was acquired immunodeficiency syndrome (AIDS) researcher Dr. David Ho, who pioneered a treatment for human immunodeficiency virus (HIV) infection that has shown promise in beating back the deadly disease. *Time* said that his work "might, just might, lead to a cure."

In 1996, 3.1 million people became HIV-infected, bringing the worldwide total to 22.6 million people living with HIV or AIDS. As long as HIV exists somewhere in the world it threatens us all (Purvis, 1997). But at last there is a ray of hope; Dr. Ho has given those with HIV and those who will be diagnosed in the near future a chance for recovery.

AIDS is tightening its grip outside the United States and Western Europe. In India, researchers estimate that by the year 2000, anywhere from 15 million to 50 million people could be HIV-positive. Half of the prostitutes in Bombay are already infected, and physicians report that the disease is spreading along major truck routes and into rural areas, as migrant workers bring the virus home. In Central and Eastern Europe, countries that had largely escaped the epidemic are seeing an explosion in the number of cases, mainly among IV drug users and their heterosexual contacts.

Across much of Africa, the disease continues to rage unchecked. Already the sub-Saharan region accounts for more than 60% of people living with HIV worldwide, or some 14 million men, women, and children. As many people will die there this year from the disease as were massacred 2 years ago in the Rwandan holocaust. The social consequences of this die-off are catastrophic. By the year 2000, nearly 2 million children in Kenya, Rwanda, Uganda, and Zambia will have lost their parents to the disease (Purvis, 1997).

The "cocktail" treatments are financially out of reach for those living in Central and Eastern Europe and Africa. A more effective alternative is prevention, through public education and safe-sex programs. Such efforts have made some progress in recent years. In Africa and in some parts of Asia, similar programs have stalled, due to a combination of poverty, official indifference, and, at times, paranoia. As a result, public understanding of even the most basic information of AIDS is still piecemeal. Most of those dying from the disease in rural parts of Africa have no clear idea of what is killing them, let alone how to prevent it.

Historical Background

The late twentieth century will be remembered as the time in which AIDS changed attitudes and beliefs of people around the world. The world is faced with many unknowns. When will a cure be discovered? Will scientists be able to create a vaccine against it? How many men, women, and children will die from AIDS and its opportunistic infections? No infectious condition of recent times has had the psychosocial impact of HIV. A near "AIDS hysteria" has developed throughout the world, as the informative as well as the sensationalist media have bombarded the public with reports about AIDS. AIDS patients must cope not only with their own adjustment to a terminal diagnosis, but also with discrimination caused by society's fear of them (Johnson, 1988).

As many as 40,000 Americans in 1996 who were defined *only* as HIV-positive woke up on New Year's Day, January 1, 1997, with a diagnosis of AIDS—the consequence of a new and more inclusive official definition that is likely to place a strain on already strapped social service agencies and add to the emotional trauma of many who are infected.

The U.S. Centers for Disease Control and Prevention, which monitor the AIDS epidemic, uses a so-called surveillance definition to determine when an HIV-positive person has developed full-blown AIDS. Under the current definition, a person who is infected with HIV is diagnosed as having AIDS when he or she develops one of 23 indicator illnesses. In 1993 the definition was expanded to include three diseases common to HIV-infected women and IV drug users: cervical cancer, pulmonary tuberculosis, and recurrent pneumonia. The expanded definition also included a fourth new indicator: a drop in the level of CD4 immune cells, also called T-cells, to $200/mm^3$ of blood, about one fifth the level of a healthy person. More so than most other diseases, AIDS also has an emotional impact on physicians who are called on to treat their AIDS patients' social, emotional, and medical problems, many of which can be overwhelming. Physicians frequently may have feelings to resolve about caring for these patients because of their own fears of contagion, homophobia, or other negative attitudes (Johnson, 1987).

Patients with AIDS, as well as those who perceive themselves to be at risk (the "worried well"), face a range of fears and concerns about AIDS (Faulstich, 1987; Holland and Tross, 1985; Johnson, 1987; Nichols, 1985). HIV infection can have devastating effects on a person's interpersonal relationships, including isolation, rejection, and overall loss of social support. Health consequences from the virus can make the basic activities of daily life difficult by causing weakness, physical debilitation, and dementia. Financial problems result from loss of job, numerous hospital and medical bills, and exhausted medical insurance. The patient may experience multiple psychological effects, including depression, anxiety, and loss of hope for the future; issues of death and dying also surface (Perry and Markowitz, 1986).

Physicians who care for these patients may feel beset by the medical, psychological, social, and other problems and may not be able to address all of these issues in a busy practice. Many communities, even smaller ones in rural areas, offer resources to which the patient can be referred for specialized AIDS-related psychosocial support. Local health departments and community mental health centers frequently can provide lists of these community services. Some health departments also provide AIDS testing. These are usually termed *alternate test sites,* and the tests and results are confidential and anonymous (AIDS Project Los Angeles, 1997).

Antibody Testing

HIV antibody testing was approved by the U.S. Food and Drug Administration in 1985 for the screening of donated blood (CDC, 1987). Since then, the test has also been used to screen persons at risk for, and those showing signs of, HIV infection. HIV antibody serological testing generally refers to a two or three test sequence. The first is an enzyme-linked immunosorbent assay (ELISA) test; if this is reactive (positive), a Western Blot test is indicated for more specificity. If this second test is also reactive, the patient should be given the immunofluorescent assay (IFA) test. If the IFA test is positive, the person is considered infectious and able to transmit the disease (APLA, 1997).

To protect the patient's confidentiality, some laboratories process HIV antibody tests differently from other laboratory work. Frequently, specimens submitted with the patient's name are not accepted; only those specimens labeled with a code number are accepted. To further protect the patient's identity, many laboratories do not directly bill insurance companies for the test. Many laboratories do not report test results over the telephone, even to the physician who ordered the test. Physicians should also direct their office or hospital practice (e.g., record keeping, staff attitudes) so that patient confidentiality is maintained (Johnson, 1988).

AIDS and HIV Counseling

Patient counseling, both before and after HIV antibody testing, has become the standard medical practice in many clinical situations. This can be done by the patient's physician, a specially trained counselor, or, before the tests, in a group setting (CDC, 1997b). All counseling involves educating the patient about HIV antibody testing. In most situations, HIV testing should be performed with informed consent, which means the patient understands that the testing is being done, the reasons for the test, and the possible implications (medical, social, and legal) of both positive and negative results. In addition, counseling should offer an environment that encourages the patient to discuss fears and feelings about AIDS. Test results should also be discussed. The clinician should assess the patient's emotional ability to handle positive or negative results and then, together with the patient, make a final decision about whether to test (Johnson, 1987).

The functions of pretest counseling are to educate the patient about AIDS and its prevention and to help the patient decide whether the test is indicated and desired. The primary purposes of posttest counseling are to inform the patient of test results and to provide emotional support. The patient should be encouraged to express feelings about the results but not be allowed to become so depressed that he can no longer function and pose a danger to himself. Some patients require a referral to mental health professionals to help them work out their feelings (Johnson, 1987).

In working with AIDS patients, therapists need to understand that the concept of family has a broader meaning than is traditionally understood. On one hand the traditional family composition is that of the nuclear family, the family of origin, or both. On the other hand is the family of choice, who are also very significant and may be included at different points in treatment. In working with the family of choice, the definition of family may include lover or life partner and close friends who may be the most significant relationships and source of support. Blending the family of choice with the family of origin is therapeutic. In doing this blending, therapists serve as models, showing that this is appropriate and needed (Appell and Blatt, 1992).

ROLE OF THE THERAPIST IN AIDS COUNSELING

In working with AIDS patients the therapist's flexibility is crucial. For those who have had more traditional training as therapists, AIDS can challenge their thinking. In addition to working on relationship and family issues, both past and present, therapists need to serve as educators, crisis counselors, and referral sources. Comfort with moving between different roles helps patients.

Many families have no experience or prior knowledge about AIDS; the therapist becomes their source of information in the beginning, educating families about transmission and addressing their fears about risks of contagion. The families' fears are real. Validating those fears and concerns is an essential step in joining with the family and helping them understand AIDS. As a therapist educates the family, AIDS is demystified.

Being available to the family is critical. Every time AIDS is discussed openly and nonjudgmentally, one serves as a role model to the family in a subtle, powerful way about open communication. Referral to support groups, helpful books, and AIDS-related agencies is part of the therapist's job that often gives the family their first connection to information about AIDS. For the therapists' well-being, they need to help their families find as many other forms of support as possible so that more than one resource is available for them.

The therapist can also use his or her role to empower patients and enhance their assertiveness or sense of control by allowing them to take the lead in bringing up issues that need to be addressed. Although this would not be always appropriate, such as in the case of unhealthy denial that created obstacles to needed treatment, generally this attitude helps preserve the autonomy of the patient, an important issue in AIDS.

BOUNDARIES OF THE THERAPIST

Boundaries for a therapist need to be defined in a way that works both ethically and therapeutically. When working with persons living with AIDS, the therapist needs to be open to seeing the patient in the context of the family or subgroup within the family. The therapist's flexibility will often be challenged. At times, patients will not be able to keep appointments and cancel at the last minute because of illness or medical appointments. Will the therapist charge? Is the schedule open enough to reschedule in the same week? Is the therapist willing to do home visits when the patient becomes too ill to travel? It is a judgment call; one should not do a house call out of one's own anxiety, but rather out of the patient's needs (Appell and Blatt, 1992).

Working with AIDS patients can be integrated into most theoretical frameworks. However, one should also focus on some of the specific issues regarding family functioning to meet effectively the unique needs of those affected by AIDS. Some family subgroups have issues that differ from those of other family subgroups. Assessing family functioning can help to develop appropriate treatment plans and goals.

Most patients wish for the family to be there and to be supportive. Therapists must assess how realistic this hope is, and how likely it is that it will be fulfilled. For instance, sometimes the disclosure of AIDS status is the first time the family has heard that the person is gay. Disclosure needs to be tailored to the specific dynamics of the family and the needs of the person (Appell and Blatt, 1992).

FAMILY SYSTEMS

When working with families, whether beginning with one person or a larger group, looking at the boundaries in the family system, and understanding what those boundaries are and how they have operated in the past as well as the present are useful. People from enmeshed (overinvolved) families may have blurred boundaries. In such families, premature disclosure of AIDS status may occur when family members are not emotionally ready to deal with it. One can assist the HIV-positive patient in containing anxiety long enough to think through the process of disclosure, including each family member's emotional preparedness and the appropriate timing for disclosure. Members of an enmeshed family could become too involved too quickly.

Understanding the style and makeup of the family system is vital for assessment and treatment. In overinvolved or enmeshed families, unity is stressed and autonomy is discouraged. Because autonomy is so important for the person who has AIDS, family members need to resist a natural tendency to overprotect the patient. The more they protect, the more helpless the patient may feel, and the less able to mobilize strength and resources. One needs to teach family members the difference between helping and rescuing. Rescuing behavior starts with the view that the patient is a victim who is hopeless and helpless. Unattended, rescuing behavior has the effect of infantilizing the client (Appell and Blatt, 1992).

If in a family few, if any, emotional connections exist, or if the family is emotionally cut off, the family is referred to as disengaged. Often in this system, AIDS disclosure may not have taken place. If it has, and if the AIDS-infected person has historically been the identified patient in the family, this may be one more reason for family members to see him or her as the identified patient and further blame the person. Because of the shame connected with HIV, this could have a devastating effect.

Depending on the level of dysfunction of the family and the emotional stability of the patient, disclosure may or may not be appropriate. Therapists have to pay attention to their own need for clients to disclose. Therapists may hold a bias that disclosure is helpful, but it may not be possible. The patients from this system are more likely to erect rigid boundaries around themselves under the stress of an AIDS diagnosis. They then might isolate themselves in unhealthy ways or may undermine, distance, or cut off relationships prematurely. If a person in this type of system wants to disclose, the therapist can help the patient prepare for disclosure by assisting in gathering other support systems and creating a more positive image. Also, repeatedly separating the virus from personhood helps take away the moral judgment that contributes to shame. If the person who has been through this process decides to disclose, he or she may be more emotionally able to handle the family's response. Sometimes in these situations, selective disclosure may work better: the person picks the safest member in the family to tell first. As in the enmeshed system, timing of disclosure is important (Appell and Blatt, 1992).

How families deal with stress and difficult news can be assessed in their level of denial. Whether healthy or unhealthy, denial can be reflected in a family's difficulty in taking in the reality of the situation, struggling with their many feelings, and eventually accepting the roller coaster ride they are about to begin. Unhealthy denial needs to be confronted, in a gentle and supportive way. Families do not unlearn denial overnight. Communication is necessary for the family to overcome their denial; otherwise, it can sabotage their chances of success in supporting one another. For therapists, confronting denial is a walk on a tightrope at best. However, not to pay attention to it is doing all a disservice.

The religious influences and beliefs of the patient and the family need to be taken into consideration. Sometimes the family and the patient are in conflict about these influences. Many gays have been cut off from their families of origin because of religious differences. These families cannot always come together and accept their differences.

Patients who are AIDS-infected sometimes want to reconnect with their original faith or find a new sense of spirituality. Some may want to explore other avenues, such as listening to meditation tapes, using crystals, or participating in other religious or spiritual organizations. Therapists must guard against personal biases and help patients define what is right for them and help the families to accept the patients' perspective (Stribling, 1990).

ISOLATION

When evaluating family systems, one should look for isolation. This isolation can be adaptive and part of the adjustment process of accepting and incorporating new information. For example, after an AIDS disclosure, some family members may distance themselves or withdraw for a short time. Therapists need to normalize this reaction so that patients do not overreact and assume that this is a permanent state.

However, isolation and withdrawal by the family may not be adaptive. People isolate for many reasons; one may be fear of contagion. Sometimes families withdraw because they feel helpless. Often family members ask, "What do I do? What do I say?" Fearing that they may make a mistake, they withdraw.

Family members may also withdraw from the AIDS member because they find it difficult to be close when they fear losing someone. They may see AIDS as an immediate death. A spouse or lover who also has AIDS may withdraw because of fears about facing his or her own mortality. Finally, family members may experience isolation and withdrawal in their own social circles because of the stigma of HIV. This adds much stress at a time when support is especially important. In all of these cases, therapists must educate, support, normalize, and validate feelings and fears. The therapist should identify isolation and intervene when necessary, and encourage open communication among family members to increase intimacy and decrease isolation (Appell and Blatt, 1992).

Grief is ongoing in working with AIDS. It is a constant adjustment process. The losses are both real and symbolic. In addition to the many losses that the patient suffers, the family experiences loss as well. Parents may be faced with losing a child. Spouses and lovers face the potential loss of a life partner. These losses are tremendous, particularly because HIV so often infects people who are quite young. So these threatened losses also challenge the hopes and future dreams of the patient and the family. Physical limitations caused by AIDS can also limit the activities the family has shared in the past. The person with AIDS and family members may also have lost other loved ones to AIDS, which decreases their support system and compounds their loss. A therapist can help people grieve by assisting them in expressing their feelings and normalizing their feelings. People often do not know how to grieve or what is normal. People often feel angry during grief; without knowing that this is normal, they may experience much guilt.

A therapist can help them talk about their feelings individually and together, as well as express regrets and remembered joys when appropriate. Not only does this help the ongoing grief process but also in the event death occurs the grief will be much less conflicted. Guilt over things unsaid makes the grief process more difficult. However, talking about loss as it occurs and death before it happens is important and healthy (Aguilera, 1997b).

Therapists must not forget their own grief. As they work with people with HIV, they care, they get attached, and they also have to let go. Therapists as caregivers should give themselves permission to grieve and get support.

DEATH

We live in a death-phobic society. The person who may be dying does the family the favor of not discussing it. The partners, in an attempt not to upset the person with AIDS, do not talk about it either. Often both parties want to talk about their feelings regarding death but are afraid. One of the most important things one can do is to help people have a peaceful closure in life. If people are not able to acknowledge or discuss death, saying good-bye when the time comes is very difficult. If one successfully facilitates these discussions, people will have the opportunity to stay connected and to say a healthy good-bye. The value of this cannot be overestimated.

Psychiatric treatment must include psychological, biological, and social approaches. The psychological sequelae of AIDS affect all people at known risk, such as homosexual men with generalized lymphadenopathy, as well as those already diagnosed with AIDS. In the AIDS patient, the impersonal aspects of the disease may be cruel and devastating. Malaise, fatigue, severe infection processes, and loss of control over excretory functions promote profound depression. This complements the intrapsychic effects of AIDS, which promote depression and anxiety, and the cognitive dysfunction, which occurs as delirious states resulting from febrile illness, meningitis, and the toxic side effects of various chemotherapeutic agents (Wise, 1986).

AIDS in the United States

AIDS is not the disease of homosexuals or intravenous drug users alone; it threatens millions of sexually active people regardless of age, gender, race, or place of residence. The disease is insidious. Transmitted during sex or through the exchange of blood (sharing needles, for example), it invades the genetic core of specific cells in the immune system. Because it directly attacks the immune system, AIDS is both daunting and deadly. Although the epidemic has spread worldwide, AIDS is an especially acute problem for all, a social and medical crisis and, according to some of the best scientific minds in the nation, a national catastrophe in the making (Conant, 1997).

The official projections for the next 10 years of the epidemic—179,000 deaths and 270,000 cumulative cases of AIDS—have been widely publicized. By the year 2000, an estimated 10 million Americans may be carrying the AIDS virus. What is less known, but vitally important, is that these projections are almost certainly low. They do not include any estimates of AIDS-related complex (ARC), a disease syndrome that is sometimes fatal in itself and almost invariably a precursor of AIDS; by most estimates, 10 times as many cases of ARC exist as cases of AIDS. Most experts in the field believe that the government's estimates of AIDS are skewed by pervasive underreporting (Conant, 1997); the real total of AIDS cases will be as much as 75% higher than the official figures. Another reason the 10-year projections may be low is that they are based on estimates of the *current* extent of the epidemic. The projections assume, perhaps unrealistically, that only those people who are already infected will develop AIDS by the year 2000 (APLA, 1997).

Who will have AIDS 10 years from now? More than 90% of the victims will be members of the two main groups, male homosexuals and intravenous drug users. However, the nation's heterosexual, drug-free majority cannot be reassured by that fact because AIDS can be transmitted through conventional sex. Heterosexual transmission is believed to have accounted for 1100 of the AIDS cases in 1986. By the year 2000, that total will probably have risen to about 7000 cases, or 9% of the epidemic caseload. Tragically, a total of 3000 infants will be born with AIDS. Babies infected with the disease at or before birth will lead short and painful lives (Frierson and Lippmann, 1987).

Many Americans have shrugged off the AIDS epidemic because it is primarily identified with homosexuals and drug addicts, an attitude that is now changing. Another reason for the nation's general complacent attitude may be the belief that science will quickly find a cure. That belief may not be warranted. Despite the optimism of many researchers and despite gains against the disease, AIDS is one of the most difficult challenges ever faced by modern medicine.

Apparently, many Americans remain confused about two key aspects of the disease. One is the relationship between infections with the AIDS virus and the onset of AIDS symptoms. For many reasons, not the least of which are human decency and compassion, many of those who are infected with the virus are told that they have a 1-in-10 to a 1-in-3 chance of contracting AIDS. The odds may be much worse; experts now believe that half of all those infected eventually develop and die of AIDS, and the actual percentage may be even higher (CDC, 1997a). The second crucial issue is transmissibility. AIDS is not easily transmitted from one person to another but it is transmitted through unprotected sexual contact, the sharing of needles, and the transfusion of infected blood. Every person who has the virus is capable of giving AIDS to someone else (Conant, 1997).

The present concern is that AIDS is on the verge of breaking out into the population at large. The source of the contagion probably will be intravenous drug users, a submerged and secretive subpopulation totaling about 1.5 million people nationwide. Intravenous drug users, most of whom are heroin addicts, are least likely to learn about controlling the spread of AIDS. Most addicts are young men with limited education, a history of criminal behavior, and only tenuous ties to the community or their families. In New York, which has the greatest concentration of heroin addicts in the nation, 60% of those addicts are believed to be infected with the AIDS virus. Assuming that most addicts are heterosexual, the next risk group will be their lovers or spouses; the infection rate among women is rising and will pass the rate of men by the year 2000 (Conant, 1997).

Those fighting against AIDS face two enemies: the epidemic itself and fear. AIDS poses profound questions to American society, and it definitely tests the nation's reserves of compassion and common sense. It has already forced millions of people to reconsider their sexual behavior and has brought the sexual revolution of the 1960s and 1970s to an abrupt halt. AIDS is raising a host of difficult legal issues about discrimination, and it may yet cause an upheaval in national politics.

The struggle against AIDS is evident daily within the nation's homosexual minority. With the disease toll mounting rapidly, homosexuals in New York, Los Angeles, San Francisco, and other cities have rallied to fight the epidemic. They have reduced their high-risk behavior—promiscuous anal sex—to a remarkable degree, and they are providing important support for AIDS victims and the worried as well. At the same time, the pall of death is omnipresent, and many homosexuals are suffering from bereavement overload (Morganthau, 1986).

Canada is far ahead of the United States in recognizing gay rights. In recent years and months, Canadian progress on homosexual rights has proceeded at such a clip that some gay activists, as well as legal scholars, say the foundations are being laid for a wholly new definition of "the family" under Canadian law, one in which men may legally marry men and women marry women, one in which same-sex couples may adopt children, receive spousal pension benefits, and generally be treated the same in all respects as traditional heterosexual couples.

"Canada is just light-years ahead of (gay-rights legal activities) in the United States," said David Pepper, an assistant to Svend Robinson, Canada's only openly gay member of Parliament. Consider the following:

- Seven of Canada's 12 provinces and territories have explicitly prohibited sexual orientation as grounds for discrimination, a high percentage compared with 7 of the 50 U.S. states that have done so.

- At a national level, Justice Minister Kim Campbell said recently that she would introduce a bill amending the Canadian Human Rights Act to proscribe discrimination against gays and lesbians. (This act has already effectively been amended by a federal court ruling.) No comparable proscription exists at the federal level in the United States, although U.S. gay activists hope that President Clinton's election heralds a long-awaited amendment of the Civil Rights Act of 1964.
- A 1990 court ruling has apparently made Canada the first country in the world to offer gays and lesbians antidiscrimination protection under national constitution.
- In October the Canadian military lifted its ban on homosexual bias in the armed forces and provided sensitivity training sessions similar to those given recruits on the sexual harassment of women.

By ending its ban on homosexuals in the military, Canada has come into step with the vast majority of armies in the Western world. It also heightened the pressure on President Clinton to make good on his campaign promise to end the Pentagon's ban on gays and lesbians in uniform (Walsh, 1992).

Homosexuals fear backlash as well. They are clinging to their gains in civil rights against an anticipated wave of prejudice, scapegoating, and stigmatization. Acutely conscious of the limits of the heterosexual majority's tolerance in the best of times, they are well aware that AIDS has reinforced their pariah status. However, the homosexual community's offensive against discrimination is going well: 33 states now include AIDS victims under laws protecting the handicapped, and others are moving in that direction. Legal experts foresee an explosion of AIDS-related lawsuits in the next 5 years (Aguilera, 1997a).

AIDS undoubtedly will become politicized; in many respects, it is the ultimate social issue, and the potential for demagogy is vast. In California, followers of the extremist Lyndon La Rouche forced an AIDS issue onto the ballot as Proposition 54, a referendum item that could have forced state public health officials to quarantine some AIDS patients. The referendum failed by better than 2 to 1, a margin that left AIDS activists cheering. However, the battle is not over. In 1988, Californians voted on two propositions whose passage may have negated the progress made against AIDS discrimination. Proposition 96, which passed, read:

Requires courts in criminal and juvenile cases, upon finding or probable cause to believe bodily fluids were possibly transferred, to order persons charged with certain sex offenses, or certain assaults on peace officers, firefighters, or emergency medical personnel to provide specimens of blood for testing for AIDS. . .

Proposition 102, which was defeated, would have required the medical community to report patients and blood donors believed to have been infected or tested positive for AIDS virus to local health authorities.

Proposition 96 could cripple the efforts of physicians, researchers, and public health officials to halt the spread of AIDS. It would only make the epidemic worse (Conant, 1997). Raising the level of public concern is essential, but it must be done without touching off hysteria.

THE AMERICANS WITH DISABILITIES ACT OF 1990

The Americans with Disabilities Act (ADA) addresses the concern that society has been inclined to segregate persons with disabilities. The ADA is a mandate to eliminate discrimination against those with physical and mental disabilities in *all* aspects of their lives. An employer, program, or healthcare provider must evaluate each person's ability to perform a given task and make *reasonable* accommodations that would allow the disabled person to perform.

Most healthcare institutions have had disability nondiscrimination. Nondiscrimination obligation can be found in Section 504 of the Vocational Rehabilitation Act passed in 1973. The ADA is modeled after Section 504 and, for the most part, the difference between Section 504 and the ADA is a change in terminology from "otherwise qualified handicapped individual" to "otherwise qualified individual with a disability."

Every court case deciding on the HIV-AIDS discrimination issue has found that people with AIDS are protected as handicapped under Section 504. Section 504 and the ADA protect not only people with actual impairments but also those with a past history of an impairment and those perceived by others as being impaired, despite the fact that the person has no past or present impairment at all (Palm, 1992). To demonstrate the extent of coverage in Section 504, Palm cites a recent AIDS discrimination case against Beth Israel Hospital. A resident teaching physician of a hospital refused to perform surgery on an HIV-infected patient. The court held that because the hospital received Medicare and Medicaid funds for services rendered, the hospital was liable under Section 504. However, the court dismissed the claim against the physician because he could not receive federal funds as a resident teaching physician. The ADA will eliminate such exclusions (Stine, 1993).

The ADA will eventually apply to all employers with 15 or more employees. It will impact nearly every local government. For large cities, the impact began in 1992; for smaller towns, in 1994. ADA will underscore the rights of the AIDS worker by utilizing the same criteria for coverage that is currently used in Section 504 of the 1973 Vocational Rehabilitation Act, but ADA goes beyond existing legislation and strengthens the rights of AIDS-infected employees in several ways. First, it is the specific intent of Congress to include HIV and AIDS as a handicap covered by ADA. Second, the legislation provides concrete examples of reasonable accommodation. Third, with the exception of drug testing, ADA will also prohibit employers from using preemployment medical examinations as a screening device. Employers will still be able to impose job-related physical examinations, but only after they have extended job offers to applicants. Moreover, AIDS-infected people will benefit from the heightened stature of ADA in that its implementation and monitoring will now fall under the auspices of the Equal Employment Opportunity Commission (Stine, 1993).

IMPACT OF AIDS ON THE HEALTHCARE SYSTEM

The expanding AIDS epidemic poses gargantuan challenges for one American institution in particular, the nation's healthcare system. Even the most conservative estimate of the 5-year outlook for active AIDS cases proves the need for changes in the delivery, financing, and character of healthcare provided to the epidemic's victims. Virtually every big city hospital in America will be treating AIDS cases by 2000, and major cities, such as New York, will be compelled to restructure their existing hospital systems to meet the rising need. At this point, real planning for the crisis that lies ahead has barely begun (Hager, 1986).

AIDS is already taking a disproportionate toll among the estimated 35 million Americans who have no medical insurance. Given the enormous expense of treating AIDS patients in the terminal phase of the disease, this gap poses three unsettling possibilities: (1) an explosive increase in billings to Medicaid, the federal safety net for the medically indigent; (2) a budget crisis for the most severely affected tax-supported big city hospitals; and (3) a drastic reduction in the level of care for most, if not all, AIDS patients (Hager, 1986).

Healthcare planners foresee much wider use of alternative-care facilities by AIDS patients, such as hospices, nursing homes, and in-home care by visiting nurses. Hospital care would be reserved for AIDS patients in acute medical crises; the epidemic's other victims would receive less intensive care. Alternative care does have its flaws. Few cities have yet established the elaborate outpatient system that will be necessary; doing so will take time, money, and effort. Nursing homes offering custodial care for the elderly are no place for young AIDS patients with Kaposi's sarcoma, and the visiting nurse programs in many cities are not equipped for the immense needs of a patient dying of AIDS-related toxoplasmosis. Many AIDS patients require 24-hour care by skilled professionals no matter where they are housed; severe nervous system impairment and dementia are commonplace when the AIDS virus invades the brain (Reese, 1986).

AIDS may well become the dominant social and political issue of the next decade, but it is first and foremost a crisis in public health, an epidemic that may be out of control. AIDS differs from other epidemic diseases in two important respects. First, as far as is known, it is fatal in every case; it may remain dormant in the body from 5 to 15 years. Second, it utterly disables the human immune system, which has always been the base of medical and public health strategies. If science cannot solve this puzzle or cannot solve it fast enough, the death toll will be enormous. Thousands have already died and thousands more will probably follow; very soon, millions of Americans will know someone who has succumbed to the disease. Without a medical miracle, tough decisions and a full measure of compassion are needed to fight this disease (Ernsberger, 1986).

Sexual Transmission of AIDS

The proportion of HIV infection and AIDS cases among the heterosexual population in the United States is now increasing at a greater rate than the proportion of HIV infections and AIDS cases among homosexuals or intravenous drug users (Friedland, 1987). In 1985, fewer than 2% of AIDS cases were from the heterosexual population; by 1989, 5% were from the heterosexual population. In 1991 7% of AIDS cases were heterosexually transmitted; that is, AIDS was transmitted during heterosexual sexual activities.

In contrast to these findings, studies in Africa, Haiti, and other Caribbean and Third World countries indicate that AIDS transmission is most prevalent among the heterosexual population. The number of men to women with AIDS in Africa is 1:1. In late 1991 the World Health Organization stated that 75% of worldwide AIDS transmission occurred heterosexually. By the year 2000, up to 90% will occur heterosexually. Homosexuality and injection drug use occur in Africa, but the incidence is reported to be very low. The high frequency of AIDS cases in Third World countries is thought to be caused by poor hygiene, lack of medicine and medical facilities, a population that demonstrates a large variety of sexually transmitted diseases (STDs) and other chronic infections, unsanitary disposal of contaminated materials, lack of refrigeration and the reuse of hypodermic syringes and needles because of supply shortages.

Transmission from men to women in Nairobi has been shown to be facilitated by common genital ulcers, the use of oral contraceptives rather than condoms, and the presence of *Chlamydia,* which probably increases the inflammatory response in the vaginal walls and increases the likelihood of having lymphocytes there that can attach to the virus and allow transmission. The damage that sexually transmitted ulcerative diseases cause to genital skin and mucous membranes may facilitate AIDS transmission. If coexisting sexually transmitted infections increase the transmission rate of AIDS, then populations with high rates of these infections are at higher risk for AIDS. Prevention and early treatment of STDs could slow AIDS transmission in the United States and in other countries.

VAGINAL AND ANAL INTERCOURSE

Among the routes of AIDS transmission, overwhelming evidence indicates that AIDS can be transmitted via anal and vaginal intercourse. In vaginal intercourse, male-to-female transmission is much more efficient than the reverse. This is believed to be caused by (1) a consistently higher concentration of HIV in semen than in vaginal secretions and (2) abrasions in the vaginal mucosa. Such abrasions in the tissue allow HIV to enter the vascular system in larger numbers than would occur otherwise, and perhaps at a single entry point.

The same reasoning explains why the receptive rather than the insertive homosexual partner is more likely to become HIV infected during anal intercourse. It appears that the membranous linings of the rectum are more easily torn than are those of the vagina. In addition, recent studies indicate the presence of receptors for HIV in rectal mucosal tissue.

Of all sexual activities, *anal intercourse* is the most efficient way to transmit AIDS (De Vincenzi and others, 1989). Information collected from cross-sectional and longitudinal (cohort) studies has clearly implicated receptive anal intercourse as the major mode of acquiring AIDS. The proportion of new AIDS infection among gay males attributable to this single sexual practice is about 90%.

Major risk factors identified with regard to AIDS transmission among gay males include anal intercourse (both receptive and insertive), active oral-anal contact, number of partners, and length of homosexual lifestyle (Kingsley and others, 1990).

Case Study   *AIDS (Heterosexual Female)*

Diane walked into a community mental health center and asked to see a therapist. She was given a brief chart to fill out and was assigned to a therapist. The therapist went out into the reception area, after reading Diane's chart, with a feeling of anger, frustration, and hopelessness, and *hoping* that it would not show.

She called Diane's name, and a very attractive young woman wearing dark glasses, approximately 5'7½" tall, slim, well dressed, with a lovely figure, stood up, walked over to the therapist, and held out her hand. They shook hands; Diane's hand was cold and slightly limp. The therapist managed to maintain her composure because she recognized her! She was a former well-known model who was doing a few small but good parts in movies and television. She asked Diane to come to her office. Diane followed her to her office.

In the office, the therapist asked Diane to have a seat. The therapist said to Diane, "I have read your chart, and it makes me angry and sad. I must let you know that I recognized you. Maybe another therapist might not know you. You may change to another therapist now if you wish."

Diane took off her dark glasses and sighed. "I really didn't think anyone would remember me. I haven't done any modeling for years, and I have only had a few very small parts in TV and a couple of movies." The therapist answered with a smile, "But you were my favorite model, your gorgeous green eyes, flowing streaked blonde hair riding a horse down a beach. I love horses!" They both laughed.

Remembering why they were there, they immediately sobered. The therapist asked Diane again, "Would you like to change to another therapist?" Diane looked at the therapist and shook her head. "No, I feel very comfortable with you and I think you like me. I don't know if anyone can help me, but if anyone can I believe it would be you." The therapist nodded her thanks and said to Diane, "Just in case someone at the clinic recognizes you we have a room upstairs where I lock your chart so no one can ever see it but me, and don't forget we have a fiduciary relationship." Diane smiled slightly and said, "Thanks."

The therapist asked, "How did you get AIDS? Didn't you use protection? Surely you know how it is transmitted." Diane said, "Let me tell you how it happened. Then maybe you won't think I'm really stupid and careless." She began talking.

She and Dave, who was also a model when they met, had been living together. She said that it was really "hate" at first sight. She felt he was conceited, all the girls chased him, and he dated first one and then another. They had a "shoot" in the Caribbean for a well-known magazine that would involve many weeks. She was thrilled that she was one of the three female models selected and Dave was one of the two men selected to go. She smiled and said that from that trip came the shot of her riding the horse on the beach. She said that when they were in the Caribbean Dave seemed so different. He was very relaxed, and he teased her. They went swimming and horseback riding, had dinner together, and were really getting to know each other. Her "hate" turned to "like" and then to "love." By the time they finished the "shoot," they were talking about living together. She said she was truly happy and he seemed happy.

When they talked about where they would live, she wanted them to live in her townhouse, but he wanted them to live in his townhouse. They were only about three blocks apart. Finally, Dave said that they could *live* in her townhouse but that he wanted to keep his townhouse. His reasons were that the "real estate market was down" and "that occasionally he liked to have his privacy." Diane said that she accepted his conditions. They moved into her house, but occasionally he would spend the night in his townhouse when he had an early morning "shoot" and she did not. They lived together in what they had agreed upon, a monogamous relationship (at least she thought they were), for a little over a year. They were both very happy. He was working more than she was. (Men can model longer than women because "they just get distinguished looking as they get older; women just get older.")

Diane said that she made an appointment with her physician because she had a discharge and it was beginning to itch. Her doctor did several lab tests on her, told her to use the suppositories he gave her, and said he would call her the next day. The next day, his nurse called her and said that the physician wanted to see her. She said that she went to his office and he told her as gently as he could that she had a yeast infection but that her blood work showed that she was HIV positive. Diane said that she could not believe it—she *knew* that she had been with only Dave.

She said she drove to her townhouse and then changed her mind and drove to Dave's. His car was in the garage, and she used her key to get in his townhouse. He was in bed with one of the new young models. "I just looked at him. Then I said, 'You bastard, you gave me AIDS.' I looked at the girl and said, 'You better get tested too!'" She said Dave got out of bed and tried to talk to her, but she said all she could think of was how stupid she had been to believe him. She said, "I really trashed his house, screaming obscenities all the time. Then I went home and started crying. I knew I had to know more about AIDS. I remembered this crisis center and I came here."

Diane needed information on AIDS. She also needed to have a buddy. Because she was probably better known than she realized, the therapist would delay getting her in a support group. She would probably intimidate the other members. She would continue seeing her in therapy until she stabilized more.

The case manager at the AIDS project was contacted and agreed to find a buddy for Diane. He also agreed with the therapist that she would probably intimidate a support group. He agreed to send all the new literature over so Diane could learn about HIV and AIDS. The therapist would remain her situational support. The main goal was to be a constant resource person to Diane, available through the exchange, day or night. She had no family and, being so beautiful, it was not easy for her to make friends.

Diane had a diagnosis of AIDS. She had been betrayed by her live-in lover. She had no situational support, this was a new situation, and she had no coping skills. She went into crisis.

Extreme remedies are very appropriate for extreme diseases.

–Hippocrates

Complete the paradigm in Figure 11-1 for this case study, then compare it with the completed one in Appendix D. Refer to the paradigms in Chapter 3 as needed.

AIDS/HIV in Adolescence

A recent survey run by *People* magazine indicated that 96% of high school students and 99% of college students knew that HIV is spreading through the heterosexual population; but the majority of these students stated that they continued to practice unsafe sex. Combined data from surveys performed in 1993 and 1996 indicate that among sexually active teenagers, only 15% used condoms. Peter Jennings stated in

CASE STUDY: DIANE

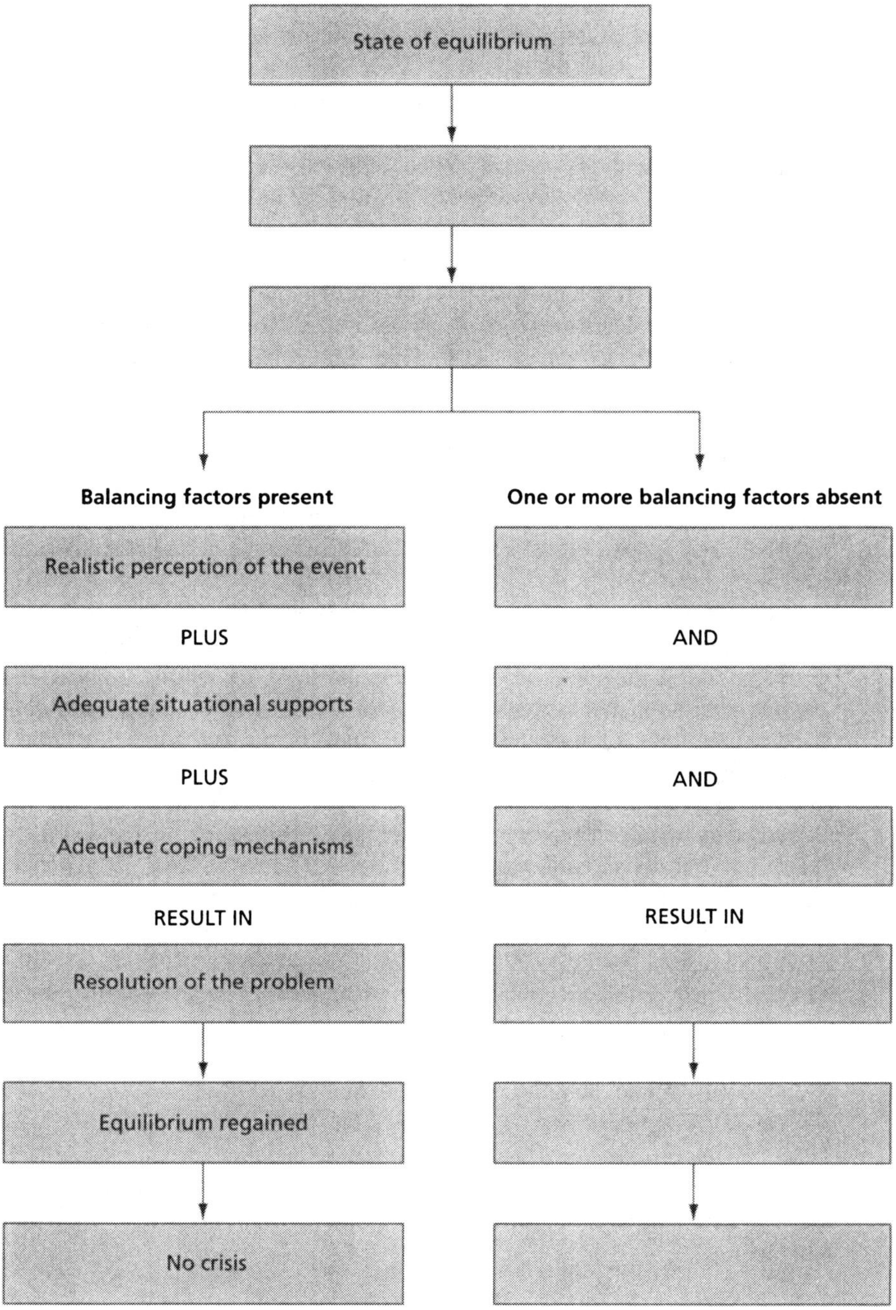

State of equilibrium

Balancing factors present

Realistic perception of the event

PLUS

Adequate situational supports

PLUS

Adequate coping mechanisms

RESULT IN

Resolution of the problem

Equilibrium regained

No crisis

One or more balancing factors absent

AND

AND

RESULT IN

Figure 11-1

a 1991 "AIDS Update" television program that 26% of American teenagers practice anal intercourse. Data such as these have prompted a number of medical and research people to express concern for the next generation. If AIDS becomes widespread among today's teenagers, a real danger exists of losing tomorrow's adults. Available data suggest that teenagers have not appreciably changed their sexual behaviors in response to HIV and AIDS information presented in their schools or from other sources (Stine, 1993).

Teenagers at high risk include some 200,000 who become prostitutes each year and others who become intravenous drug users. About 1% of high school seniors have used heroin, and many from junior high on up have tried cocaine (Stine, 1993). A large number of children from age 10 consume alcohol. Is it possible that too much hope is being placed on education to prevent the spread of AIDS? Through the end of June 1992, teenagers made up about 0.5% of 225,000 AIDS cases, or 1125 cases. Teenagers must be convinced that they are vulnerable to AIDS infection and death. Until then, it only happens to someone else. Jonathan Mann, past director of the World Health Organization, estimates that between 1 and 2 million teenagers are AIDS-infected worldwide.

Teenagers, like adults, must be convinced of their risk of infection but not with scare tactics. Behavior modification as a result of a scare is short-lived. However the information is given, it must be internalized if it is to be of long-term benefit (Stine, 1993).

Teenagers feel invulnerable. Their hormones are flooding their systems, and they are inclined to believe that they know it all. Too young to indulge legally in drinking, smoking, and having sex, they still indulge in these behaviors. It makes them feel mature, grown up, and very macho. They brag to their peers about how many beers they had, how many cigarettes they have smoked, and how many girls they "made it with." Ironically, smoking is increasing in the younger population as it is decreasing in the older population.

Statistics indicate that even though sex education classes in schools stress abstinence and the use of condoms, this education is ignored. Adolescents want to test their limits in the forbidden areas of life to prove to themselves and their peers that they are not afraid of anything (even AIDS) or anyone. The majority of teenagers do not use condoms. Why should they? After all, they know the people they are having sex with; they have been going to school together for years. Even though they may have a condom with them at the time, perhaps the last beer clouded their judgment, and they do not use it. Then they develop strange and uncomfortable symptoms, they begin to miss school, and their friends tell them they are not looking too good.

The following case study is how Jack, age 14, contracted AIDS. He trusted his older brother, Bill, so he discussed his symptoms and asked for his advice. Bill called the AIDS hot line and got the address of an anonymous test site. Jack was tested, and the test came back HIV-positive. The test center sent him to the crisis center for assessment.

Case Study   AIDS (Adolescent)

The therapist was given Jack's chart and went to the reception area to meet him. Jack's brother Bill was with him. They both looked as if they were in a complete state of shock. The therapist introduced herself to Jack; he nodded and asked if his brother Bill could go to her office with them. She replied, "Of course." They walked to the therapist's office.

After Jack and Bill sat down, the therapist said to Jack, "I see that you were referred to the crisis center by the AIDS hot line. Have you been tested?" Jack replied that he had been tested for AIDS and he was HIV-positive. He was asked if he knew the source of his infection. Jack answered, "It could only be one of three girls. I haven't been with any more." He was told that they should be notified by the health department so they could be tested for AIDS.

His brother Bill had been quiet, but he spoke up and in anger and sadness said to Jack, "How many times have I told you to *always* protect yourself. That's what condoms are for! How are we going to tell Mom and Dad?"

Jack answered, "I know I have been stupid, but I've known all three of the girls for years. I also always have a condom with me but I *hate* using the damn thing. Most of the time, I've had a few beers and the girls don't like me to use condoms anymore than I like to—so I don't." Bill replied in anger, "Yeah, and look where it got you!"

The therapist interrupted them and said to Jack, "What do you know about being HIV-positive?" He looked puzzled and said, "It means I've got AIDS and there is no cure." The therapist said, "You are HIV-positive but you don't have any of the ARC symptoms. You could go 15 years and never get AIDS. This means you can pass the AIDS virus to someone else so you will have to always use a condom or abstain."

It was obvious that he had tuned out his sex education classes. He obviously needed more in-depth knowledge of AIDS. Because Jack apparently had problems believing "adults" or authority figures, the therapist believed he could learn and relate better to his own peer group. His brother Bill was trusted by Jack, and he could be an important supporter and mediator with their parents. She planned to meet with their parents.

The therapist contacted the AIDS project and the case manager. She discussed Jack's situation and asked about informal classes with a peer support group for him. The case manager told her that he had two ongoing support groups and one that started the next day that sounded perfect for Jack. He added that they were all approximately Jack's age and all were still in a state of shock and disbelief.

The main goal was to maintain contact with Jack and Bill to determine if Jack was following through with the peer group classes at the AIDS project. She would be available to him if he had any questions. She would also meet with his family, have them come for therapy, and be their situational support.

Jack was a 14-year-old adolescent with a recent diagnosis of HIV positive. He had little knowledge of AIDS. He did not know anyone his age who had AIDS. This was a totally new situation and he had no coping skills, his anxiety and depression increased, and he entered a state of crisis.

Golden lads and girls all must
As chimney sweepers, come to dust.

–*William Shakespeare*

Complete the paradigm in Figure 11-2 for this case study, then compare it with the completed one in Appendix D. Refer to the paradigms in Chapter 3 as needed.

CASE STUDY: JACK

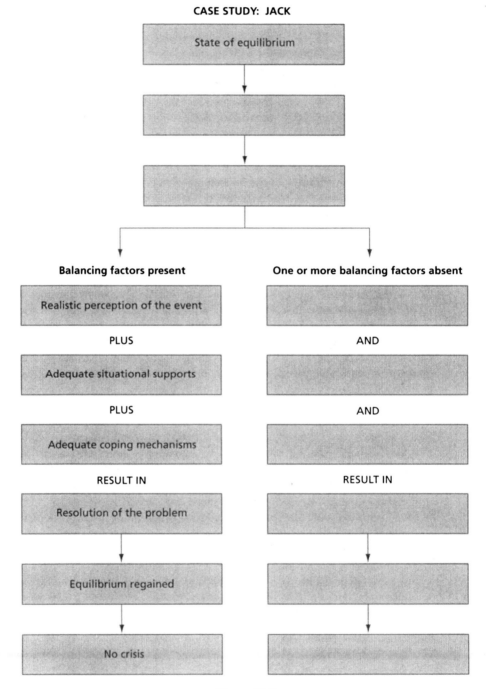

Figure 11-2

Common Questions About AIDS

AIDS is a frightening disease, but it is hard to catch and can be avoided. The following questions and answers will provide a working knowledge of the disease and how people can protect themselves, their families, and their friends from AIDS (APLA, 1997).

WHAT IS AIDS?

AIDS is the acronym for acquired immune deficiency syndrome, which results from a viral infection and most often causes death. The AIDS virus does its damage by breaking down the body's shield against disease, its *immune system*. Because they have lost this natural shield against disease, people with AIDS contract diseases that usually do not seriously harm those with intact immune systems. These diseases are called *opportunistic diseases*. Some of the opportunistic diseases occurring most often in people with AIDS include the following:

- Kaposi's sarcoma (KS), a type of skin cancer
- *Pneumocystis carinii* (PC), an organism that causes a kind of pneumonia
- Toxoplasmosis, a disease caused by a parasite that infects the brain and the central nervous system and can cause pneumonia
- Cryptosporidiosis, caused by an intestinal parasite that causes extreme diarrhea
- Candidiasis, caused by a fungus that coats the intestinal tract and is seen most often in the throat as hard, white patches of growth
- Cytomegalovirus (CMV), a virus of the digestive tract
- Herpes simplex, a virus causing the ulceration of mucous membranes as well as of the digestive and circulatory systems
- Lymphoma, a cancer that, in AIDS, affects the brain
- Cryptococcal meningitis

WHAT CAUSES AIDS?

The AIDS virus is a newly discovered type of virus called a *retrovirus*. Retroviruses are difficult for scientists to understand because these viruses continually develop new structures. This ability to change structure complicates the development of medical treatment for AIDS and frustrates the search for a vaccine to prevent it. Whether HIV is the direct cause of AIDS or if its ability to produce an AIDS infection results from a damaged immune system is not yet known. One or both of these possibilities may be true.

Scientists do not know why most of the people exposed to the AIDS virus have not yet developed symptoms. In fact, scientists believe that most of those exposed may never develop symptoms. However, scientists think that those who have no symptoms (are asymptomatic) may carry the virus for many years following their exposure to it. Some people who are exposed to the AIDS virus but do not develop full-blown cases of AIDS may develop a less life-threatening condition of ARC.

HOW IS AIDS SPREAD?

The AIDS virus does not survive easily outside the human body, and it is not transmitted through air, food, or water. People can contract the virus only by having certain body fluids (blood and semen) that are contaminated with the virus come into contact with their own bloodstreams. Infection most commonly occurs by:

- Having sexual intercourse with a person who carries the AIDS virus (this includes anal intercourse, oral-anal contact, and oral-genital contact).
- Sharing hypodermic needles and syringes with people who carry the AIDS virus.
- Receiving transfusions of blood or blood products donated by someone who carries the AIDS virus.
- Being born to a woman who contracted the AIDS virus before or during pregnancy.
- Contaminating open wounds or sores with HIV-infected bodily fluids.
- Receiving organs from an HIV-infected donor.

WHAT ARE THE SYMPTOMS OF AIDS?

Symptoms of the opportunistic diseases associated with AIDS may include:

- Swelling or hardening of the glands located in the throat, groin, or armpit
- The appearance of a thick, whitish coating on the tongue or mouth, called *thrush,* which may also be accompanied by a sore throat
- Increasing shortness of breath
- Periods of continued deep, dry coughing that are not the result of other illnesses or smoking
- Periods of extreme and unexplainable fatigue that may be accompanied by headaches, light-headedness, or dizziness
- Rapid loss of more than 10 pounds of weight that is not the result of increased physical exercise or dieting
- Bruising more easily than normal
- Unexplained bleeding from growths on the skin, from mucous membranes, or from any opening in the body
- Repeated occurrences of diarrhea

Whether or not such symptoms prove to be AIDS-related, a physician should be consulted if any of these symptoms occur.

HOW IS AIDS DIAGNOSED?

Diagnosis is based on factors that include the state of a person's immune system, the presence of AIDS antibodies, and the presence of opportunistic infections and diseases associated with AIDS.

HOW CAN PEOPLE AVOID GETTING AIDS?

To avoid getting AIDS, the following precautions should be taken:

1. Abstain from having unsafe sex.
2. When having sex, follow "safe sex" guidelines.
   - Know your partner's health status and whether he or she has other sex partners.
   - Do not exchange blood and semen.

- Limit your number of sex partners (preferably to one person who has also had no other sex partners).
- Use latex condoms.
3. Never share needles when using intravenous drugs (boiling does not guarantee sterility).
4. Do not share toothbrushes, razors, or other personal items that could be contaminated with blood.
5. Maintain a strong immune system.
   - Eat well.
   - Get enough rest and exercise.
   - Avoid recreational use of illicit drugs.
   - Avoid heavy use of alcohol and tobacco.
   - Have regular medical checkups.

People with AIDS, people who are at risk for AIDS, and people who carry the AIDS virus must not donate blood, plasma, sperm, body organs, or other tissues.

SHOULD MOTHERS EXPOSED TO THE AIDS VIRUS BREASTFEED THEIR INFANTS?

No. Breastfeeding may spread AIDS from the mother to her child.

IS A TEST AVAILABLE TO DETERMINE IF A PERSON HAS BEEN EXPOSED TO AIDS?

Blood tests that determine whether a person has been exposed to the AIDS virus are available through private physicians, hospital clinics, and blood banks, as well as most local, state, and federal health departments. The tests are designed to detect antibodies to the AIDS virus. The presence of AIDS antibodies in a person's blood means that he or she has been exposed to the AIDS virus; it does not mean that the person has or will have AIDS. Although they are highly accurate, AIDS antibody tests are not reliable in detecting infections that have been present for less than 4 months.

WHO SHOULD BE TESTED FOR ANTIBODIES TO AIDS?

Several things should be considered before deciding to be tested for antibodies to AIDS. For example:
- Testing positive for AIDS antibodies does not mean that the person has or will develop AIDS.
- Test results cannot distinguish persons who have developed an immunity to AIDS from those who have not.
- Positive test results, if leaked to an employer or insurance company, can lead to serious and prejudicial consequences.
- Use of birth control pills, alcoholism, and other factors may cause false-positive results.

However, confidential testing may be appropriate for people at risk for AIDS and/or for their partners who:
- Are considering parenthood

- Are considering enlisting in the armed forces
- Have been exclusively monogamous for a number of years and wish to disregard safer sex guidelines

WHAT IS THE RISK OF GETTING AIDS BY DONATING BLOOD?

None. Blood banks and other blood collection centers use sterile disposable needles and syringes that are used only once.

HOW IS AIDS TREATED?

Currently, no cure exists for AIDS and no vaccine can prevent it. Therapies are available to treat each of the many opportunistic diseases affecting patients with AIDS; success of these therapies varies from one patient to another.

It is possible to ease the burdens of this frightening, tragic, and often lengthy illness. Many people with AIDS, their families, friends, neighbors, and healthcare workers have made major strides by coming to terms with the feelings of fear, helplessness, and inadequacy that surround AIDS. Learning to cope with the overwhelming personal catastrophe of AIDS has also led to the recognition that other nonmedical elements are essential in the treatment of AIDS victims.

People with AIDS require not only the most advanced medicines and chemical therapies but also psychologically positive environments. The latest medical research indicates a direct relationship between a person's psychological outlook and the function of his or her immune system. The ingredients for maintaining the healthy outlook of a person with AIDS are those of any normal and healthy life. They include the following:

- Companionship
- Access to a job
- Access to social, educational, and recreational facilities
- Access to a place of worship in the community

WHAT CAN ONE DO?

The first thing is abstinence. The second thing is to practice safer sex. Know one's partner's health status and whether he or she has other sex partners. Limit the number of sexual partners, and always use condoms. A wide range of lubricants commonly used in conjunction with condoms—including Wesson Oil, Nivea hand cream, Vaseline Intensive Care Lotion, and baby oil—can cause condoms to break within 60 seconds. Safe lubricants include water-based preparations such as KY jelly and generic contraceptive gels that contain spermicide nonoxynol-9 (Parachini, 1989).

One can help prevent families, friends, and neighbors from contracting AIDS by making sure that they are informed about the disease and the way in which it is spread. If they already have AIDS, one can do everything possible to make the rest of their lives dignified and rewarding (APLA, 1997).

REFERENCES

Aguilera BA (Vice President/General Counsel, The Mirage, Las Vegas): Personal communication, January 1997a.

Aguilera CS (Chief Investigator, Orange County Health Care Agency, Public Health and Medical Services): Personal communication, January 1997b.

AIDS Project Los Angeles (APLA): Personal communication, January 1997.

Appell T, Blatt T: How HIV has changed traditional therapy, *Pacific Center J* 4:1, 1992.

Associated Press: Man of the year: 1996, *Los Angeles Times,* December 22, 1996.

Centers for Disease Control and Prevention: Update: acquired immunodeficiency syndrome—United States, *MMRW* 34:245, 1987.

Centers for Disease Control and Prevention: Personal communication, December 1997a.

Centers for Disease Control and Prevention: Public health service guidelines for counseling and antibody testing to prevent HIV infection and AIDS, *MMWR* 36:509, 1997b.

Chua-Eoan H: The Tao of Ho, *Time,* p 69, December 30, 1996/January 6, 1997.

Cohen B: The AIDS epidemic: future shock, *Newsweek,* November 24, 1986.

Conant M (Chairperson, AIDS Leadership Committee, State of California): Personal communication, January 1997.

DeVincenzi I and others: Risk factors for male to female transmission of HIV, *BMJ* p 298, 1989.

Ernsberger R Jr: The AIDS epidemic: future shock, *Newsweek,* November 24, 1986.

Faulstich ME: Psychiatric aspects of AIDS, *Am J Psychiatry* 144:551, 1987.

Friedland G: Fear of AIDS, *NY State J Med* 87(5):260, 1987.

Frierson R, Lippmann S: Psychologic implications of AIDS, *Am Fam Physician* 35:109, 1987.

Hager M: The AIDS epidemic: future shock, *Newsweek,* November 24, 1986.

Holland JC, Tross S: The psycho social and neuropsychiatric sequelae of the acquired immunodeficiency syndrome and related disorders, *Ann Intern Med* 103:760, 1985.

Johnson J: Psychiatric aspects of AIDS: overview for the general practitioner, *JAOA* 87:99, 1987.

Johnson J: AIDS-related psychosocial issues for the patient and the physician, *JAOA* 88:94, 1988.

Kingsley LA and others: Sexually transmission efficiency of hepatitis B virus and human immunodeficiency virus among homosexuals, *JAMA* 264:230, 1990.

Morganthau T: The AIDS epidemic: future shock, *Newsweek,* November 24, 1986.

Nichols SE: Psycho social reactions of persons with the acquired immunodeficiency syndrome, *Ann Intern Med* 103:765, 1985.

Palm LL: Americans with Disabilities Act (ADA): Take the first steps now, *AIDS Newsline: Mountain Plains Regional AIDS Education and Training Center,* 3:8, 1992.

Parachini A: Condom failure stressed by panel, *Los Angeles Times,* February 28, 1989.

Perry SW, Markowitz J: Psychiatric interventions for AIDS-spectrum disorders, *Hosp Community Psychiatry* 37:1001, 1986.

Purvis A: The global epidemic, *Time,* p 76, December 30, 1996/January 6, 1997.

Reese M: The AIDS epidemic: future shock, *Newsweek,* November 24, 1986.

Stine GJ: *Acquired immune deficiency syndrome,* Englewood Cliffs, NJ, 1993, Prentice Hall.

Stribling TB: *Love broke through: a husband, father, and a minister tells his own story,* 1990, Grand Rapids, Mich, Zondervan Books.

Walsh M: *Los Angeles Times,* p 1, December 29, 1992.

Wise TN: Psychiatric aspects of acquired immunodeficiency syndrome, *Psychiatr Med* 4:79, 1986.

ADDITIONAL READING

Bor R and others: The relevance of a family counseling approach in HIV/AIDS: discussion paper, *Patient Education Counseling* 17:235, 1991.

Cameron P, Playfair WL: AIDS: intervention works, "education" is questionable, *Psychol Rep* 68:467, 1991.

Centers for Disease Control and Prevention: *HIV/AIDS surveillance report* 7(1):1, 1995.

Centers for Disease Control and Prevention: Update: acquired immunodeficiency syndrome— United States, *MMWR* 34:245, 1995.

Gorman C: Invincible AIDS, *Time,* p 30, August 3, 1992.

Holtzman S and others: Changes in HIV-related information services, instruction, knowledge, and behaviors among U.S. high school students, 1989-1990, *Am J Public Health* 84(3):388, 1994.

Hunter CE, Ross MW: Determinants of health-care workers' attitudes toward people with AIDS, *J Appl Soc Psychol* 21:947, 1991.

Kessler RC and others: Stressful life events and symptom onset in HIV infection, *Am J Psychiatry* 148:733, 1991.

Mastojanni CM, Liuzzi GM, Riccio P: AIDS dementia complex: on the relationship between HIV-1 infection, immune-mediated response and myelin damage in the brain, *Acta-Neurol (Napoli)* 1:184, 1991.

Maugh H II, Times medical writer: New AIDS tests may predict disease course, *Los Angeles Times,* July 11, 1996.

Moffatt B and others, editors: *AIDS: a self-care manual,* Los Angeles, 1992, AIDS Project Los Angeles.

Moore SM, Barling NR: Developmental status and AIDS attitudes in adolescence, *J Genet Psychol* 152:5, 1991.

O'Dowd MA and others: Characteristics of patients attending an HIV related psychiatric clinic, *Hosp Community Psychiatry* 42:615, 1992.

Olsen JA, Jensen LC, Greaves PM: Adolescent sexuality and public policy, *Adolescence* 25:419, 1991.

Owen N, Mylvaganam A: AIDS prevention: epidemiologic and behavioral perspectives, *Aust Psychol* 26:11, 1991.

Power R, Dale A, Jones S: Toward a process evaluation model for community-based initiatives aimed at preventing the spread of HIV amongst injecting drug users, *AIDS Care* 3:123, 1991.

Salisbury D: AIDS psychosocial implications, *J Psychosoc Nurs Ment Health Serv* 24, 1986.

Shilts R: *And the band played on,* New York, 1987, St. Martin's Press.

Simonton SM: *The healing family: the Simonton approach for families facing illness,* New York, 1984, Bantam.

Skinner A, Walls L, Brown LS: Aids related behavioral research and nursing, *J Nat Med Assoc* 83:585, 1991.

Snell WE, Finney PD: Interpersonal strategies associated with the discussion of AIDS, *Ann Sex Res* 3:425, 1990.

Stolberg S: New AIDS definition to increase tally, *Los Angeles Times,* p 1, December 31, 1992.

Wallack JJ and others: An AIDS bibliography for the general psychiatrist, *Psychosomatics* 32:243, 1991.

Williams RJ, Stafford WB: Silent casualties: partners, families and spouses of persons with AIDS, *J Counsel Dev* 69:423, 1991.

Zimet GD and others: Knowing someone with AIDS: the impact on adolescents, *J Pediatr Psychol* 16:287, 1991.

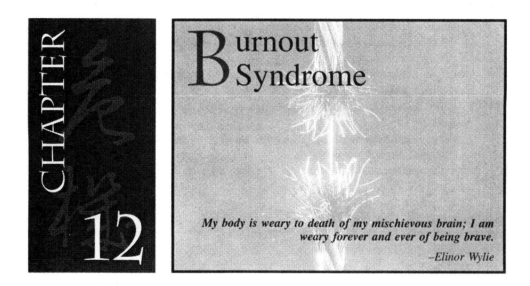

CHAPTER

12

Burnout Syndrome

My body is weary to death of my mischievous brain; I am weary forever and ever of being brave.

–Elinor Wylie

Burnout syndrome and its effects have been extensively studied; however, research has generally focused on individual response to people-based stimuli in a care-giving environment. Although Freudenberger's (1975) first definition of burnout was failure, wearing out, or exhaustion from the demands of the organization on a person's strength, energy, and resources, which suggest work environment involvement, the focal point of the burnout syndrome became the individual. His definition evolved to include loss of concern for the recipients of one's care, and emotional exhaustion (Maslach and Pines, 1977; Rogers, 1984). These dimensions have been sustained through the theoretical development of the burnout syndrome.

As many definitions of *burnout* have been proposed as are authors writing about it. Freudenberger (1974), an authority on burnout, says it is "a depletion of energy experienced by those in helping professions when they feel overwhelmed by other problems." Maslach's Burnout Inventory is an excellent verifiable instrument developed to test the degree of burnout that occurs when staff nurses show indications that they are suffering from the burnout syndrome. Nurses who work in high-stress areas such as the emergency room, intensive care unit, coronary care unit, AIDS wards, and hospice facilities should be very aware of their vulnerability (Raphael, 1983).

More recently, burnout has been defined as a syndrome of emotional exhaustion, depersonalization of others, and perceptions of reduced personal accomplishment, resulting from intense involvement with people in a care-giving environment (Garden, 1989; Maslach and Jackson, 1986; Pines and Aronson, 1981). The environment in which the work is done has received far less attention in the literature than either the individual response to pressures or job-specific aspects of the burnout syndrome (Turnipseed, 1994).

Freudenberger (1974) has identified personality types most prone to burnout:
- The dedicated and committed worker who tends to take on too much for too long and too intensely
- The staff member who is overcommitted to work and whose outside life is unsatisfactory
- The authoritarian worker who relies on authority and obedience to control others
- The administrator who is usually genuinely overworked but begins to view himself as indispensable
- The professional who tends to overidentify with those he is working with and for

Burnout and the Work Environment

Emotional exhaustion is negatively linked to peer cohesion and job structure and positively related to work pressure in the work environment. The importance of social support with respect to stress is widely acknowledged in the literature and illustrates a negative impact of support (peer cohesion) on emotional exhaustion and, thus, on burnout. Feelings of emotional exhaustion are a logical result of working in an environment that has little camaraderie or feeling of mutual support. This may be especially true for work characterized by close, constant peer interaction, such as nursing. A workplace lacking in peer support may produce emotional exhaustion whether or not it has other contributing factors, such as people-care job stresses.

Job structure and communication are also negatively related to emotional exhaustion. Constant uncertainty may contribute to emotional exhaustion. Poor or conflicting communications regarding rules, policies, or other pertinent elements of the job may aggravate the effects of the uncertainty or may themselves be emotionally draining. An uncertain work environment and a lack of stabilizing support (peer cohesion) may be sufficiently unsettling to cause exhaustion. Also, a lack of peer cohesion may alter a person's susceptibility to other negative stimuli in the workplace (Tighe, 1991).

The influence of work pressure on emotional exhaustion may be explained by mental preoccupation with the stress that is causing the pressure. A person will make conscious and unconscious attempts to reduce or remove such stressors, and, that failing, emotional exhaustion may result as time and mental resources are expended combating the stress. Work pressure may directly cause emotional exhaustion, or it may reduce the ability to cope with other workplace stimuli, which leads to exhaustion.

The work environment stress considered here is not stress of the job, but the degree to which the press of work and time urgency dominate the work climate. Consequently, for a given person, the contribution of work pressure to emotional exhaustion may be reduced or alleviated by changing jobs in the same profession. Pressure is an inescapable part of many jobs, but perhaps with careful assessment, some amount of that work pressure could be removed (e.g., reduce paperwork, reassign nonessential job duties). Also, intervention attempts to enhance coping strategies may reduce emotional exhaustion. This suggests that supervisory behavior is quite important in burnout, as supervisors have some degree of control over clarity and, albeit perhaps limited, overwork pressure in the organization.

The negative relationship of supervisor support and autonomy to burnout through depersonalization bolsters the idea that supervisory behavior is a force in the work environment/burnout pathway. Employees may view any negative supervisory behavior (or a lack of positive behavior) as a detriment to the work process. The worker may react by depersonalizing the care recipient in a defense-type reaction to insulate and protect the psyche from the person who, in the worker's opinion, is receiving suboptimal care from poor or inadequate management. Also, the worker may depersonalize the care recipient because of a lack of acceptable ways to attack the supervisor. A corollary explanation is that the workers feel a disequilibrium in their personal input/output ratio, and purposefully reduce the patients' outcomes by depersonalizing to balance the perceived deficit in the inputs of the organization (the poor supervision).

Supervisors have considerable control over the autonomy allowed; thus a lack of autonomy may be perceived as a lack of support, a lack of confidence, or a reluctance by the supervisor to relinquish any control. Workers experiencing a lack of autonomy, and attributing it to any of these reasons, may have negative feelings toward the supervisor. Depersonalization of patients may result from displacement of their anger or dissatisfaction (Turnipseed, 1994).

The importance of autonomy is explained by its positive linkage with personal accomplishment, which is a contradimension in the burnout triad (increasing amounts of personal accomplishment reduce burnout). The degree of autonomy allowed is a partial function of supervisor decisions; other determinants may include the training and competency of the worker. When management allows or fosters autonomy, it communicates a message of personal worth and competency to the worker, suggesting that at least part of any success experienced is a result of personal abilities and efforts of the employee. Also, autonomy allows workers to pursue their optimal approach to the job, with the possible benefit of increased quantity and quality of output. Logically, feelings of personal accomplishment will follow.

With the exception of work pressure, the work environment factors linked to burnout are those of job structure (clarity and autonomy) and relationships (peer and supervisory relationships), which may be relatively easily altered. They are also factors that a worker may believe should be present, positive, and supportive. When they are lacking, emotional exhaustion and depersonalization may result, at least in part, from attempts to cope with or to rationalize this difficulty.

Under the right conditions, anyone can experience burnout in his job situation. It could be a staff nurse, supervisor, psychotherapist, social worker, or anyone in a helping profession.

Stressors in Hospice and AIDS Care

HOSPICE CARE

Stressors include those factors that are part of the work environment as compared with stressors that are a function of a person's own experience. They include five important facts: (1) all hospice patients are dying; (2) their disease process presents staff with many distressful symptoms; (3) the work itself is physically and emotionally demanding; (4) many aspects of care cannot be controlled in the home because of the family; and (5) the process of integrating hospice into a healthcare system can be difficult.

The most obvious stressor is the nature of terminal illness itself. Dying patients and their families are under a tremendous amount of stress, which significantly affects the hospice staff. Most families have little experience in caring for a gravely ill person and are, therefore, apprehensive, unsure, anxious, and in need of a tremendous amount of support and assurance from the hospice caregiver. In addition, their own feelings about the impending death of a family member generates many emotions and potential difficulties with interpersonal relationships.

Although death is the ultimate loss, in the course of a terminal illness the patient and family experience many other losses. Coping with each successive one often becomes increasingly difficult for the family, as well as for the patient. Their emotional reactions are often exacerbated by previous experiences with grief and loss that may or may not have been resolved (Friel and Tehan, 1980). The needs of patients at the terminal stage are also great. Not only do they have physical symptoms to alleviate but also psychological, spiritual, emotional, and financial needs to meet.

Recognizing the impact of working with patients at only one end of the health-illness continuum is essential. The staff know and interact with families at a most difficult time in their lives. They have had no opportunity to participate in the curative treatment phase when a more positive or hopeful atmosphere prevailed. In short, the staff has no other perspective from which to work with this family. Although many rewards are associated with this work, the pain and suffering of patients and families occupy a significant portion of the staff's day. Consequently, the innumerable problems a staff member faces in caring for a terminally ill patient become major contributors to burnout in hospice care.

Organizational factors may also be considered as stressors. Hospice care requires the availability of 24-hour coverage, 7 days a week. The work is never predictable; although a team member schedules regular visits, emergencies and crises are a way of life. This translates into long workdays to accommodate unexpected needs. Flexibility and adaptability are essential personal characteristics of hospice team members.

In most home care situations, the patient is cared for by family members who, for the most part, are inexperienced and untrained. Although hospice care is predicated on the team approach, the nurse remains responsible for the coordination of care with no other shift taking over after he leaves the home. All aspects of care, including supplies and personnel, must be arranged by the staff.

The number of patients assigned to a hospice staff member, as well as the acuity level of each patient-family unit, influences the amount of stress a hospice staff member experiences. In short, the size of the caseload must be considered in relation to the severity of the needs and problems of each particular family unit.

AIDS CARE

With the prevalence of AIDS in the United States today, healthcare providers are at great risk for experiencing burnout because of many stressors: (1) fear of contagion and mortality, (2) the young age of those afflicted, (3) the inevitability of the patient's death, (4) deterioration of the patient's physical condition and psychological state, (5) the need for extra precautions, and (6) being the target of the patient's anger. The emotional and educational needs of the patient's significant others also place a burden on the health professional. Additional stress may be experienced if the healthcare worker becomes placed in the role of mediator between the patient, the patient's family, and the patient's lover (Salisbury, 1986).

Healthcare workers who have adverse feelings toward homosexuality, bisexuality, or AIDS experience additional stress. The strain is compounded when the professional tries to suppress personal feelings and attitudes to deliver care in a nonjudgmental fashion. Healthcare providers may be shunned by their families, friends, the community, and other professionals for their work with AIDS patients. They may try to protect their personal and professional lives by concealing the nature of their jobs from others. The combined stressors involved in working with AIDS patients result in an increased potential for burnout among health professionals (Nichols, 1985).

Indicators of Burnout

No one stressor is apt to cause burnout. One must look instead at the number of stressors experienced by a staff member and the extent to which individual stressors impact the caregivers. One does not suddenly "burn out"; rather, he undergoes a process marked by physical, emotional, and behavioral indicators that can be easily recognized. *Physically,* the staff member may describe a never-ending sense of exhaustion and fatigue; often, he shows symptoms of frequent headaches, gastrointestinal disturbances, respiratory problems, loss of appetite, weight changes, sleeplessness, and continual colds. He may also increase the normal use of alcohol, cigarettes, or drugs.

Emotionally, the staff member may be described as depressed, irritable, or paranoic, often with a negative self-image because he does not like what is happening or how he feels. A person may describe a sense of powerlessness and a lack of appreciation. An overall feeling of negativity prevails about changes that may be occurring within the job or about the work in general. Overall, job satisfaction is decreasing because the rewards do not nearly balance the problems.

Observable *behavioral* changes occur that include increased absenteeism, inability or unwillingness to be as productive as previously, irritability with patients and other staff members, and an attitude of omnipotence or "I can do it alone," accompanied by increasing isolation from co-workers. Nightmares about patients or about the job may occur to the point where it interferes with sleep. In the staff member's personal life, spouse, friends, or children may complain about being ignored; a major change may precipitate in these relationships. Often, the burned-out person complains about not being able to relax (Friel and Tehan, 1980).

BURNOUT PROGRESSION

Two factors are most likely to create conditions under which burnout may progress. First, therapists are vulnerable when they fail to adhere to the psychological boundaries that separate their lives from their patient's lives or when these boundaries are poorly or unrealistically defined. When boundaries fail, therapists adopt into their personal lives the emotional responses—grief, anger, fear—that patients bring to the counseling session. Although identifying with their work is often productive for therapists, psychological boundaries also protect their personal lives from being substituted by work (Tighe, 1991).

Second, unrealistic goals and expectations set the stage for frustration and burnout. Therapists are limited in what they can achieve at antibody test sites during one session; for example, if they see success as entirely changing a person's risk-taking behaviors or totally eliminating the transmission of AIDS, they will fail. A related factor is the perception that an inadequate healthcare system can never fully satisfy patient needs and therefore leaves them to therapists to resolve. By contrast, expectations of failure—for example, thinking that patients will not be able to get appropriate treatment despite referrals offered by therapists—may lead therapists to feel hopeless and powerless (Stine, 1993).

A therapist's emotional state and job performance may offer warning signs of burnout. During the early stages of burnout, therapists often report that outside work, they are listless and inactive, inclined to meet only minimal responsibilities imposed on them by friends and family, and apt to sleep longer. They are more likely to participate in addictive behaviors, such as eating, smoking, drinking, and recreational drug use.

STAGES OF DISILLUSIONMENT

The most definitive work on burnout syndrome is the text by Edelwich and Brodsky (1980). According to the authors, the four stages of disillusionment that occur are (1) enthusiasm, (2) stagnation, (3) frustration, and (4) apathy. Each of these stages of disillusionment is discussed briefly, and a fifth stage, that of hopelessness, is included, as well as some intervention techniques.

Enthusiasm.   Enthusiasm is the initial period of high hopes, high energy, and unrealistic expectations. During this period, the person does not need anything in life but the job because the job promises to be everything. Overidentification with clients and excessive and inefficient expenditure of one's own energy are the major hazards of this stage.

People go into the human services to make a living but not to make money. Although the full extent of the inequities in salaries between publicly funded service positions and jobs in the private sector may become apparent only after a person has invested years of training and work in a helping profession, the person is generally aware that such professions do not pay especially well. The motivation is a desire to "help" people. These workers become "helpers" because they really enjoy working with people and they want to make a difference in people's lives. Those who are genuinely involved far outnumber those who are cynical and self-seeking.

An important factor in bringing people into the human services is the example of others in the field. People want to be like those who have helped them. This is especially common in teaching and medicine because every young person is exposed to teachers and physicians, some of whom are inspiring models.

In other human services fields, the experience of being a patient often engenders the desire to be a helper (Edelwich and Brodsky, 1980). The experience of being helped provides the strongest demonstration of the value of helping. At the same time, it creates expectations of what it would be like to assume the role of helper.

People who have been counseled unsuccessfully do not become counselors. The people who become counselors are those who have been counseled successfully, and their experiences as cooperative patients who have benefitted from the services offered them may give them unrealistic expectations. They may expect all patients to be as receptive and resourceful as they were and all counselors to be as competent and caring as those who counseled them.

Enthusiasm comes not only from high initial motivation but also from early successes and satisfactions on the job. The new counselor or social worker, needing a certain amount of structure and supervision, tends to be put to work in environments that are safer and more rewarding than those they will face later. When the social worker has moved out into tougher, more demanding environments and has exhausted the capacity for self-reinforcement as well, he tends to look back on those halcyon days with a certain wistful nostalgia. In the stage of enthusiasm, it is commonly believed that the job is the person's whole life and that all gratifications are coming from the job. This unbalanced existence comes about by a kind of vicious cycle. On the one hand, an inflated conception of the job tends to obliterate personal needs and concerns. On the other hand, glorification of work may arise from deficiencies in a worker's personal life. The cycle of overcommitment is self-fulfilling because the longer the personal life is neglected, the more it deteriorates. The helper is thus left in a highly vulnerable position when the job ceases to furnish the rewards it once did (Edelwich and Brodsky, 1980).

Overidentification with patients is a major link in the chain that stretches from enthusiasm to burnout, both because it leads the helper to act in ways that are detrimental to patients and because it makes the helper's emotional well-being dependent on the patient's living up to unrealistic expectations. Overidentification stems from an excess of energy and dedication, a lack of knowledge and experience in the field, and a confusion of personal needs with those of patients. It manifests itself as a lack of clarity in role definitions between patient and helper. It leads well-meaning professionals and paraprofessionals to make themselves available to receive telephone calls at home at all hours of the night, a degree of accessibility that can have damaging effects on the helper's life.

The problem facing those who are dedicated to human services is to be realistic enough to cope with discouraging conditions without suffering a total loss of idealism and concern. This is also the lesson that needs to be conveyed to students and trainees. This is the area where intervention is the most crucial, especially when a person reflects that an initial lack of realism is what leaves him most vulnerable to eventual disillusionment.

Stagnation. According to Edelwich and Brodsky (1980) *stagnation* refers to the process of becoming stalled after an initial burst of enthusiasm. It is the loss of the momentum of hope and desire that originally brought the person into the helping professions.

No sharp distinction can be drawn between stagnation and frustration or, indeed, between any two of the four stages of burnout. The progression through the four stages cannot be traced in precise chronological sequence in any given instance.

When accomplishments are reduced to a human scale, minor annoyances such as low pay and long hours begin to be noticed. The frustrations that occur at this point are not enough to question doing the job, but they are enough to question doing nothing but the job. In stagnation a person is still doing the job, but the job can no longer make up for the fact that personal needs—to earn a decent living, to be respected on and off the job, to have satisfying family and social relationships, and to have some leisure time in which to enjoy them—are not being met. If those needs remain unmet, that person will not be able to keep on doing the job for very long.

Stagnation often begins with the discovery that one cannot as easily as anticipated see, let alone assess, the results of one's labors. Initially, it is experienced not as a source of active discontent but as a kind of bewilderment that leaves a person wondering why the job is not quite what it appeared to be. At the heart of stagnation lies the feeling that one's career is at a dead end (Edelwich and Brodsky, 1980).

Frustration.   In the stage of frustration, helpers who have set out to give others what they need find that they themselves are not getting what they want. They are not doing the job they set out to do. In essence, they are not really "helping." Besides the low pay, long hours, and low status, a more basic frustration in the helping professions becomes evident: people are extremely difficult to change, especially under negatively perceived working conditions.

The sensation of powerlessness is felt at many levels by people in the helping professions. Most obvious is the powerlessness felt by front-line workers who occupy the lowest positions in the decision-making hierarchy, for example, the therapist who has no way to compel his crisis patients to keep their appointments with him. Powerlessness is relative to a person's position. A frequent complaint of supervisors is that their subordinates credit them with more power than they actually have (Larson and others, 1978).

The feeling of powerlessness is universal; it goes beyond hierarchical status. Its broader implications are the inability to change the system and the inability to control patients, subordinates, superiors, or the agency. This is the frustration that leads directly to burnout.

Notwithstanding the idealism that motivates people to enter the helping professions, issues of power and control are central to the helping relationship. Some people complain that they do not have enough power; others complain that they have too much power. The unresponsiveness of the system to the people working in it is seen as a lack of appreciation. Workers who are not given responsibility, are not consulted about decisions, and are generally overlooked by the bureaucratic system will certainly believe they are not appreciated by their supervisor or by the organization as a whole.

Appreciation from patients is what enables the worker to go on despite lack of institutional support. A person can take the stress from the supervisor when appreciated and receiving positive feedback from patients. When patients, too, become unappreciative, a worker begins to question the whole purpose of being there.

The effects of frustration and of stagnation on the quality of services rendered to patients are all too evident. Implicit and explicit in the accounts of overwork, inadequate funding, staff polarization, bureaucratic sluggishness, and other sources of discouragement and demoralization among staff members is the almost inevitable conclusion that the patient is the one who suffers.

The importance of frustration in burnout lies in what a person does with it. Reaction to frustration has a great deal to do with whether the worker will fall deeper into burnout and, ultimately, leave the field. A person can respond to frustration in three ways: (1) use it as a source of negative energy, (2) use it as a source of positive energy, or (3) just withdraw from the situation.

Frustration no doubt creates energy. When it is an energy of willful denial, a frenzy of activity aimed at evading the reality of frustration or doing away with the causes of frustration that are among the givens of the situation, then it is a self-destructive, negative energy. The energy of frustration can also be directed into a constructive effort. By taking responsibility, confronting issues, and taking actions that may bring about change, a person can release some of the emotional tension created by frustration. Frustration can be a major turning point in the progression through the stages. A person who misses this turn is likely to descend into apathy.

Probably the most common response to frustration is to not express it at all, but to internalize it and withdraw from the threatening situation. The helper avoids patients, disliking or resenting them, despairs of being unable to do anything for them, or is physically exhausted. Some walk away from their jobs and from their idealism and concern. Then they may get angry, assert themselves, and get back into the center of things. Others, unfortunately, drift into the fourth and last stage of burnout—apathy (Edelwich and Brodsky, 1980).

Apathy. Apathy takes the form of a progressive emotional detachment in the face of frustration. The starting point is the enthusiasm, the idealism, and overidentification of the beginner. If one is to come down from the clouds and work effectively, some detachment is desirable and inevitable, but most people do not have ideal learning conditions and sympathetic guidance to help them reach an optimum level of detachment. Frustration comes as it will, sometimes brutally, and the detachment that develops in its wake is less a poised emotional distancing than a kind of numbness. In turning off to frustrating experiences, a person may well turn off to people's needs and to his own caring. Apathy can be felt as boredom. The once idealistic helper can trace the erosion of a previous desire to help and the feeling of involvement with patients. People who started out caring about others end up caring mainly about their own health, sanity, peace of mind, and survival.

The most severe and saddest form of apathy is experienced when a person remains at a job for one reason only—because the job is needed for survival. The person has seen what is going on but has no inclination to try to change it. Certainly, no risks are taken when the worker can just go along, protecting the position while doing as little as possible. Security has become the prime concern. Of all the stages of burnout, apathy is the hardest to overcome and the one against which intervening successfully is most difficult. It is the most settled and the most deep-seated stage, the one that takes the longest to arrive at, and it lasts the longest. It stems from a decision, reached over a period of time and reinforced by one's peers, to stop caring. In the absence of a major personal upheaval, vastly changed conditions on the job, or a concerted intervention, it can last forever.

Hopelessness.   Edelwich and Brodsky (1980) did not discuss hopelessness as a stage in the process of disillusionment; it is, however, implicitly evident in their stages of stagnation, frustration, and apathy. According to Horney (1967), hopelessness is the ultimate product of unresolved conflicts. It is a looking forward to an event or an occurrence with the deeply held belief that the anticipated will not occur.

When hope is lost, a person may be in the stage of stagnation, frustration, or apathy. Hopelessness may fluctuate throughout the stages, diminishing at times and then returning full force to make the person feel like giving up the role of helper. With hopelessness, the helper has a tendency to deny or to avoid revealing any personal thoughts or feelings that could be considered "unprofessional" and to behave instead as if in control of the situation and doing well. Failing to share true feelings with others leads to the erroneous assumption of being the only one having such problems. This error is further enhanced by the fact that the helper who believes he is alone in having these feelings will be especially careful not to reveal this response to others and will maintain the facade of professionalism (McConnell, 1982).

Avoiding Burnout

A first useful step in managing or avoiding burnout is to acknowledge the difficulties and limitations of the therapist's job: seeing patients for short periods of time, soliciting information that many consider private, and being charged with providing risk-reduction education and counseling as well as emotional support. The second step is to acknowledge the complexity of patient's lives, the fact that all of their needs and emotional concerns cannot be resolved during a single session, and the fact that therapists cannot compensate for all of the inadequacies of the healthcare and social service systems. Therapists should not excessively scrutinize themselves about what they are unable to do. Instead, they should give themselves credit for the positive work they can accomplish (Miller and others, 1990).

Therapists state that "taking care of yourself" is the most important way to maintain a healthy approach to work. This requires satisfying personal needs, which may include independence, acceptance, support, and emotional expression, as well as feeling good about oneself and one's work. Patients' needs for social services, emotional support, and information are important during therapy, but therapists should not carry their patients' burdens away from the test site. To accomplish this, therapists must set explicit psychological boundaries and review their work and behavior to make sure that they are not exceeding these boundaries.

Institutions and organizations that deal with AIDS patients have a responsibility to be aware of these stressors and to take action to prevent burnout. Weekly meetings with the staff can assist in stress management by encouraging members to express their feelings. The meetings can decrease anxiety, provide for an exchange of mutual support, and allow acceptance of the situation. The sessions can occur in the form of staff meetings or support groups. Other techniques that may prove useful in preventing burnout include relaxation exercises, assignment rotation, and scheduled time off for "mental health days."

Educational needs of healthcare workers should be strongly considered. Access to current information about AIDS and instructions on mental status examinations should be readily available. Institutions and organizations caring for AIDS patients can provide optimal care only when they take optimal care of their health professionals (Salisbury, 1986).

INTERVENTION

Intervention may be self-initiated, or it may occur in response to an immediate frustration or threat. It may be fueled in part by a person's own strength and in part by support and guidance from peers, supervisors, family and friends, or whoever else is important in his life. It may be a temporary stopgap or a real change. Intervention can and should occur at any of the four stages of disillusionment. One of the major tasks of trainers and supervisors should be to help staff members experience the four stages with greater awareness and thus be less subject to violent swings of emotion. In reality, however, intervention most often takes place at the stage of frustration, when it is almost too late. In the stage of enthusiasm, people are having too good a time to see any need for intervention. Stagnation does not usually provide the energy required to change course, although interventions in the areas of further education, skill development, and career advancement are sometimes initiated at this stage. As for apathy, that stage is already a long way toward disillusionment, and the road back up is a long, hard one that some people negotiate successfully but many never attempt.

More often, frustration moves a person off center and impels changes. Frustration is effective when it gets people angry enough to break out of a bad situation instead of becoming apathetic.

Nothing is more important in handling burnout than to know what responsibilities the worker does and does not have. Professionals are not responsible for patients or for the institution but are responsible for themselves. This does not mean that professionals do not become involved with patients or do not try to change the way the institution is run. It simply means that they are responsible for their own actions and remain responsible for their own actions regardless of what patients do or do not do.

When other systems in life are strengthened, the worker gains strength for coping with work as well. The things people do to strengthen their outside lives and create a larger world to live in vary from individual to individual. An important first step is to make a clear separation between work and other areas of life by limiting off-hours socializing with co-workers or others in the same field and controlling the tendency toward extracurricular preoccupation with job-related issues. The number of hours required at work is usually set, but the rest of the day is controlled by the person. The professional can, however, refuse to give friends and relatives free professional assistance with their personal problems. The benefits of giving a home telephone number to clients to be available to them in an emergency must be weighed against the costs.

Probably the most important way of enlarging a person's world is through close personal and family relationships. Developing and maintaining these relationships requires and, in turn, creates time commitments and emotional commitments that keep the person from being devoured by the job. It may take a lot of work to negotiate with family and close friends the space needed for commitment to the job and the space all concerned need to be together and to be away from constant reminders of the job, but by making this effort, an identity independent of the job is created. Of course, many other reasons exist for wanting to have a fulfilling personal life. With regard to burnout, however, the importance of close personal ties is clear and crucial. When one is loved and appreciated by the family, whether one is loved and appreciated by patients or supervisors is no longer a life-or-death matter. When deep and constant support of family and friends is enjoyed, a person's whole self is not put on the line every morning.

Other interventions could include the technique of planned, temporary social isolation. At a minimum, professionals need times when they can get away from those who are often the direct source of job stress—the recipients and, in some cases, the administrators. This can be accomplished through physical and psychological withdrawals and long vacations (Edelwich and Brodsky, 1980).

Another alternative is a "decompression routine" between leaving work and arriving home, a time in which they can engage in some solitary activity, preferably physical and noncognitive, in order to unwind and relax. By being alone for a while, they are then more ready to be with people again, especially with those people who are close to them.

Some helping professionals deliberately use some of their off-duty hours to engage in activities with people who are normal, healthy, and functioning well. By having pleasant and successful interactions with these people, professionals can counteract the development of negative attitudes about clients and about their ability to work well with clients.

Case Study   *Burnout*

Sabrina, a 34-year-old registered nurse, came to a community mental health center. She completed the brief chart and was told she would be able to see a therapist later that afternoon, in approximately 3 hours. Sabrina told the volunteer she would go out for coffee and come back later—maybe. The volunteer told the therapist assigned to Sabrina that she seemed "very angry."

Sabrina did return and leafed through every magazine, throwing them on the table carelessly; if they fell, she just let them lay. The therapist came out and called Sabrina. Sabrina stood up rather defiantly and looked at the therapist. The therapist introduced herself, and they shook hands. The therapist looked at the magazines on the floor and then at Sabrina, smiled, and asked, "Did you throw those magazines on the floor?" Sabrina put her chin up and said, "Yes, I did." The therapist smiled again and said firmly, "Then please pick them up and we can go to my office and begin therapy. We only have an hour and you are wasting my time." Sabrina looked slightly shocked and began to pick up the magazines. When she was through, she looked at the therapist, smiled slightly, and said, "My friends call me Bree. You can call me Bree." They walked to the therapist's office.

The therapist asked Bree to sit down, and picked up her chart. The therapist had read Bree's chart. She knew that she was 34, married, had a 6-year-old son, Brian, and was a registered nurse. Until 3 days ago she had worked as a charge nurse at a hospice. She was of average height and weight and attractive, with large gray eyes and auburn hair. In answer to the question "Why are you here?" she had written on her chart, *"I can't take it anymore!!!"*

The therapist told Bree that she had read her chart and asked, "What can't you take anymore?" Bree looked up with tears in her eyes and said, "I can't take the dying. . . not anymore, I just can't!" The therapist asked Bree to tell her what had happened 3 days ago. Bree answered angrily, "It was more than 3 days ago. I don't *know* when it began. I just walked out 3 days ago and told them I would not be back!"

The therapist asked Bree how long she had worked at the hospice. Bree said that she had been the first nurse to go to the hospice when it had opened 3 years ago. The therapist asked her how she had liked working at the hospice. Bree answered, "It was wonderful. I really *felt* like a nurse, not just a paper pusher! It was so rewarding to be able to be in that lovely hospice. The rooms were just like a bedroom in a home, not at all like a cold, sterile hospital room! The families and friends, even pets, could visit any time they wanted to; I truly loved working there. It was sad when someone died, but all the staff supported each other; we never felt that we were grieving alone." She paused and then said, "I am a good nurse, a very good nurse. I honestly think no one is a better nurse than me." She started to cry. The therapist handed her a tissue and let her cry. She finally stopped and apologized for crying. The therapist said there was no need to apologize.

Bree looked at the therapist and began talking again. She said that she did not know what was wrong with her. Lately, she had been so irritable. She said that at home "she wasn't fit to live with" and that a week ago her husband asked her to take some time off so they could go away for a few days. She said that she had lost her temper and told him that she could not take any time off because she was needed. She said he became angry and said, "We need you, too. Do you realize that we haven't had a single day to ourselves since you started at the hospice?"

The therapist asked if this was true, and Bree reluctantly said that she had been too busy. So much needed to be done at the hospice, and a charge nurse was the only one who could do it.

The therapist asked Bree, "Why do you think you are the only nurse that can take care of *everything* at the hospice? Are you omnipotent? Everyone can be replaced in their job, even you or me. Don't you care about your family? Bree, surely you have heard of burnout. It sounds to me as if you are in burnout now. No job is worth the happiness and love you have with your husband and son."

Bree had listened to the therapist quietly and thoughtfully. She then said, "I know you are right. I am so exhausted, I've been having nightmares. I wonder if I gave Mr. A or Mrs. C their pain medication so I go back to the hospice to check, and I *had* given them their meds. It's just that I hate to fail! I have never failed before."

The therapist said, "Bree, you have not failed. I doubt if many nurses could work in a hospice as long as you did; 3 years is a long time. I know *I* couldn't. Bree, could you take a 3-month leave of absence from nursing, and that includes the hospice? You need a good rest, and you need to get to know your family. You are young, and you need to have some fun in your life. Would you go home and talk to your husband about it? Call me and let me know what he says, and I'll see you next week. Try taking a brisk 2-mile walk every day to relieve your excess energy."

Bree said, "I don't know what I would do with 3 months off. I'll talk to Patrick and then call you." The therapist said, "Good, let's make an appointment for next week!" They walked out of the office together, talking as they went, to schedule an appointment for Bree.

Bree was apparently suffering from burnout. She needed time off from the hospice and nursing. She was concerned that no one could take her place. It was felt that meeting and talking with her husband to get feedback from him was important. It was essential to find out how he felt about her taking a 3-month leave of absence.

Bree called the therapist and said that she had talked with Patrick and that he wanted to talk to the therapist. The therapist said, "Fine, Bree, put him on the telephone." Patrick took the phone and said hello to the therapist. He then said, "I can't believe that anyone could convince Bree that the hospice would not fall apart without her. I have got to meet you!" The therapist laughed and replied, "You read my mind. Could you come in with Bree next week?" Patrick said, "You can bet on it!"

The therapist continued to see Bree and Patrick together for the remaining sessions. Patrick had been very concerned about Bree and agreed with the therapist that she was suffering from burnout. Eventually, Bree began to relax. She began spending more time with their son, Brian, and he began to bloom with her attention, as did Patrick. At their last session, Bree said happily, "I have asked for a transfer out of the hospice—and I'm going to be working a 'normal' shift in pediatrics. I told my supervisor that I would work in the hospice for 1 week at a time—if I was needed and only if I was needed."

Both Bree and Patrick were told that they could return to the center around any future crisis. The therapist cautioned Bree about becoming so involved with her work that it controlled her life completely. Bree agreed and said that she loved going into pediatrics. She was reminded to continue taking her 2-mile walks, as often as possible, to help her burn off her excess energy.

Bree did not recognize her symptoms of burnout. She refused the support of her husband. Her coping mechanisms were ineffective in this situation. Her anxiety and depression increased. She had burnout and went into a crisis.

Take rest; a field that has rested gives a bountiful crop.

–Ovid

Complete the paradigm in Figure 12-1 for this case study, then compare it with the completed one in Appendix D. Refer to the paradigms in Chapter 3 as needed.

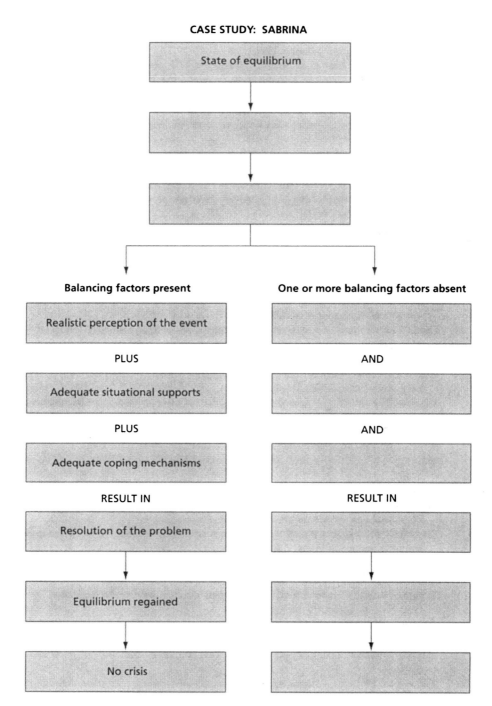

Figure 12-1

REFERENCES

Cameron M: The moral and ethical component of nurse-burnout, *Nurs Manage* 17:42B, 1986.

Edelwich J, Brodsky S: *Burn-out: stages of disillusionment in the helping professions,* New York, 1980, Human Sciences Press.

Freudenberger HJ: Staff burn-out, *J Soc Issues* 30:159, 1974.

Freudenberger HJ: The staff burnout in alternative institutions, *Psychother* 12:73, 1975.

Friel M, Tehan C: Counteracting burn-out for the hospice care-giver, *Cancer Nurs* 3:258, 1980.

Fulton R, Fulton J: A psychosocial aspect of terminal care: anticipatory grief, *Omega* 2:91, 1971.

Garden AM: Burnout: the effect of psychological type on research findings, *J Occup Psychol* 62:223-235, 1989.

Horney K: *Feminine psychology,* New York, 1967, WW Norton.

Larson C, Gilbenson D, Powell J: Therapist burn-out: perspectives on a critical issue, *Soc Casework* 59:563, 1978.

Maslach C, Jackson SE: Burned out cops and their families, *Psychol Today* 12:59, 1979.

Maslach C, Pines A: The burnout syndrome in the day care setting, *Child Care Q* 6:100, 1977.

McConnell E: *Burnout in the nursing profession,* St. Louis, 1982, Mosby.

Miller EN and others: Neuropsychological performance in HIV-1 infected homosexual men: the Multicenter AIDS Cohort Study (MACS), *Neurology* 40:197, 1990.

Nichols SE: Psychological reactions of persons with the acquired immunodeficiency syndrome, *Am Intern Med* 103:765, 1985.

Parkes CM: Terminal care: evaluation of in-patient care at St. Christopher's Hospice, *Postgrad Med J* 55:517, 1979.

Pines AM, Aronson E: *Burnout,* New York, 1981, Free Press.

Rando T: A comprehensive analysis of anticipatory grief. In *Loss and anticipatory grief,* Lexington, Mass, 1986, Heath.

Ransford E, Smith M: Grief resolution among the bereaved in hospice and hospital wards, *Soc Sci Med* 32:295, 1991.

Raphael B: *The anatomy of bereavement,* New York, 1983, Basic Books.

Rogers DP: Helping employees cope with burnout, *Business* 22:3, 1984.

Salisbury DM: AIDS psychosocial implications, *J Psychosoc Nurs Ment Health Serv* 24:13, 1986.

Stine G: *Acquired immune deficiency syndrome,* Englewood Cliffs, NJ, 1993, Prentice Hall.

Tighe JB: Taking control, focus: a guide to AIDS research and counseling, *California Department of Health Services* 6:2, 1991.

Turnipseed DL: An analysis of the influence of work environment variables and moderators on the burnout syndrome, *J Appl Soc Psychology* 24(9):782, 1994.

ADDITIONAL READING

Bruning-Nealia S: Gender differences in burnout: observations from an "unbiased" researcher, *Can Psychol* 32(4):575, 1991.

Cherniss C: Long-term consequences of burnout: an exploratory study, *J Organ Behav* 13(11):1, 1992.

Day HI, Chambers J: Empathy and burnout in rehabilitation counselors, *Can Rehab* 5(1):33, 1991.

Eichinger J, Heifetz LJ, Ingraham C: Situational shifts in sex role orientation: correlates of work satisfaction and burnout among women in special education, *Sex Roles* 25(7-8):425, 1991.

Green DE, Walkey FH, Taylor AJ: The three-factor structure of the Maslach Burnout Inventory: a multicultural, multinational confirmatory study, *J Soc Behav Pers* 6(3):453, 1991.

Greenglass BR: Burnout and gender: theoretical and organizational implications, *Can Psychol* 32(4):562, 1991.

Jayaratne S, Himle DP, Chess WA: Job satisfaction and burnout: is there a difference? *J Appl Soc Sci* 15(2):245, 1991.

Kruger LJ, Botman HI, Goodenow C: An investigation of social support and burnout among residential counselors, *Child Youth Care Forum* 20(5):335, 1991.

Leiter M: The dream denied: professional burnout and constraints of human service organizations, *Can Psychology* 32(4):547, 1991.

Naisberg-Fennig S and others: Personality characteristics and proneness to burnout: a study among psychiatrists, *Stress Med* 7(4):201, 1991.

Revenson TA, Cassel BJ: An exploration of leadership in a medical mutual help organization, *Am J Community Psychol* 19(5):683, 1991.

Rosse JG and others: Conceptualizing the role of self-esteem in the burnout process, *Group Organization Stud* 16(4):428, 1991.

Seidman SA, Zager J: A study of coping behaviours and teacher burnout, *Work Stress* 5(3):205, 1991.

POSTSCRIPTUM

Patients and mental health professionals in the next century can look forward to not only bright hopes but also many challenges and confrontations. No, I do not have a crystal ball. What I do have are some solid predications from impeccable sources—Harvard University and the World Health Organization.

Richmond and Harper (1996)* state that the following needs for child and adolescent psychiatry will be priorities for the next generation of professionals. *First*, a commitment to equity is necessary so that all children and families have access to services. *Second*, a greater emphasis on health promotion and prevention is in order. Professional activities that apply knowledge are needed to influence not only healthcare policy but also social policy recommendations as well, since much of prevention and health promotion requires improving the environments of children and families. *Third*, an awareness of resource limits will be needed by those who seek to improve the lives of children. *Fourth*, research support must continue if interventions are to improve. Research is the engine of change.

Professional organizations will have to reaffirm their social responsibilities by emphasizing priorities and social roles:

- The maintenance of professional standards and ethics
- Social conscience; individual strategies must become essential to preserve professional ethical standards
- Advocacy for the whole child, for an integrated biopsychosocial approach, and for community interventions
- Partnership in advocacy; alliances with groups that represent the public interest will make for more effective advocacy

Our Children Are Our Future

A 5-year study by an international team at Harvard University School of Public Health stated that the causes of death and disability will change dramatically by the year 2020 (Maugh, 1996†). The study is called "The Global Burden of Disease" by the World Health Organization. When the study is completed, they are projecting ten volumes. The first two volumes of results compares the statistics of death in 1990 with the projected statistics of 2020.

---

*Richmond J, Harper G: Child and adolescent psychiatry: toward the twenty first century, *Harvard Rev Psychiatry* 4(2):51, 1996.

†Maugh TH II, Times medical writer: World-wide study finds big shift in causes of death, Los Angeles Times, September 16, 1996.

For comparison the first two diseases are listed below.

1990 RANK	DISEASE OR INJURY	2020 RANK	DISEASE OR INJURY
1	Lower respiratory infections	1	Ischemic heart disease
2	Diarrheal disease	2	Unipolar major depression

It should be apparent why only two comparisons were necessary. Unipolar major depression is the number two disease predicted for future professionals to work with.

Let us not forget our *hopes:* the gene theories and therapies that are even now being discovered and utilized in identifying and preventing multitudes of diseases and the brain that rules the body in finally giving up its secrets. Pharmaceutical companies are working day and night to find medications that will prevent, cure, or inoculate against every known illness.

Our challenges and confrontations will occur when as mental health professionals we become entrepreneurs and have our own offices and care for patients with minimal supervision of physicians. We will be collaborators; we will work *with* them not *for* them. It is possible to work together with other professionals; we do research with them now on equal terms.

Our major confrontation will be managed healthcare providers. They will either be the only providers or the public will demand that we return to individual care from our physicians. They will either continue to proliferate and function as a closed "union" or they will be eliminated because of lack of care and financial abuses. It is strongly anticipated that the public will begin to demand that payment for mental healthcare be equated with that for physical healthcare.

We will eventually be accepted by managed healthcare providers. We will receive not only acceptance but also recognition that our expertise is worthy of a quality standard salary.

> *O magic sleep! O comfortable bird,*
> *That broodest o'er the troubled sea of the mind*
> *Till it is hush'd and smooth!*
>
> *–John Keats*

APPENDIX A

Disciplinary Key

ACCUSATION

refers to the formal document or pleading that officially initiates the licensing board's action against the respondent and specifies the unprofessional conduct alleged. The accusation is served on the respondent after an investigation by the Department of Consumer Affairs' Division of Investigation and after a review of the investigative report by the board and the attorney general's office.

DECISION

refers to the written decision of the administrative law judge who decides the case and imposes the discipline, if any, after the hearing has been held and the testimony of all witnesses have been received.

DEFAULT DECISION

refers to the situation whereby the respondent, after being served with the accusation, fails to respond by filing the required notice of defense, therefore resulting in a decision by the administrative law judge. Additionally, a default decision can also occur when the respondent, after filing the notice of defense, fails to attend the administrative hearing.

NO CONTEST

refers to the response to an accusation that neither admits nor denies the charges but simply says that the respondent does not wish to contest or argue with the charges. No contest usually results in the imposition of disciplinary action through a stipulated agreement. The major purpose of entering a no contest *(nolo contendere)* response is to avoid future civil liability based on the board's action.

NON-ADOPTED DECISION

refers to the situation whereby the administrative law judge has rendered a decision, but the board later votes not to adopt the judge's decision. The board may thereafter decide the case and impose the penalties that they believe are appropriate under the circumstances.

PUBLIC REPROVAL

refers to the situation where the board has not imposed any period of suspension of the license but has decided to make public the fact that the respondent has been disciplined for some usually minor form of unprofessional conduct or for misconduct that is mitigated by other facts and circumstances.

RESPONDENT

refers to the licensee or registrant who is charged with unprofessional conduct.

REVOCATION

refers to the most severe action that can be taken by the licensing board. Once a license is revoked, the respondent may get the license back only by petitioning the board for reinstatement after the passage of a specific amount of time and with a sufficient showing of rehabilitation.

STAYED (STAY)

refers to an action that puts the imposition of the penalty on hold, provided that the respondent complies with certain probationary terms. "Revocation stayed" therefore means that the license is not actually revoked, but if the respondent violates the terms or conditions of probation, the stay can be lifted and the imposition of the revocation can then occur.

STIPULATION

refers to a written agreement between the respondent and the licensing board that settles the matter. The stipulation typically includes an admission of wrongdoing by the respondent to one or more charges and also includes the specific disciplinary action (punishment) to be imposed.

SURRENDER OF LICENSE

refers to the situation whereby a licensee decides to surrender the license. The surrender of license usually results in the licensing board dropping the charges before any hearing is held. Surrendered licenses cannot be restored through the petition process, and generally, once surrendered, the license is gone forever.

SUSPENSION

refers to the temporary loss of license or registration for the time specified. Once the period of suspension has expired, the license or registration is automatically restored. The respondent does not have to petition the board for reinstatement.

APPENDIX B

Descriptive Terms Applicable To A Mental Status Examination

Characteristics	Normal	Abnormal
APPEARANCE AND BEHAVIOR		
Posture	Normal	Rigid, limp, ill-at-ease, bizarre
Gestures	Appropriate	Hyperactive, agitated, fidgeting, hand-wringing, picking, touching, violent, purposeless, tics, twitches, clumsy, bizarre
Grooming (hair, nails)	Neat and well groomed	Slovenly, meticulously clean
Dress	Appropriate, casual but clean	Careless, seductive, dirty, inappropriate, bizarre
Facial expression	Appropriate	Dazed, perplexed, grimacing, poor eye contact, staring, lip smacking
Speech		
Pace	Normal	Pressured, retarded, halting, blocking, mute, stuttering
Volume	Normal	Very loud or soft, monotonous
Form	Logical, coherent	Illogical, rambling, incoherent, tangential, circumstantial
Clarity	Clear	Slurred, garbled
Content	Normal, unremarkable	Flight of ideas, word salad, loose associations, rhyming, echolalia neologisms, obscene
ATTITUDE AND SENSORIUM		
Attention	Normal span, alert	Short span, hyperalert, fluctuating, drowsy, easily distracted
Mood	Cheerful, friendly, happy	Elated, euphoric, agitated, fearful, anxious, panicky, hostile, apathetic, sad
Affect	Appropriate	Inappropriate, intense, shallow, flat, blunted, labile, indifferent
PERCEPTION AND THOUGHT		
Hallucinations		
Auditory		Own voice, another's, many; talking to/about patient; flattering, accusatory, directive

Continued

287

Characteristics	Normal	Abnormal
PERCEPTION AND THOUGHT—CONT'D		
Hallucinations—cont'd		
Visual		Shadows, lights, halos, forms, figures
Tactile/		
Somatesthetic		
Gustatory		
Olfactory		
Delusions		Paranoid/persecutory, grandeur, reference, alien control, guilt, nihilism, thought insertion/broad cast/withdrawal
Illusions		Visual, auditory
Other		Derealization, autistic thinking, phobias, ambivalence, obsessions, compulsions, ruminations, suicidal/homicidal ideation or plans
ORIENTATION	Oriented × 3	Disoriented to time, place, and person (others, familiar others, self)
JUDGMENT	Intact	Impaired
COGNITION		
Memory, short-term	Intact	Impaired
Immediate recall	Good	Poor (digit span of 5 or less)
Reversals	Good	Poor (digits backward of 4 or less)
Concentration	Good	Poor
Calculations	Good	Poor
ABSTRACTION		
Similarities	Handled well	Poor, bizarre responses
Absurdities	Recognized	Not recognized, poorly handled
Proverb interpretation	Good, appropriate	Literal, semiconcrete, concrete, bizarre
INSIGHT	Good, excellent	Fair, poor, absent

APPENDIX C

Parent Support Groups

National Self-Help Clearinghouse
CUNY Graduate Center, 1206A
33 West 42nd Street
New York, NY 10036
(212) 840-1259

Provides the best means of finding national self-help, mutual-aid groups.

SHARE, c/o Sister Jane Marie Lamb
Saint John's Hospital
800 East Carpenter Street
Springfield, IL 62769
(217) 544-6464, ext. 5275

Provides a list of national groups for parents who have experienced miscarriage, stillbirth, or newborn loss.

The Compassionate Friends, Inc.
PO Box 3696
Oak Brook, IL 60522-3696
(313) 323-5010

Provides a list of self-help groups for bereaved parents who can help each other after the loss of an infant or an older child.

Pregnancy-Loss Peer-Support Program
National Council of Jewish Women (New York Section)
9 East 69th Street
New York, NY 10021 (212) 535-5900, ext. 16

A nonsectarian support service for parents who have suffered pregnancy loss or stillbirth. Parent support groups meet weekly for 6 weeks and are facilitated by trained volunteers who have also experienced pregnancy loss. Telephone counseling is also available.

Bereavement Clinic
c/o Sharon Pentel
Downstate Medical Center
450 Clarkson Avenue
Brooklyn, NY 11203

Offers monthly support groups, led by a professional, for parents who have suffered stillbirth.

Pastoral Care
c/o Sister Mary Alice
Mercy Hospital
North Village Avenue
Rockville Center, NY 11570

A bereavement group that meets twice monthly for 8 to 10 weeks for parents who have suffered miscarriage or stillbirth.

Pregnancy and Infant Loss Center
1415 East Wayzata Blvd, #2
Wayzata, MN 55391
(612) 473-9372—24-hour Help Line (612) 292-1184

A nonprofit organization offering support, resources, and education on miscarriage, stillbirth, and infant death; publishes a newsletter, "Loving Arms."

Reach Out to Parents of an Unknown Child
c/o Health House
555 North Country Road
Saint James, NY 11780
(516) 862-6743

Offers voluntary support groups of parents who have experienced unexpected loss through miscarriage, stillbirth, or infant death. Groups are also available for a subsequent pregnancy. Telephone contacts are also available.

RESOLVE, Inc.
5 Water Street
Arlington, MA 02174
(617) 643-2424

A nonprofit organization offering counseling, referral, and support groups to people with problems of infertility and miscarriage. Telephone counseling is available. Based in Boston, RESOLVE has 46 affiliated chapters nationwide.

COPING
Santa Barbara Birth Resource Center
2255 Modoc Road
Santa Barbara, CA 93101
(805) 682-7529

Their goal is to offer comfort to people suffering from intrauterine and neonatal grief; they also provide support for those who are experiencing a loss and for those planning or going through a subsequent pregnancy.

UNITE (Understanding Newborns in Traumatic Experiences)
Jeannes Hospital
7600 Central Avenue
Philadephia, PA 19111
(215) 728-2082, or -3777

Offers support groups for parents within the area who have experienced miscarriage or infant death. For copies of their quarterly newsletter, send $5 to Department of Social Services at the address above.

ICU (Intensive Caring Unlimited)
c/o Diane Sweeney
1844 Patricia Avenue
Willow Grove, PA 19090

Offers support groups for parents of children born premature or at high risk or for those who have lost a child. They publish a newsletter and send out a packet of reprint articles for parents who have experienced miscarriage, stillbirth, and loss of a baby or child.

DAD (Depression after Delivery)
Contact: Nancy Berchtold
PO Box 1282
Morrisville, PA 19067
(215) 295-3994

Offers parent support groups for those experiencing postpartum depression or depression after miscarriage or infant loss. A nationwide referral service and telephone counseling are available.

Grieving Process Group
Booth Maternity Center
6051 Overbrook Avenue
Philadelphia, PA 19131
(215) 878-7800, ext. 658

Other Related Support Groups and Services

Sudden Infant Death Syndrome (SIDS)
Regional Center
School of Social Welfare
HSC L2 Room 099
SUNY at Stony Brook
Stony Brook, NY 11794
(516) 246-2582

SIDS Counseling Program
520 First Avenue
New York, NY 10016
(212) 868-8854

National SIDS Clearinghouse
1555 Wilson Boulevard, #600
Rosslyn, VA 22209
(703) 528-8480

Bereavement and Loss Center of New York
170 East 83d Street
New York, NY 10028
(212) 879-5655

Perinatal Loss
2116 NE 18th Avenue
Portland, OR 97212
(503) 284-7426

Hot Lines

Pregnancy/Environmental Hot Line National Birth Defects Center
Kennedy Memorial Hospital
Boston, Massachusetts

They will accept calls from practitioners nationally: 800-322-5014
(Massachusetts only) 617-787-4957

Pregnancy Exposure Information Service
University of Connecticut Health Center
Farmington, Connecticut only: 800-325-5391

Washington State Poison Control Network
University of Washington
Seattle: 800-732-6985
(Washington only) 206-526-2121

APPENDIX D

Completed Case Study Paradigms

CASE STUDY: JENNINE

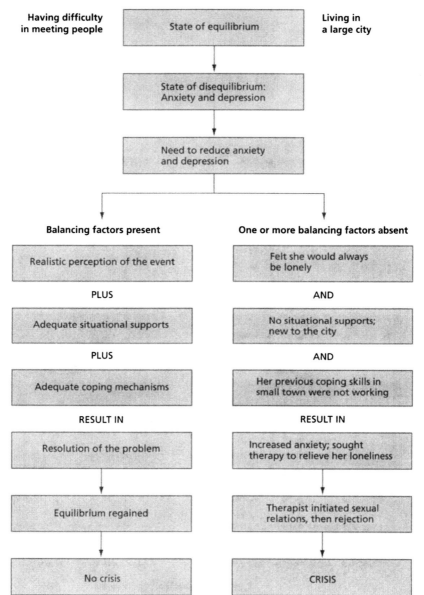

Having difficulty in meeting people — State of equilibrium — **Living in a large city**

State of disequilibrium: Anxiety and depression

Need to reduce anxiety and depression

Balancing factors present

Realistic perception of the event

PLUS

Adequate situational supports

PLUS

Adequate coping mechanisms

RESULT IN

Resolution of the problem

Equilibrium regained

No crisis

One or more balancing factors absent

Felt she would always be lonely

AND

No situational supports; new to the city

AND

Her previous coping skills in small town were not working

RESULT IN

Increased anxiety; sought therapy to relieve her loneliness

Therapist initiated sexual relations, then rejection

CRISIS

Corresponds with Figure 4-1

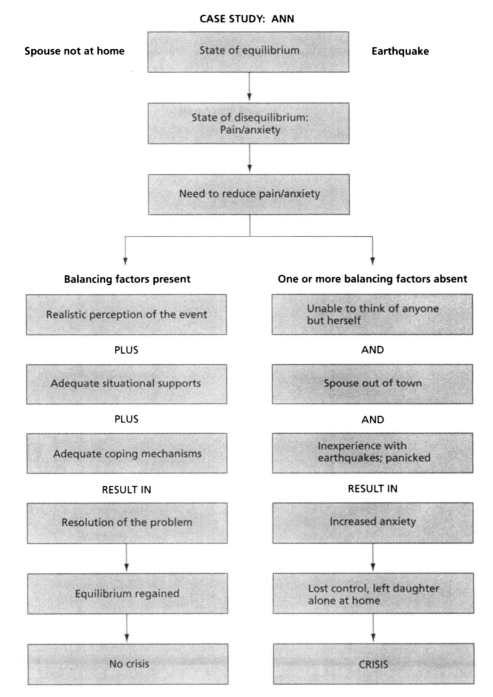

CASE STUDY: ANN

Spouse not at home — State of equilibrium — Earthquake

State of disequilibrium: Pain/anxiety

Need to reduce pain/anxiety

Balancing factors present

Realistic perception of the event

PLUS

Adequate situational supports

PLUS

Adequate coping mechanisms

RESULT IN

Resolution of the problem

Equilibrium regained

No crisis

One or more balancing factors absent

Unable to think of anyone but herself

AND

Spouse out of town

AND

Inexperience with earthquakes; panicked

RESULT IN

Increased anxiety

Lost control, left daughter alone at home

CRISIS

Corresponds with Figure 5-1

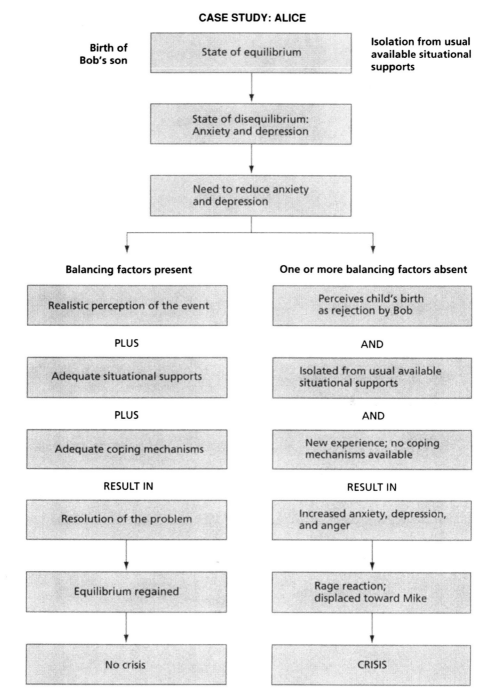

CASE STUDY: ALICE

Birth of
Bob's son

State of equilibrium

Isolation from usual
available situational
supports

State of disequilibrium:
Anxiety and depression

Need to reduce anxiety
and depression

Balancing factors present

Realistic perception of the event

PLUS

Adequate situational supports

PLUS

Adequate coping mechanisms

RESULT IN

Resolution of the problem

Equilibrium regained

No crisis

One or more balancing factors absent

Perceives child's birth
as rejection by Bob

AND

Isolated from usual available
situational supports

AND

New experience; no coping
mechanisms available

RESULT IN

Increased anxiety, depression,
and anger

Rage reaction;
displaced toward Mike

CRISIS

Corresponds with Figure 6-1

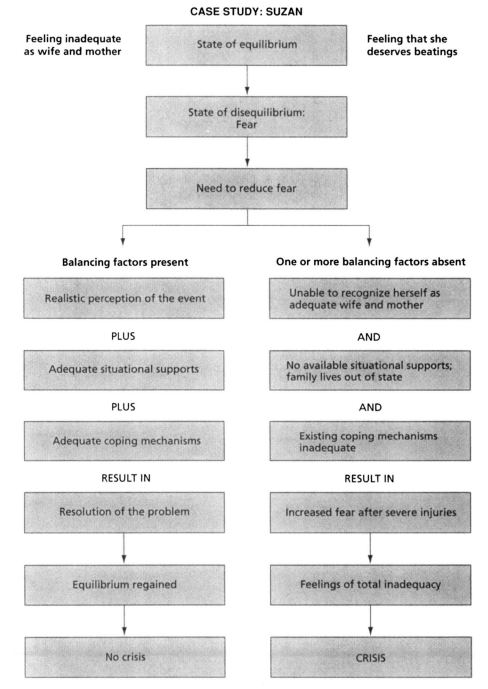

CASE STUDY: SUZAN

Feeling inadequate
as wife and mother

State of equilibrium

Feeling that she
deserves beatings

State of disequilibrium:
Fear

Need to reduce fear

Balancing factors present

Realistic perception of the event

PLUS

Adequate situational supports

PLUS

Adequate coping mechanisms

RESULT IN

Resolution of the problem

Equilibrium regained

No crisis

One or more balancing factors absent

Unable to recognize herself as
adequate wife and mother

AND

No available situational supports;
family lives out of state

AND

Existing coping mechanisms
inadequate

RESULT IN

Increased fear after severe injuries

Feelings of total inadequacy

CRISIS

Corresponds with Figure 6-2

CASE STUDY: RICARDO

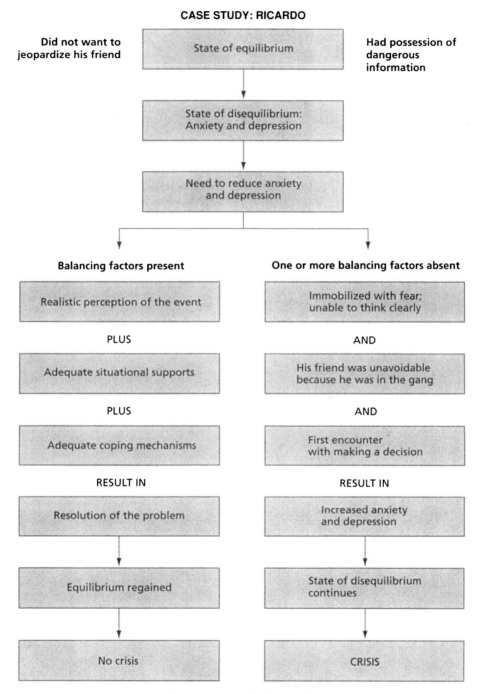

Did not want to jeopardize his friend

State of equilibrium

Had possession of dangerous information

State of disequilibrium:
Anxiety and depression

Need to reduce anxiety
and depression

Balancing factors present

Realistic perception of the event

PLUS

Adequate situational supports

PLUS

Adequate coping mechanisms

RESULT IN

Resolution of the problem

Equilibrium regained

No crisis

One or more balancing factors absent

Immobilized with fear;
unable to think clearly

AND

His friend was unavoidable
because he was in the gang

AND

First encounter
with making a decision

RESULT IN

Increased anxiety
and depression

State of disequilibrium
continues

CRISIS

Corresponds with Figure 6-3

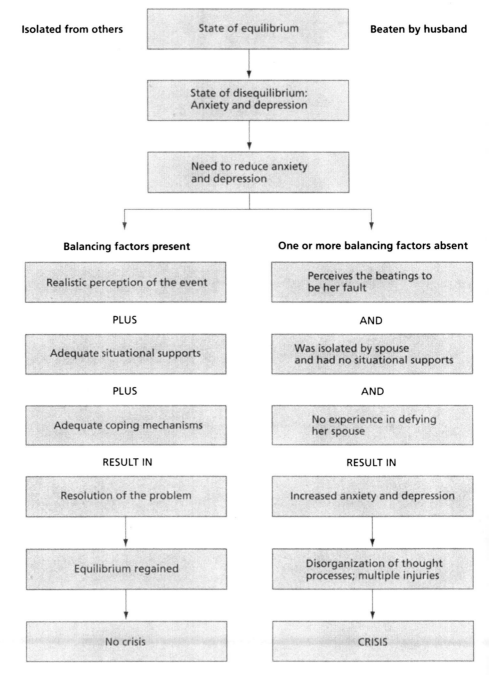

CASE STUDY: HATTIE

Isolated from others · State of equilibrium · Beaten by husband

State of disequilibrium:
Anxiety and depression

Need to reduce anxiety
and depression

Balancing factors present · One or more balancing factors absent

Realistic perception of the event · Perceives the beatings to be her fault

PLUS · AND

Adequate situational supports · Was isolated by spouse and had no situational supports

PLUS · AND

Adequate coping mechanisms · No experience in defying her spouse

RESULT IN · RESULT IN

Resolution of the problem · Increased anxiety and depression

Equilibrium regained · Disorganization of thought processes; multiple injuries

No crisis · CRISIS

Corresponds with Figure 6-4

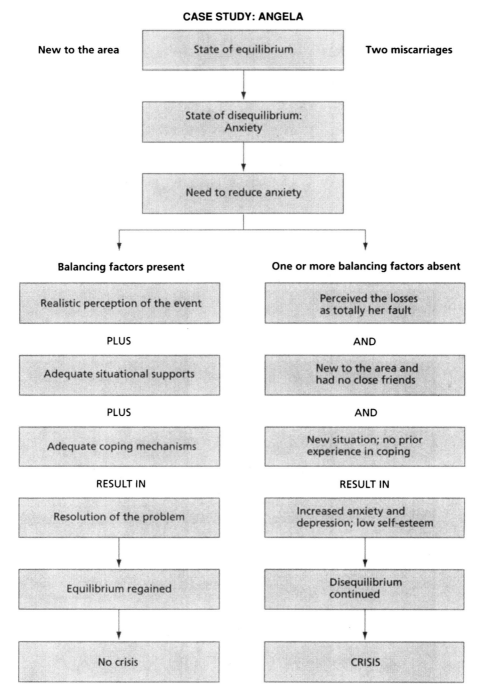

CASE STUDY: ANGELA

New to the area

State of equilibrium

Two miscarriages

State of disequilibrium:
Anxiety

Need to reduce anxiety

Balancing factors present

Realistic perception of the event

PLUS

Adequate situational supports

PLUS

Adequate coping mechanisms

RESULT IN

Resolution of the problem

Equilibrium regained

No crisis

One or more balancing factors absent

Perceived the losses
as totally her fault

AND

New to the area and
had no close friends

AND

New situation; no prior
experience in coping

RESULT IN

Increased anxiety and
depression; low self-esteem

Disequilibrium
continued

CRISIS

Corresponds with Figure 7-1

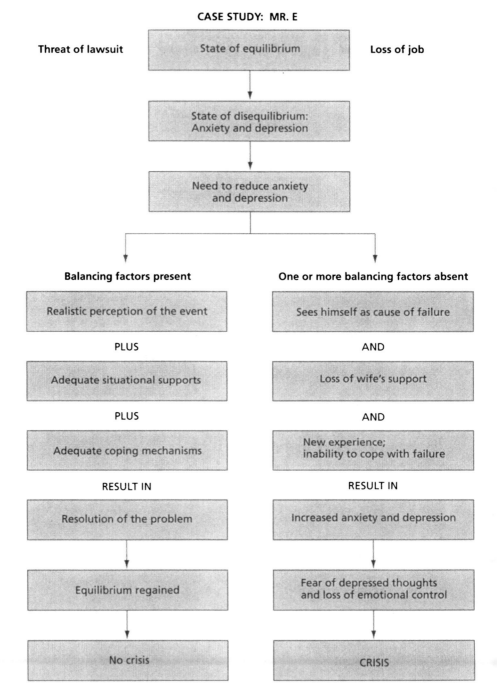

CASE STUDY: MR. E

Threat of lawsuit — State of equilibrium — Loss of job

State of disequilibrium:
Anxiety and depression

Need to reduce anxiety
and depression

Balancing factors present

Realistic perception of the event

PLUS

Adequate situational supports

PLUS

Adequate coping mechanisms

RESULT IN

Resolution of the problem

Equilibrium regained

No crisis

One or more balancing factors absent

Sees himself as cause of failure

AND

Loss of wife's support

AND

New experience;
inability to cope with failure

RESULT IN

Increased anxiety and depression

Fear of depressed thoughts
and loss of emotional control

CRISIS

Corresponds with Figure 8-1

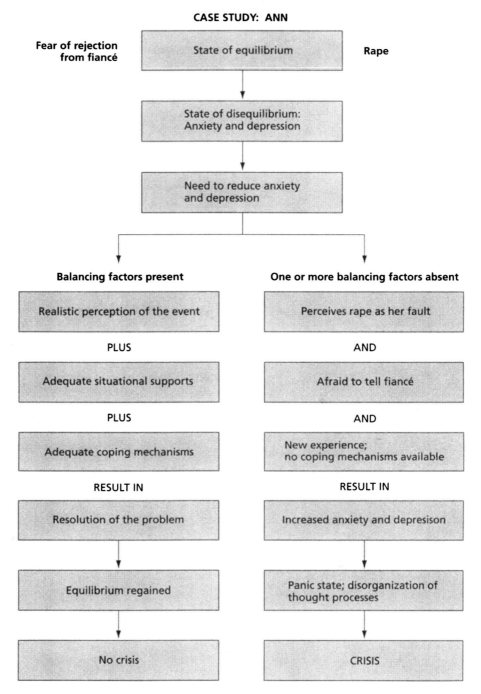

CASE STUDY: ANN

Fear of rejection from fiancé — State of equilibrium — Rape

State of disequilibrium: Anxiety and depression

Need to reduce anxiety and depression

Balancing factors present

Realistic perception of the event

PLUS

Adequate situational supports

PLUS

Adequate coping mechanisms

RESULT IN

Resolution of the problem

Equilibrium regained

No crisis

One or more balancing factors absent

Perceives rape as her fault

AND

Afraid to tell fiancé

AND

New experience; no coping mechanisms available

RESULT IN

Increased anxiety and depresison

Panic state; disorganization of thought processes

CRISIS

Corresponds with Figure 8-2

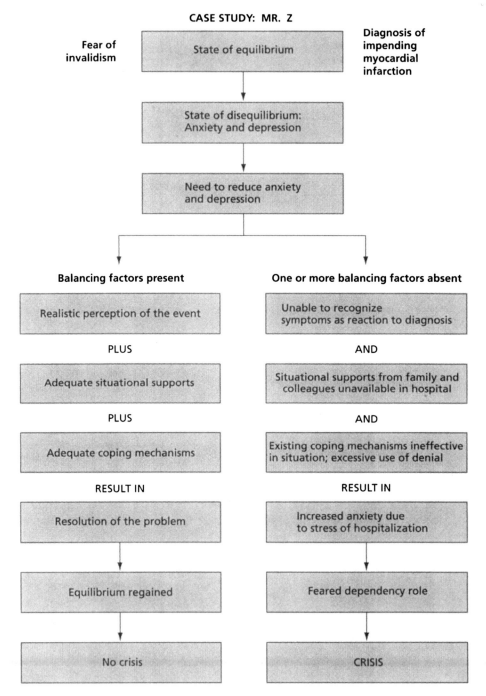

Corresponds with Figure 8-3

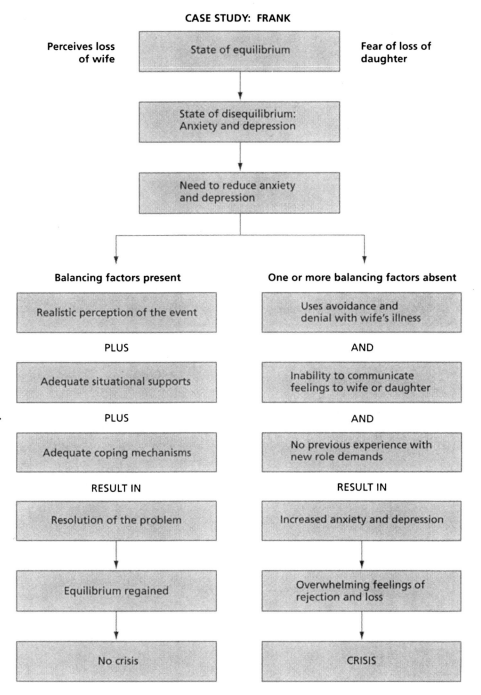

CASE STUDY: FRANK

Perceives loss of wife

State of equilibrium

Fear of loss of daughter

State of disequilibrium: Anxiety and depression

Need to reduce anxiety and depression

Balancing factors present

Realistic perception of the event

PLUS

Adequate situational supports

PLUS

Adequate coping mechanisms

RESULT IN

Resolution of the problem

Equilibrium regained

No crisis

One or more balancing factors absent

Uses avoidance and denial with wife's illness

AND

Inability to communicate feelings to wife or daughter

AND

No previous experience with new role demands

RESULT IN

Increased anxiety and depression

Overwhelming feelings of rejection and loss

CRISIS

Corresponds with Figure 8-4

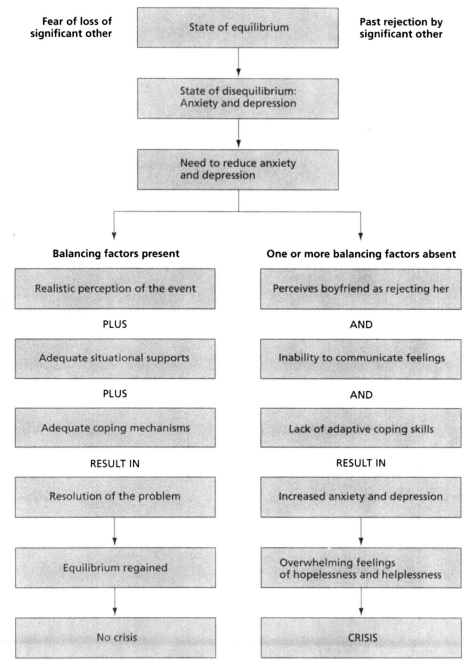

CASE STUDY: CAROL

Corresponds with Figure 8-5

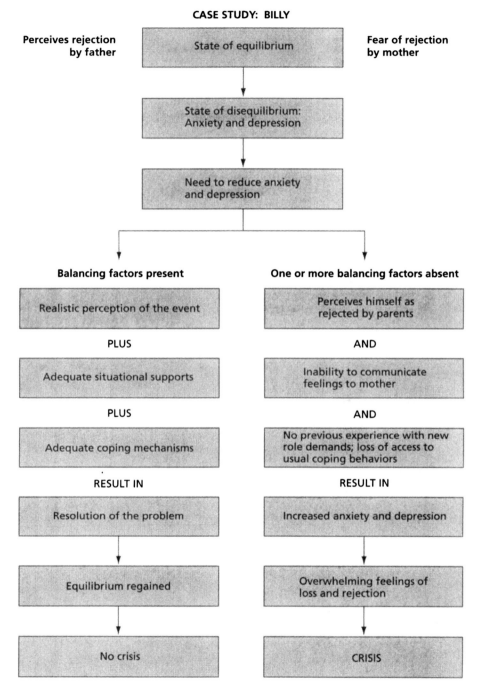

CASE STUDY: BILLY

Perceives rejection by father

State of equilibrium

Fear of rejection by mother

State of disequilibrium: Anxiety and depression

Need to reduce anxiety and depression

Balancing factors present

Realistic perception of the event

PLUS

Adequate situational supports

PLUS

Adequate coping mechanisms

RESULT IN

Resolution of the problem

Equilibrium regained

No crisis

One or more balancing factors absent

Perceives himself as rejected by parents

AND

Inability to communicate feelings to mother

AND

No previous experience with new role demands; loss of access to usual coping behaviors

RESULT IN

Increased anxiety and depression

Overwhelming feelings of loss and rejection

CRISIS

Corresponds with Figure 9-1

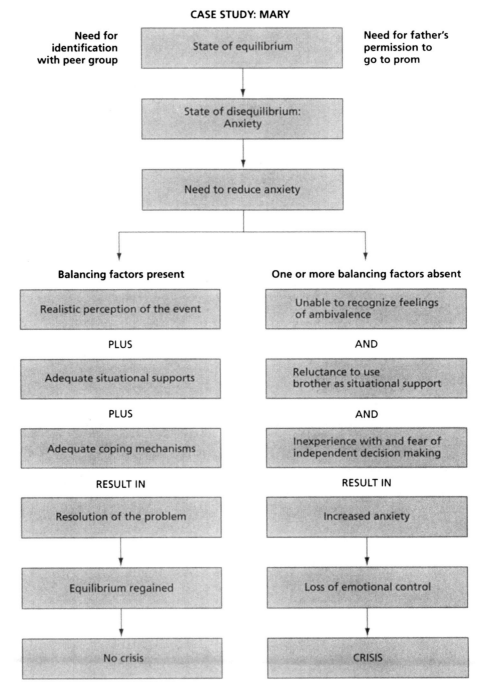

CASE STUDY: MARY

Need for identification with peer group

State of equilibrium

Need for father's permission to go to prom

State of disequilibrium: Anxiety

Need to reduce anxiety

Balancing factors present

Realistic perception of the event

PLUS

Adequate situational supports

PLUS

Adequate coping mechanisms

RESULT IN

Resolution of the problem

Equilibrium regained

No crisis

One or more balancing factors absent

Unable to recognize feelings of ambivalence

AND

Reluctance to use brother as situational support

AND

Inexperience with and fear of independent decision making

RESULT IN

Increased anxiety

Loss of emotional control

CRISIS

Corresponds with Figure 9-2

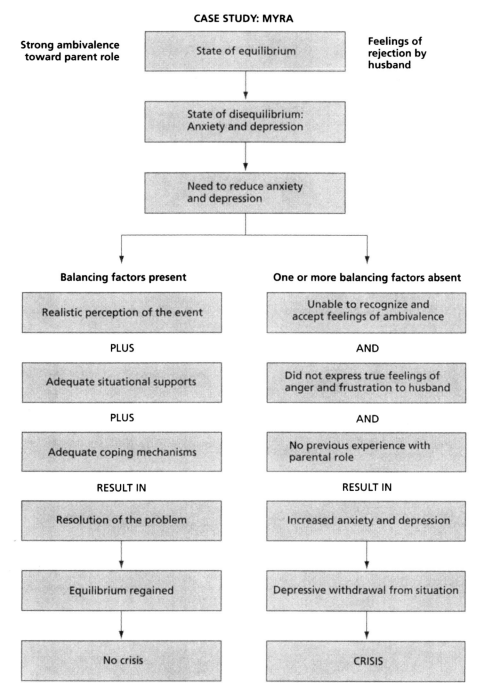

Corresponds with Figure 9-3

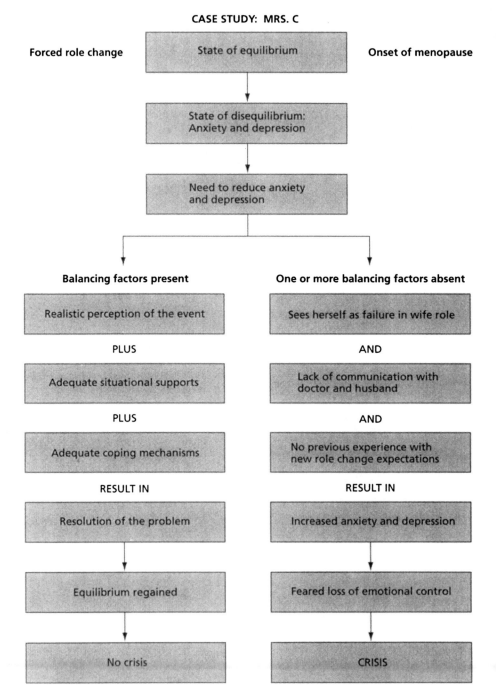

CASE STUDY: MRS. C

Forced role change

State of equilibrium

Onset of menopause

State of disequilibrium:
Anxiety and depression

Need to reduce anxiety
and depression

Balancing factors present

Realistic perception of the event

PLUS

Adequate situational supports

PLUS

Adequate coping mechanisms

RESULT IN

Resolution of the problem

Equilibrium regained

No crisis

One or more balancing factors absent

Sees herself as failure in wife role

AND

Lack of communication with
doctor and husband

AND

No previous experience with
new role change expectations

RESULT IN

Increased anxiety and depression

Feared loss of emotional control

CRISIS

Corresponds with Figure 9-4

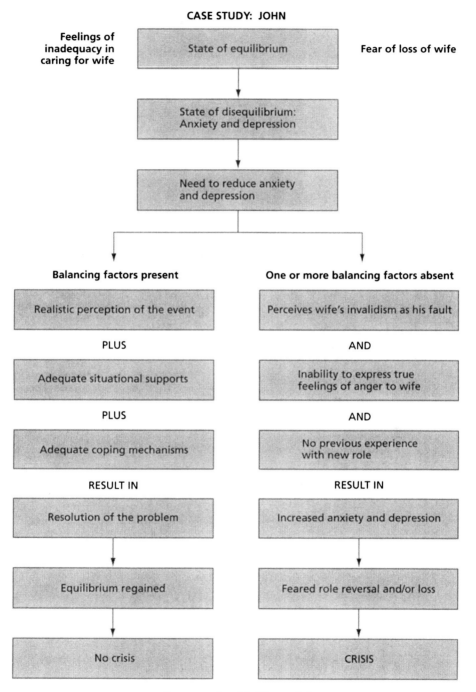

CASE STUDY: JOHN

Feelings of inadequacy in caring for wife

State of equilibrium

Fear of loss of wife

State of disequilibrium:
Anxiety and depression

Need to reduce anxiety
and depression

Balancing factors present

Realistic perception of the event

PLUS

Adequate situational supports

PLUS

Adequate coping mechanisms

RESULT IN

Resolution of the problem

Equilibrium regained

No crisis

One or more balancing factors absent

Perceives wife's invalidism as his fault

AND

Inability to express true
feelings of anger to wife

AND

No previous experience
with new role

RESULT IN

Increased anxiety and depression

Feared role reversal and/or loss

CRISIS

Corresponds with Figure 9-5

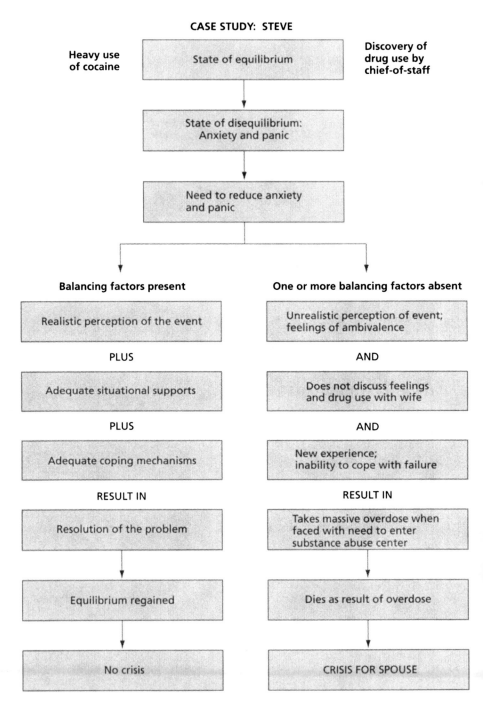

CASE STUDY: STEVE

Heavy use of cocaine

Discovery of drug use by chief-of-staff

State of equilibrium

State of disequilibrium: Anxiety and panic

Need to reduce anxiety and panic

Balancing factors present

Realistic perception of the event

PLUS

Adequate situational supports

PLUS

Adequate coping mechanisms

RESULT IN

Resolution of the problem

Equilibrium regained

No crisis

One or more balancing factors absent

Unrealistic perception of event; feelings of ambivalence

AND

Does not discuss feelings and drug use with wife

AND

New experience; inability to cope with failure

RESULT IN

Takes massive overdose when faced with need to enter substance abuse center

Dies as result of overdose

CRISIS FOR SPOUSE

Corresponds with Figure 10-1

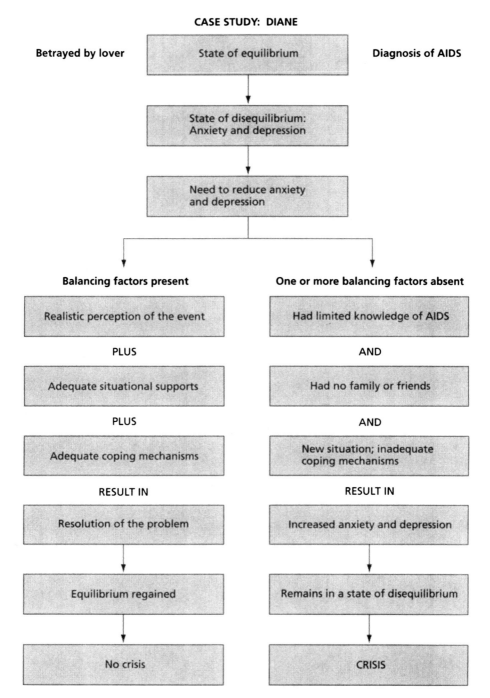

CASE STUDY: DIANE

Betrayed by lover — State of equilibrium — Diagnosis of AIDS

State of disequilibrium: Anxiety and depression

Need to reduce anxiety and depression

Balancing factors present

Realistic perception of the event

PLUS

Adequate situational supports

PLUS

Adequate coping mechanisms

RESULT IN

Resolution of the problem

Equilibrium regained

No crisis

One or more balancing factors absent

Had limited knowledge of AIDS

AND

Had no family or friends

AND

New situation; inadequate coping mechanisms

RESULT IN

Increased anxiety and depression

Remains in a state of disequilibrium

CRISIS

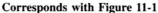

Corresponds with Figure 11-1

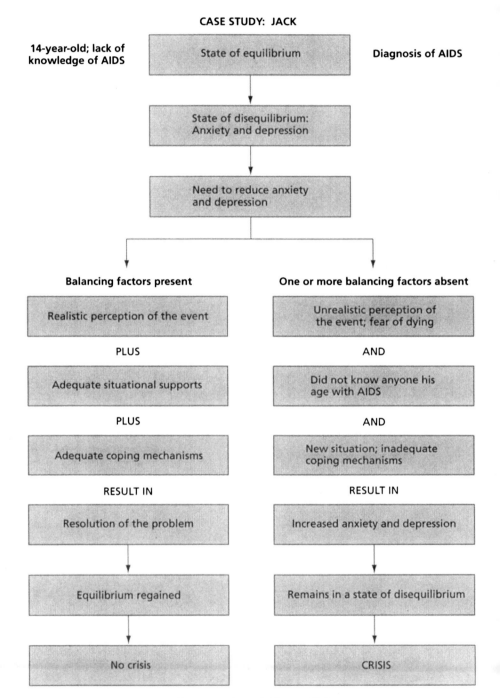

CASE STUDY: JACK

14-year-old; lack of knowledge of AIDS

State of equilibrium

Diagnosis of AIDS

State of disequilibrium: Anxiety and depression

Need to reduce anxiety and depression

Balancing factors present

Realistic perception of the event

PLUS

Adequate situational supports

PLUS

Adequate coping mechanisms

RESULT IN

Resolution of the problem

Equilibrium regained

No crisis

One or more balancing factors absent

Unrealistic perception of the event; fear of dying

AND

Did not know anyone his age with AIDS

AND

New situation; inadequate coping mechanisms

RESULT IN

Increased anxiety and depression

Remains in a state of disequilibrium

CRISIS

Corresponds with Figure 11-2

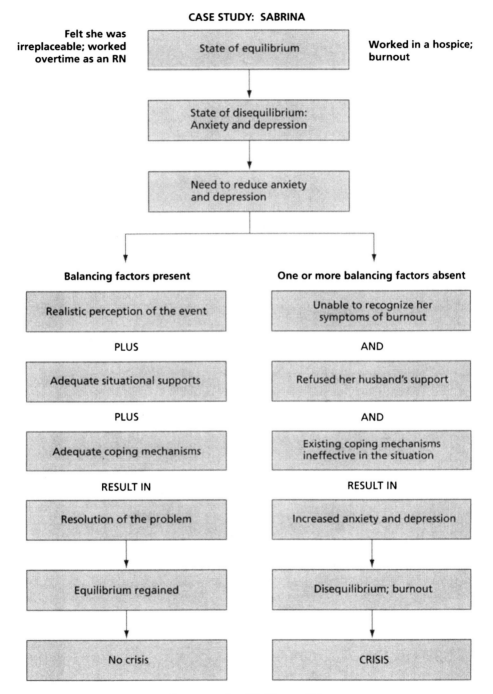

CASE STUDY: SABRINA

Felt she was irreplaceable; worked overtime as an RN

Worked in a hospice; burnout

State of equilibrium

State of disequilibrium: Anxiety and depression

Need to reduce anxiety and depression

Balancing factors present

Realistic perception of the event

PLUS

Adequate situational supports

PLUS

Adequate coping mechanisms

RESULT IN

Resolution of the problem

Equilibrium regained

No crisis

One or more balancing factors absent

Unable to recognize her symptoms of burnout

AND

Refused her husband's support

AND

Existing coping mechanisms ineffective in the situation

RESULT IN

Increased anxiety and depression

Disequilibrium; burnout

CRISIS

Corresponds with Figure 12-1

APPENDIX E

Authors Quoted in This Book

Addison, Joseph   1672-1719
Bierce, Ambrose Gwinett   1842-1914
Byron, George Gordon (6th Baron: Byron of Rochdale, called Lord
   Byron)   1788-1824
Cicero, Marcus Tullius   106-43 BC
Dickinson, Emily Elizabeth   1830-1886
Disraeli, Benjamin   1804-1881
Duc de La Rochefoucauld, Francois   1613-1680
Emerson, Ralph Waldo   1803-1882
Epictetus   circa AD 55-circa 135
Franklin, Benjamin   1706-1790
Gandi, Mohandas K.   1869-1948
Gilbran, Kahil   1883-1931
Goethe, Johann Wolfgang von   1749-1832
Goldsmith, Oliver   1728-1774
Hippocrates   460-377 BC
Holy Bible, King James Version
Horace (Quintus Horatius Flaccus)   65-8 BC
Houseman, Alfred Edward   1859-1936
Keats, John   1795-1821
Kennedy, John Fitzgerald   1917-1963
Ovid, P. Ovidius Naso   43 BC-17 AD
Retz, Cardinal de   1614-1679
Roux, Joseph   1834-1905
Saki (pseudonym of HH Muno)   1870-1916
Shakespeare, William   1564-1616
Sophoceles   496-406 BC
Stevenson, Robert Louis   1850-1894
Wordsworth, William   1770-1850
Wylie, Elinor   1885-1928
Young, Edward   1623-1765

INDEX

CPSIA information can be obtained at www.ICGtesting.com

228592LV00001B/2/P

9 780815 126041